Marine Natural Products as Anticancer Agents 3.0

Marine Natural Products as Anticancer Agents 3.0

Guest Editors

Celso Alves
Marc Diederich

MDPI

Basel • Beijing • Wuhan • Barcelona • Belgrade • Novi Sad • Cluj • Manchester

Guest Editors
Celso Alves
MARE—Marine and Environmental Sciences Centre
Polytechnic University of Leiria
Peniche
Portugal

Marc Diederich
Department of Pharmacy
Seoul National University
Seoul
Republic of Korea

Editorial Office
MDPI AG
Grosspeteranlage 5
4052 Basel, Switzerland

This is a reprint of the Special Issue, published open access by the journal *Marine Drugs* (ISSN 1660-3397), freely accessible at: https://www.mdpi.com/journal/marinedrugs/special_issues/841OM8M7Q0.

For citation purposes, cite each article independently as indicated on the article page online and as indicated below:

Lastname, A.A.; Lastname, B.B. Article Title. *Journal Name* **Year**, *Volume Number*, Page Range.

ISBN 978-3-7258-6608-3 (Hbk)
ISBN 978-3-7258-6609-0 (PDF)
https://doi.org/10.3390/books978-3-7258-6609-0

Contents

About the Editors

Celso Alves

Celso Alves holds a PhD in Marine Science, Technology, and Sea Management (Do*Mar), awarded in 2019 by the University of Aveiro, Portugal. He is currently a Senior Researcher at MARE—Marine and Environmental Sciences Centre, ESTM, Polytechnic University of Leiria. His scientific career has been dedicated to the exploration of marine biodiversity, including seaweeds, bacteria, fungi, jellyfish, sponges, and other marine organisms, as a source of novel natural bioactive compounds. His research focuses on the discovery and characterization of molecules with biotechnological and therapeutic potential, contributing to innovation in the blue bioeconomy and sustainable marine resource valorization.

Marc Diederich

Marc Diederich earned his PhD in molecular pharmacology in 1994 from the University Henri Poincaré Nancy 1, France. After training at the University of Cincinnati, USA, he focused his research on cancer and leukemia cell signaling pathways and gene expression mechanisms triggered by natural compounds with epigenetic, anti-inflammatory, and cell-death-inducing potential. He directed the Laboratory for Molecular and Cellular Biology of Cancer (LBMCC) in Luxembourg until 2025. In 2012, he was appointed Professor of Biochemistry at the College of Pharmacy of Seoul National University. Prof. Diederich's research focuses on exploring new combination treatments for cancer, including natural marine compounds.

marine drugs

Editorial

Marine Natural Products as Anticancer Agents 3.0

Celso Alves [1,]* and Marc Diederich [2,]*

1 MARE—Marine and Environmental Sciences Centre/ARNET-Aquatic Research Network, ESTM, Polytechnic University of Leiria, 2520 630 Peniche, Portugal
2 Department of Pharmacy, College of Pharmacy, Seoul National University, 1 Gwanak-ro, Gwanak-gu, Seoul 08826, Republic of Korea
* Correspondence: celso.alves@ipleiria.pt (C.A.); marcdiederich@snu.ac.kr (M.D.)

Keywords: cytotoxicity; semi-synthesis; apoptosis; immunotherapy; in vivo; mitochondrial dysfunction; motility; co-administration; anticancer

Cancer represents a major global health challenge, with 20 million new cases and 9.7 million deaths reported in 2022. By 2050, the number of new cancer cases will exceed 35 million [1]. Cancer is commonly understood as a single disease, but it comprises over 100 distinct pathological conditions, each with unique characteristics. This complexity makes it difficult to develop universal, effective treatments and classify cancer as a uniformly treatable condition. The therapeutic strategy for each type of cancer may differ depending on the nature and stage of the disease and often requires the combination of multiple therapeutic approaches, including radiotherapy, chemotherapy, hormone therapy, anti-angiogenic therapy, immunotherapy, and stem cell transplantation [2]. Consequently, the development of precise, individualized treatments and increased investment in cancer drug research are essential to fight this burden and reduce global cancer mortality. Despite the availability of large libraries of synthesized compounds, they have not been as successful in producing new drugs as many had hoped. In contrast, natural products, including those of marine origin, continue to play a key role in the discovery and development of novel anticancer medicines. They offer several advantages in drug discovery and development, such as remarkable structural diversity, the potential for multi-target effects, the ability to overcome drug resistance, and the specificity to interact with key targets associated with carcinogenesis [3].

The Special Issue "Marine Natural Products as Anticancer Agents 3.0" comprises eleven publications, three reviews, and eight original research articles, focusing on the anticancer activities of marine natural or derived compounds. The original research articles in this collection study the effects of these substances in silico, in both 2D and 3D in vitro cellular and in vivo models, across a range of solid and non-solid tumors. Forty-one marine natural or derived compounds classified as terpenes, alkaloids, polyketides, polyether phycotoxins, and quinazolinones were examined. In addition, one extract enriched in 13-acetoxysarcocrassolide and salmon oil enriched in omega-3 polyunsaturated fatty acids were also explored. These substances impacted cell viability across various in vitro and in vivo cancer models derived from diverse tissues, including the lung, prostate, breast, colorectal, stomach, skin, lymphatic system, kidney, and hematological malignancies such as leukemia and myeloma. These natural or derived marine compounds have been shown to target various biological biomarkers involved in cancer development and progression by activating distinct intracellular signaling pathways. These include mechanisms related to apoptosis, oxidative stress, mitochondrial dysfunction, and DNA fragmentation and condensation, as well as cell proliferation, cell migration, motility, invasion, and immune system activation.

In Contribution 1, Giani and co-workers critically review the biological activities of the rare C_{50} carotenoid called bacterioruberin (BR) and its derivatives, monoanhydrobacterioruberin and bisanhydrobacterioruberin. These compounds are produced by extreme halophilic microorganisms that inhabit hypersaline environments, where they are constantly exposed to ionic and oxidative stress due to saturated salt concentrations and high levels of UV radiation. These compounds demonstrated immunomodulatory, anti-inflammatory, and cytotoxic activities on various cellular models, and have been shown to modulate intracellular signaling pathways involved in key biological processes related to cancer, such as apoptosis and cell adhesion. The critical reflection conducted by Garcia and colleagues in Contribution 2 is focused on the potential of marine-derived compounds to disrupt hypoxic signaling pathways, inhibiting hypoxia-inducible factors (HIF-1 and HIF-2), given their critical roles in tumor metastasis and angiogenesis. Eighty-seven marine natural compounds were identified as being effective in modulating HIF activity. However, despite their potential, some of these compounds exhibit significant toxicity, and their mechanisms of action and validation in disease-relevant models remain limited. Therefore, further efforts are needed to optimize their efficacy, minimize toxicity, and improve pharmacokinetic profiles. In turn, in Contribution 3, Jiang and co-workers present a critical review focused on the discovery and development of novel variable new antigen receptors (VNARs), emphasizing shark VNARs as promising agents for the treatment and early diagnosis of tumors, particularly solid tumors. The VNAR from shark immunoglobulin novel antigen receptor (IgNAR) offers various advantages for anticancer development, including small size, high stability, high affinity, and distinct structural and functional characteristics. However, further research is needed to understand better the unique characteristics and therapeutic potential of IgNAR/VNAR in clinical and oncological applications.

The number of newly reported compounds of marine origin has grown over the last few decades. According to Faulkner, Blunt, and their collaborators, between 1977 and 2019, sponges (30.93%) were the leading source of new marine natural compounds, followed by microorganisms (20.53%) and seaweeds (10.44%) [4]. In 2023, more than 1200 new compounds were reported as having been isolated from marine microorganisms and phytoplankton; green, brown, and red algae; sponges; cnidarians; bryozoans; mollusks; tunicates; echinoderms; mangroves; and other intertidal plants. These molecules exhibited various activities, including cytotoxic and antiproliferative effects, as well as the ability to modulate intracellular signaling pathways relevant to therapeutic targets for the treatment of oncological diseases [5]. Herein, the compounds and marine-derived compounds studied were either isolated from or inspired by various marine sources, including algae, soft corals, fish, bacteria, and sponges. In Contribution 4, Lin and colleagues studied the anticancer potential of extracts from soft coral cultivated in aquaculture, focusing on their ability to interact with topoisomerase II, HDAC, and tubulin polymerization targets. Among the one hundred eighty ethyl acetate extracts tested, the *Lobophytum crassum* extract (LCE) displayed the smallest IC_{50} values on prostate cancer cells and significantly inhibited tubulin polymerization. Its effects on cell viability seemed to be mediated by apoptosis. In vivo, the extract was able to suppress tumor growth and reduce the tumor volume and weight. The LCE also displayed the ability to modulate various intracellular signaling pathways and biological events related to cell migration and invasion. Chemical analysis identified 13-AC (13-acetoxysarcocrassolide) as the major component of the LCE. In Contribution 5, Anh and co-workers explored the chemical diversity of compounds isolated from the culture broth of the marine-derived bacterium *Salinispora arenicola*, identifying five known (2–5 and 8) and three new (1, 6, and 7) rifamycin-related polyketide derivatives.

After structural elucidation, the cytotoxic effects of these compounds were evaluated on several malignant cell lines. The rifamycin derivatives exhibited moderate to weak cytotoxicity, with evidence suggesting that the aromatic moiety plays an important role in their activity, particularly for the compound 1 that displayed the highest activity with GI_{50} values ranging from 2.36 to 9.96 μM.

In Contribution 6, Pulat and colleagues isolated a new quinazolinone derivative, actinoquinazolinone (**1**), from the culture of *Streptomyces* sp. CNQ-617, along with two known compounds. The new compound exhibited the strongest antitumor activity, demonstrating the ability to suppress invasion in AGS cells by modulating EMT and STAT3 signal pathways and the expression of various genes related to cell motility. In Contribution 7, Kim and co-workers investigated the anticancer effects of palytoxin, one of the most potent biotoxins, on various leukemia and solid tumor cell lines. The biotoxin isolated from the soft coral *Palythoa aff. Clavate* mediated selective cell death in leukemia cell lines, modulating the expression of several biological biomarkers related to apoptosis. In vivo, palytoxin inhibited the tumor formation on a zebrafish xenograft model at pM concentrations.

On the other hand, in Contribution 8, Tsai and colleagues evaluated the immunotherapeutic effects of crassolide, a cembranolide isolated from the Formosan soft coral *Lobophytum michaelae*, on in vitro/in vivo breast cancer models. This compound has been demonstrated to reduce the viability of human breast malignant cells and murine mammary carcinoma cells while also inducing immunogenic cell death (ICD) and decreasing the expression levels of CD24 on 4T1-luc2 cells. One of the major inducers of ICD is endoplasmic reticulum (ER) stress, in which the p38 MAPK signaling pathway plays a critical role. Crassolide upregulates the phosphorylation of p38α and downregulates the phosphorylation of NF-κB, STAT1, and EIK-1, key downstream effectors of the p38α signaling cascade. These findings suggest that crassolide may act as a novel p38 catalytic inhibitor.

Despite the potential of marine natural products as anticancer agents, the translation from laboratory findings to clinical trials has been limited, particularly due to low stability, bioavailability, water solubility, efficacy, pharmacokinetics, etc. [6]. Over the past few decades, various strategies have been developed to overcome these limitations, including the synthesis or hemi-synthesis of structurally related analogs. These modified molecules are designed to enhance the potency and efficacy of the original molecules as well as to mitigate their drawbacks. Accordingly, in Contribution 9, Alves and co-workers conducted the semi-synthesis of six novel sphaerococcenol A derivatives through reactions on the enone function group via thiol-Michael addition and enone reduction. These modifications did not contribute to potentiating the cytotoxic effects of the original compound. Of the analogs, compound (**1**) exhibited similar effects to those of sphaerococcenol A, accompanied by an increase in reactive oxygen species levels, changes in mitochondrial membrane potential, and the activation of apoptosis. In Contribution 10, Orfanoudaki and colleagues investigated the antitumor effects of twenty-four compounds from a library of naturally occurring and semi-synthetic discorhabdins on the viability of Merkel cell carcinoma cells. These compounds do not seem to induce apoptosis, but a rapid loss of cellular reducing potential and mitochondrial membrane potential suggests that they trigger mitochondrial dysfunction, leading to non-apoptotic cell death.

Chemoresistance, whether inherent or acquired, remains one of the major challenges in effective cancer treatment. It is often responsible for cancer recurrence, treatment failure, and, ultimately, patient death. Therefore, beyond the discovery and development of new molecules with anticancer activity and novel mechanisms of action, exploring their potential to enhance the efficacy of existing medicines is also relevant. Combination strategies may contribute to overcoming the limitations of single-agent therapies and contribute to more successful clinical outcomes [7]. In Contribution 11, Pettersen and co-workers explored the antitumor effects of salmon oil OmeGo (Hofseth BioCare), rich in fatty acids, including the n-3 PUFAs docosahexaenoic acid (DHA) and eicosahexaenoic acid (EPA), in colorectal malignant cell lines alone and in combination with the chemotherapeutic agent 5-fluorouracil (5-FU). OmeGo displayed to decrease the cell viability and potentiate the effects of 5-FU, suggesting that this strategy holds promise for further studies as an alternative treatment approach for patients with colorectal cancer.

Together, the eleven publications featured in this volume provide a compelling overview of the huge potential of marine natural products as scaffolds for developing next-generation therapeutic agents to fight cancer through various strategies. As Guest Editors, we sincerely acknowledge the valuable contributions of all researchers and reviewers involved in this Special Issue and the support from the editorial board and the *Marine Drugs* editorial office. Our special thanks go to Dr. Grace Qu for her dedicated assistance.

Funding: Marc Diederich was supported by the National Research Foundation of Korea (NRF) grants [2022R1A2C1013141], the 4th phase of the Brain Korea 21 (BK21) Program, the Creative-Pioneering Researchers Program at SNU [Funding number: A0433-20230100], the "Recherches Scientifiques Luxembourg" asbl, and the "En Häerz fir kriibskrank Kanner" asbl. Celso Alves acknowledges support from the Portuguese Foundation for Science and Technology (FCT) through strategic projects awarded to MARE—Marine and Environmental Sciences Centre (UIDP/04292/2020, DOI.org/10.54499/UIDP/04292/2020 and UIDB/04292/2020, DOI.org/10.54499/UIDB/04292/2020) and the Associate Laboratory ARNET (LA/P/0069/2020), as well as through his FCT researcher contract (doi.org/10.54499/CEECINST/00060/2021/CP2902/CT0004). Additional support was provided by the European Union, co-funding the BEAP-MAR project (EAPA_0032/2022) through the Interreg Atlantic Area program.

Conflicts of Interest: The authors declare no conflicts of interest.

List of Contributions:

1. Giani, M.; Pire, C.; Martínez-Espinosa, R.M. Bacterioruberin: Biosynthesis, Antioxidant Activity, and Therapeutic Applications in Cancer and Immune Pathologies. *Mar. Drugs* **2024**, *22*, 167.
2. Garcia, M.R.; Andrade, P.B.; Lefranc, F.; Gomes, N.G.M. Marine-Derived Leads as Anticancer Candidates by Disrupting Hypoxic Signaling through Hypoxia-Inducible Factors Inhibition. *Mar. Drugs* **2024**, *22*, 143.
3. Jiang, X.; Sun, L.; Hu, C.; Zheng, F.; Lyu, Z.; Shao, J. Shark IgNAR: The Next Broad Application Antibody in Clinical Diagnoses and Tumor Therapies? *Mar. Drugs* **2023**, *21*, 496.
4. Lin, H.Y.; Tsai, T.N.; Hsu, K.C.; Hsu, Y.M.; Chiang, L.C.; El-Shazly, M.; Chang, K.M.; Lin, Y.H.; Tu, S.Y.; Lin, T.E.; et al. From Sea to Science: Coral Aquaculture for Sustainable Anticancer Drug Development. *Mar. Drugs* **2024**, *22*, 323.
5. Van Anh, C.; Kang, J.S.; Yang, J.W.; Kwon, J.H.; Heo, C.S.; Lee, H.S.; Shin, H.J. Rifamycin-Related Polyketides from a Marine-Derived Bacterium *Salinispora arenicola* and Their Cytotoxic Activity. *Mar. Drugs* **2023**, *21*, 494.
6. Pulat, S.; Kim, D.A.; Hillman, P.F.; Oh, D.C.; Kim, H.; Nam, S.J.; Fenical, W. Actinoquinazolinone, a New Quinazolinone Derivative from a Marine Bacterium *Streptomyces* sp. CNQ-617, Suppresses the Motility of Gastric Cancer Cells. *Mar. Drugs* **2023**, *21*, 489.
7. Kim, J.; Ji, S.; Lee, J.Y.; Lorquin, J.; Orlikova-Boyer, B.; Cerella, C.; Mazumder, A.; Muller, F.; Dicato, M.; Detournay, O.; Diederich, M. Marine Polyether Phycotoxin Palytoxin Induces Apoptotic Cell Death via Mcl-1 and Bcl-2 Downregulation. *Mar. Drugs* **2023**, *21*, 233.
8. Tsai, K.C.; Chen, C.S.; Su, J.H.; Lee, Y.C.; Tseng, Y.H.; Wei, W.C. The Blockade of Mitogen-Activated Protein Kinase 14 Activation by Marine Natural Product Crassolide Triggers ICD in Tumor Cells and Stimulates Anti-Tumor Immunity. *Mar. Drugs* **2023**, *21*, 225.
9. Sousa, D.; Fortunato, M.A.G.; Silva, J.; Pingo, M.; Martins, A.; Afonso, C.A.M.; Pedrosa, R.; Siopa, F.; Alves, C. Sphaerococcenol A Derivatives: Design, Synthesis, and Cytotoxicity. *Mar. Drugs* **2024**, *22*, 408.

10. Orfanoudaki, M.; Smith, E.A.; Hill, N.T.; Garman, K.A.; Brownell, I.; Copp, B.R.; Grkovic, T.; Henrich, C.J. An Investigation of Structure-Activity Relationships and Cell Death Mechanisms of the Marine Alkaloids Discorhabdins in Merkel Cell Carcinoma Cells. *Mar. Drugs* **2023**, *21*, 474.
11. Pettersen, C.H.H.; Samdal, H.; Sætrom, P.; Wibe, A.; Hermansen, E.; Schønberg, S.A. The Salmon Oil OmeGo Reduces Viability of Colorectal Cancer Cells and Potentiates the Anti-Cancer Effect of 5-FU. *Mar. Drugs* **2023**, *21*, 636.

References

1. Bray, F.; Laversanne, M.; Sung, H.; Ferlay, J.; Siegel, R.L.; Soerjomataram, I.; Jemal, A.J.C. Global cancer statistics 2022: GLOBOCAN estimates of incidence and mortality worldwide for 36 cancers in 185 countries. *CA Cancer J. Clin.* **2024**, *74*, 229–263. [CrossRef] [PubMed]
2. Xia, Y.; Sun, M.; Huang, H.; Jin, W.-L. Drug repurposing for cancer therapy. *Signal Transduct. Target. Ther.* **2024**, *9*, 92. [CrossRef] [PubMed]
3. Chunarkar-Patil, P.; Kaleem, M.; Mishra, R.; Ray, S.; Ahmad, A.; Verma, D.; Bhayye, S.; Dubey, R.; Singh, H.N.; Kumar, S. Anticancer Drug Discovery Based on Natural Products: From Computational Approaches to Clinical Studies. *Biomedicines* **2024**, *12*, 201. [CrossRef] [PubMed]
4. Silva, J.; Alves, C.; Soledade, F.; Martins, A.; Pinteus, S.; Gaspar, H.; Alfonso, A.; Pedrosa, R. Marine-Derived Components: Can They Be a Potential Therapeutic Approach to Parkinson's Disease? *Mar. Drugs* **2023**, *21*, 451. [CrossRef] [PubMed]
5. Carroll, A.R.; Copp, B.R.; Grkovic, T.; Keyzers, R.A.; Prinsep, M.R. Marine natural products. *Nat. Prod. Rep.* **2025**, *42*, 257–297. [CrossRef] [PubMed]
6. Seyhan, A.A. Lost in translation: The valley of death across preclinical and clinical divide—Identification of problems and overcoming obstacles. *Transl. Med. Commun.* **2019**, *4*, 18. [CrossRef]
7. Ramos, A.; Sadeghi, S.; Tabatabaeian, H. Battling Chemoresistance in Cancer: Root Causes and Strategies to Uproot Them. *Int. J. Mol. Sci.* **2021**, *22*, 9451. [CrossRef] [PubMed]

marine drugs

Review

Bacterioruberin: Biosynthesis, Antioxidant Activity, and Therapeutic Applications in Cancer and Immune Pathologies

Micaela Giani [1], Carmen Pire [1,2] and Rosa María Martínez-Espinosa [1,2,*]

[1] Multidisciplinary Institute for Environmental Studies "Ramón Margalef", University of Alicante, Ap. 99, E-03080 Alicante, Spain; micaela.giani@ua.es (M.G.); carmen.pire@ua.es (C.P.)

[2] Biochemistry and Molecular Biology and Edaphology and Agricultural Chemistry Department, Faculty of Sciences, University of Alicante, Ap. 99, E-03080 Alicante, Spain

* Correspondence: rosa.martinez@ua.es; Tel.: +34-965903400 (ext. 1258 or 8841)

Abstract: Halophilic archaea, also termed haloarchaea, are a group of moderate and extreme halophilic microorganisms that constitute the major microbial populations in hypersaline environments. In these ecosystems, mainly aquatic, haloarchaea are constantly exposed to ionic and oxidative stress due to saturated salt concentrations and high incidences of UV radiation (mainly in summer). To survive under these harsh conditions, haloarchaea have developed molecular adaptations including hyperpigmentation. Regarding pigmentation, haloarchaeal species mainly synthesise the rare C_{50} carotenoid called bacterioruberin (BR) and its derivatives, monoanhydrobacterioruberin and bisanhydrobacterioruberin. Due to their colours and extraordinary antioxidant properties, BR and its derivatives have been the aim of research in several research groups all over the world during the last decade. This review aims to summarise the most relevant characteristics of BR and its derivatives as well as describe their reported antitumoral, immunomodulatory, and antioxidant biological activities. Based on their biological activities, these carotenoids can be considered promising natural biomolecules that could be used as tools to design new strategies and/or pharmaceutical formulas to fight against cancer, promote immunomodulation, or preserve skin health, among other potential uses.

Keywords: bacterioruberin; haloarchaea; C_{50} carotenoids; antioxidant; immunomodulation; antitumoral

1. Introduction

Most moderate and extreme halophilic microorganisms require salt concentrations above 1 M to be alive and metabolically active, although several species can endure a spectrum of saline conditions, ranging from low-salt to salt saturation concentrations (around 4 M) [1]. Based on the ionic strength required by the cells for stability and metabolic activity, microbial halophilic microorganisms are mainly classified into the following categories: slight halophiles (0.34 to 0.85 M), moderate halophiles (0.85 to 3.4 M), and extreme halophiles (3.4 M to saturation point) [2].

Studies based on microbial ecology and microbial biodiversity in salty aquatic environments confirmed that halophilic archaea species (also termed "haloarchaea") constitute the predominant populations, especially at high salt concentrations (2–4 M), apart from some bacterial genera like *Salinibacter* [3]. At significantly high salt concentrations, halophilic archaea belonging to the families *Halobacteriaceae* and *Haloferacaceae* (phylum Euryarchaeota within the Archaea domain) are the most abundant populations [4]. These halophilic archaea are widely distributed in saline environments, such as marshes or brackish ponds, which serve as sources of NaCl for human consumption [5]. Halophilic archaea primarily thrive in aerobic conditions, although certain species exhibit the capability to grow under microaerobic or even anaerobic conditions, utilising nitrate and/or nitrite as the final electron acceptors through denitrification processes [6]. Additionally, a noteworthy characteristic of these archaea is that most of them typically show a distinctive red/orange pigmentation, thus providing these kinds of colours to the salted ponds where they live all together with pigmented yeast and microalgae like *Dunaliella salina* [7]. These pigmented halophilic archaea have mainly been isolated from water column and sediment sampling at hypersaline environments such as hypersaline lakes such as the Great Salt Lake in Utah, USA; salt marshes; coastal wetlands; or solar salterns like those located in the south and southeast of Spain (Alicante, Murcia, or Huelva) [5].

Haloarchaea have attracted global scientific attention due to their unique features related to the molecular machinery of nitrogen, biodegradable polymers, and carotenoid metabolism; their easy manipulation; their reduced space requirements for cultivation compared to other organisms like microalgae or yeast from which highly marketed compounds can be obtained; and their capacity to produce a wide array of biomolecules and metabolites with potential biotechnological applications compared to plants, bacteria, fungi, or eukaryotic algae [8,9]. Their remarkable resilience and functionality even in the face of challenging environmental conditions, including high salinity, intense ultraviolet (UV) radiation, elevated ion concentrations, and extreme temperatures and pH, make them good model organisms to be used as cell factories for different purposes compared to their bacterial counterparts [10–12].

Among the biomolecules or metabolites of biotechnological interest synthesised by haloarchaea, small proteins and peptides, enzyme bioplastics, carotenoids, and nanoparticles can be highlighted. The carotenoids found in haloarchaea have garnered significant attention in various industries due to their versatility, serving as antioxidants, anticancer agents, antimicrobials, anti-inflammatory compounds, and food colourants, thus offering numerous biotechnological and biomedical applications [13–15]. Bacterioruberin (BR), the main carotenoid pigment synthesised by halophilic archaea, has demonstrated notable biological activity, particularly in antioxidant properties [14,16–20]. Understanding its biosynthesis pathways and structural features can provide insights into its potential therapeutic applications. This review focuses on the multifaceted biological activity of BR obtained from haloarchaea due to their better characterisation and the abundance of literature available on these microorganisms. BR, known for its characteristic red colouration, exhibits remarkable antioxidant properties owing to its ability to scavenge reactive oxygen species (ROS) and mitigate oxidative stress [21–23]. Additionally, recent studies have unveiled its potential immunomodulatory effects, suggesting a role in modulating immune responses and inflammation [24,25]. Therefore, advances in the comprehension of the pharmacological relevance of bacterioruberin hold promise for developing novel therapeutic interventions targeting oxidative-stress-related disorders, immune system dysregulation, and potentially other pathological conditions.

2. Characteristics of Haloarchaeal Carotenoids and Their Biological Roles

2.1. Chemical Composition and Structure

The literature concerning carotenoids synthesised by haloarchaea is still scarce compared to the literature available on carotenoids from other living beings, such as plants, algae yeast, and fungi [26–32]. The first reported studies on carotenoids isolated from haloarchaea date back to the 1970s, using *Halobacterium cutirubrum* as a model microorganism [33,34]. At that time, it was confirmed that the major carotenoid produced by the cells is the rare C_{50} BR followed by monoanhydrobacterioruberin (MABR) at the expense of lycopene and bisanhydrobacterioruberin (BABR); both MABR and BABR are precursors of BR [33,34]. Other carotenoids have been identified in haloarchaeal carotenoid extracts but at lower percentages, including β-carotene, lycopene, and some xanthophylls [35,36]. Structurally, BR is very unique among carotenoids (being considered a "rare C_{50} carotenoid" by several authors), consisting of a primary conjugated isoprenoid chain that contains 13 conjugated double bonds and four hydroxyl groups arising from the terminal ends. Table 1 displays the chemical structure of BR and its precursors (Table 1) [37].

Table 1. Structures and common and scientific names of bacterioruberin (BR) and its precursors.

Common Name	Molecular Formula	Chemical Structure (Stereoisomers)
Bacterioruberin	$C_{50}H_{76}O_4$	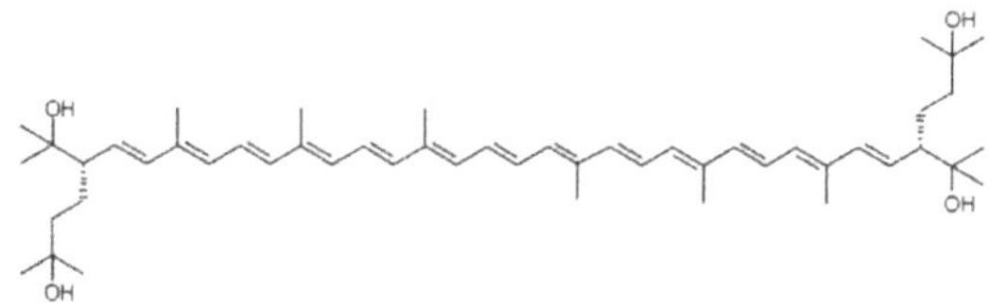 (2*S*,2′*S*)-2,2′-bis(3-hydroxy-3-methylbutyl)-3,4,3′,4tetrahydro-γ,γ-carotene-1,1′-diol
Monoanhydrobacterioruberin	$C_{50}H_{74}O_3$	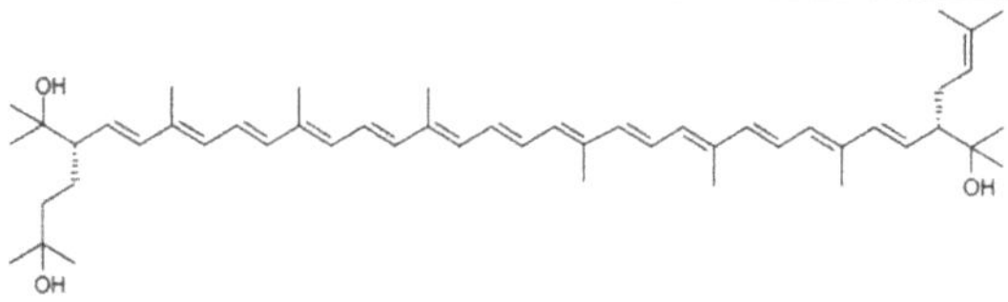 (3*S*,4*E*,6*E*,8*E*,10*E*,12*E*,14*E*,16*E*,18*E*,20*E*,22*E*,24*E*,26*E*,28*E*,30*S*)-30-(2-hydroxypropan-2-yl)-2,6,10,14,19,23,27,33-octamethyl-3-(3-methylbut-2-en-1-yl)tetratriaconta-4,6,8,10,12,14,16,18,20,22,24,26,28-tridecaene-2,33-diol
Bisanhydrobacterioruberin	$C_{50}H_{72}O_2$	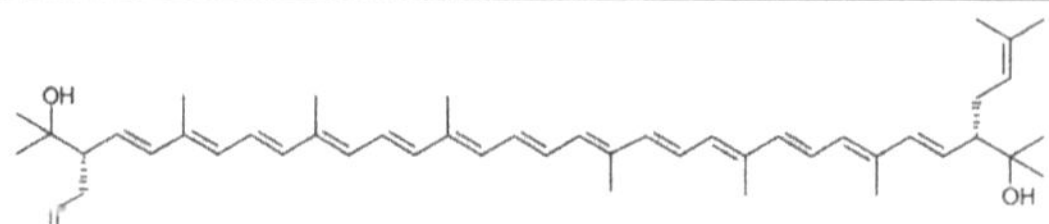 (3*S*,4*E*,6*E*,8*E*,10*E*,12*E*,14*E*,16*E*,18*E*,20*E*,22*E*,24*E*,26*E*,28*E*,30*S*)-2,6,10,14,19,23,27,31-octamethyl-3,30-bis(3-methylbut-2-en-1-yl)dotriaconta-4,6,8,10,12,14,16,18,20,22,24,26,28-tridecaene-2,31-diol

Although BR is produced almost exclusively by haloarchaea, some studies confirmed that few bacterial species showing extreme phenotypes like the Antarctic psychrotrophic bacterium *Micrococcus roseus* and *Arthrobacter* species are also able to synthesise it [38–40].

2.2. Carotenogenesis and Biological Role of Carotenoids in Haloarchaeal Cells

The synthesis of carotenoids (also termed "carotenogenesis") and its regulation have not been studied as deeply in haloarchaea [26,41–44] as they have in bacteria, yeasts, or plants [27,45–52]. In brief, haloarchaea use the mevalonate pathway to produce the carotenoid precursor isopentenyl pyrophosphate. Then, it is converted into trans-phytoene, which leads to ζ-carotene which is further converted to neurosporene. Neurosporene is transformed into lycopene, from which most carotenoids derive, including β-carotene with ϒ-carotene as an intermediate compound. Bacterioruberin is also synthesised from lycopene [26,41]. The main reaction involved is the addition of C_5 isoprene units to each end of the lycopene structure. However, in contrast to other secondary metabolites, the enzymes related to carotenogenesis are not always encoded within the same gene cluster [41] and some paralogs do not serve functional roles, as recently reported by Mishra and collaborators [53]. This circumstance poses a challenge in accurately identifying complete carotenogenesis pathways in each strain. Although other xanthophylls, including cantaxanthin and astaxanthin, have been detected in carotenoid extracts obtained from haloarchaeal cells [36,54], the genes coding for enzymes involved in their synthesis have not been identified in haloarchaeal genomes [41]. More recently, Serrano and collaborators reported that β-carotene could be converted to canthaxanthin by the action of a β-carotene ketolase protein. Through genome analysis, the authors identified a crtO candidate in one of the six circular plasmids in *Haloterrigena turkmenica*, which suggests that this species can produce canthaxanthin from β-carotene [26]. CrtO ketolases are structurally related to CrtI phytoene desaturases [55,56]. In consequence, haloarchaea without CrtO-like genes could still be producing canthaxanthin expressing one of their sometimes multiple CrtI genes [26]. Alternative unidentified pathways for the synthesis of these carotenoids could be a possible explanation.

Among all the carotenoids mentioned, BR is the most abundant natural carotenoid produced by haloarchaea. It is responsible for the intense pink colour since it is located in the cell membrane of the haloarchaea that synthesise it [57]. Its long hydrocarbon chain makes it able to fit in between the glycerolipids forming the bilayer, with the hydroxyl group facing outwards and inwards. Haloarchaeal pigments play a pivotal role in membrane stability, acting as a protection mechanism against the harsh conditions usually present in the natural environment of these extremophilic microorganisms, such as high oxidative and osmotic stress and elevated radiation [21,39,57,58]. BR protects cells from oxidative damage by acting as an antioxidant thanks to the electron transport between the pairs of conjugated double bonds. Since bacterioruberin presents a longer hydrocarbon chain and a higher number of conjugated double bonds than other carotenoids, such as β-carotene (C_{40} carotenoid, nine conjugated double bonds), it has extraordinary scavenging activity [14,16,18,59–62].

In addition, the presence of bacterioruberin in the cell membrane increases the rigidity and decreases water permeability, while allowing oxygen to enter inside the cell [63]. Thus, cells are capable of modulating membrane rigidity in a wide range of temperatures as well as in a concrete range of salinity conditions.

Finally, BR contributes to maintaining the structural stability of rhodopsin complexes. More specifically, some studies have demonstrated that it is associated with archaerhodopsin, which is a complex formed by a retinal protein and a carotenoid, identified in some haloarchaeal species, including *Halobacterium salinarum* [64–66].

3. Antioxidant Properties of Bacterioruberin and Its Precursors

Advances in the knowledge of the biological activities of BR have revealed that it could be of interest in several industrial and biomedical sectors due to its high antioxidant activity [14, 15,25,59–61,67,68]. Based on the chemical composition and structure of BR, it was initially assumed that this natural carotenoid has strong antioxidant properties as it was quantified later compared to one of the most marketed carotenoids, β-carotene [14,16,18,59–61,69,70]. This is probably the biological activity that is better characterised in the case of BR (Table 2).

A recent study has reported how the modification of the nutritional conditions of *Haloferax mediterranei* during growth can lead to changes in the carotenoid extract composition and, in consequence, its properties and antioxidant capacity [14]. The combination of 2.5% (*w*/*v*) glucose with 12.5% (*w*/*v*) salinity led to a carotenoid extract with an IC_{50} value of 0.03 µg/mL in the ABTS (2,2′-Azinobis-(3-Ethylbenzthiazolin-6-Sulfonic Acid) assay. This value was lower than the one obtained for ascorbic acid [14], coinciding with other reported results and confirming the remarkable antioxidant properties of these complex extracts [19,20]. Other researchers have explored the activity of carotenoid extracts of *Haloarcula hispanica* and *Halobacterium salinarum*, observing that they could scavenge DPPH (2,2-diphenyl-1-picrylhydrazyl) (2.05 µg/mL and 8.9 µg/mL) and ABTS radicals (3.89 µg/mL and low activity for *H. salinarum*) and reduce ferrocyanide and chelate copper, but not scavenge NO radicals or chelate iron [60]. Carotenoid extracts from *Halococcus morrhuae* and *H. salinarum* presented IC_{50} values of 0.85 µg/mL and 0.84 µg/mL for the ABTS assay [18]. *Haloferax* sp. ME16, a haloarchaeal strain isolated from Algerian salt lakes, displayed significantly higher antioxidant power than ascorbic acid in both the DPPH and ABTS assays [69]. Recently, carotenoid extracts from *Halorhabdus utahensis* exerted their scavenging power in a set of different antioxidant assays (DPPH, FRAP, and Superoxide Scavenging Activity assays), confirming that haloarchaeal carotenoids have a broad range of modes of action against oxidants [14,17]. A similar approach (ABTS, FRAP, and DPPH) was chosen to evaluate the antioxidant activity of *Natronoccoccus* sp. TC6 and *Halorubrum tebenquichense* carotenoid extracts. Although the extracts were efficient in all tests, they showed a dominating capacity of hydrogen and single electron transfer [68]. In summary, there are notable differences in the antioxidant activity of carotenoid extracts from different haloarchaeal species. There are different possible explanations for the variability in the results. It is possible that halophilic archaea could synthesise antioxidant compounds of different natures and polarities that contribute independently to the total antioxidant activity of the extracts, and this might be dependent on the haloarchaeal species but also influenced by the growth conditions. However, if this is the case, the concentration of those compounds should be significantly low because they cannot be easily detected by standard chromatographic-based approaches, at least those used in the case of *Haloferax mediterranei* extracts. One of the greatest difficulties when comparing current studies is that although they all agree that the all-trans-BR isomer is the most abundant, not all of them include the percentages of the different components of the extract, which in turn could be one of the factors influencing the antioxidant activity. Aside from that, there are experimental differences that might also influence the results obtained in the antioxidant tests, such as the organic solvent used for the extraction of carotenoids.

In addition, BR and intracellular KCl in *Halobacterium salinarum* and *Halobacterium* sp. strain NRC1 act as a protective mechanism against oxidative DNA damage induced by UV radiation. Therefore, this carotenoid might have potential applications in medicine and cosmeceuticals focused on the mitigation of DNA damage and the preservation of cellular integrity [71,72]. Understanding these protective mechanisms could inspire the development of novel therapies and skincare products targeting oxidative-stress-induced DNA damage, offering promising applications in healthcare and cosmetic industries.

Table 2. Antioxidant activity of BR with potential applications in food, cosmetics, and pharmacy.

Species	Aim of the Research	Reference
Halorubrum ruber	Optimisation of BR production and analysis of the effect of its antioxidant activity on the survival rate of *Caenorhabditis elegans* under oxidative stress conditions	[23]
Halorubrum ezzemoulense	Description of the effects of BR on the thermal and oxidative stabilities of fish oil	[22]
Haloarcula japonica *Haloarcula salaria* *Halococcus morrhuae* *Halobacterium salinarium* *Haloferax alexandrinus* GUSF-1 *Haloferax* sp. ME16 *Halogeometricum* sp. ME3 *Haloarcula* sp. BT9 *Halorhabdus utahensis* *Halorubrum chaoviator* *Halorubrum lipolyticum* *Halorubrum sodomense* *Halorubrum* sp. BS2 *Halorubrum tebenquichense* SU10 *Haloterrigena turkmenica* *Natronoccoccus* sp. TC6	Isolation and characterisation of the total carotenoid extract and antioxidant activity quantification	[16–19,68–70,73]

4. Immunomodulatory/Anti-Inflammatory Activities of BR Collectively with Antioxidant Activity

In connection with the antioxidant activity, recent studies have described the anti-inflammatory activities and immunomodulatory benefits of BR on human commercial cell lines. For example, *Haloarcula* sp. isolated from Odiel Saltworks (south of Spain) was used as the source of a carotenoid extract which is rich in BR and C_{18} fatty acids. This extract showed potent antioxidant capacity using the ABTS assay. This study further demonstrates that pretreatment with this carotenoid-rich extract of lipopolysaccharide (LPS)-stimulated macrophages resulted in a reduction in ROS production, a decrease in the pro-inflammatory cytokines TNF-α and IL-6 levels, and an upregulation of the factor Nrf2 and its target gene heme oxygenase-1 (HO-1), supporting the potential of the carotenoid extract as a therapeutic agent in the treatment of oxidative-stress-related inflammatory diseases [24].

Similarly, another study carried out with BR from *Halorubrum tebenquichense* suggested that the carotenoid in combination with dexamethasone (Dex) in ultra-small macrophage-targeted nanoparticles could act as a potential intestinal repairing agent [25]. The ultra-small structures in which BR and dexamethasone were embedded were extensively captured by macrophages and Caco-2 cells and displayed high anti-inflammatory and antioxidant activities on a gut inflammation model made of Caco-2 cells and lipopolysaccharide-stimulated THP-1-derived macrophages, reducing 65% and 55% of TNF-α and IL-8 release, respectively, and 60% of reactive oxygen species production. The ultra-small structures also reversed the morphological changes induced by inflammation and increased the transepithelial electrical resistance, partly reconstituting the barrier function. The main conclusion was that this nanostructure containing BR and Dex deserves further exploration as an intestinal-barrier-repairing agent [25].

In summary, while the evidence published until now suggests the therapeutic potential of bacterioruberin (BR) in mitigating oxidative-stress-related inflammatory diseases and promoting intestinal repair, it is important to note that the current body of research is limited, and further studies are needed to establish robust conclusions. These initial studies underscore BR's antioxidant capacity and its potential anti-inflammatory and immunomodulatory effects. The utilisation of BR-rich extracts or BR in combination with drugs within innovative nanostructures shows promise for addressing several pathologies. Nonetheless, the existing findings highlight the need to further research and develop BR-based formulations, elucidate underlying mechanisms, and assess the safety and efficacy of BR in clinical settings.

5. Antitumoral Properties of Bacterioruberin and Its Precursors

The effect of BR on tumoral cells has been recently explored. Thus, carotenoids (0.2–1.5 μM) from a haloarchaeal strain (M8) could reduce up to 50% hepatoma cell line (HepG2) viability in a concentration-dependent way. In addition, hepatoma cells treated with haloarchaeal carotenoids were less sensitive to oxidative stress generated by H_2O_2, thus exerting a protective effect [59]. The antiproliferative effect on hepatoma cells was also reported for extracts obtained from *Halogeometricum limi* and *Haloplanus vescus* [61]. These extracts also presented antihemolytic activities against H_2O_2-induced hemolysis in mouse erythrocytes [61]. The anticancer effect of *Natrialba* sp. M6 carotenoid extract was reported again for hepatoma cells (HepG2) as well as for other types of cancer cell lines, including Caco-2 (colon cancer), MCF-7 (breast cancer), and HeLa (cervical cancer) [74]. In the case of MCF-7 commercial cell lines, a real-time PCR technique was used to monitor the expression of genes specific for apoptosis, in the presence or absence of BR-rich carotenoid extract. Both early and late apoptosis were increased significantly by about 10% and 39%, respectively, due to the upregulation of CASP3, CASP8, and BAX gene expression in the MCF-7 cell line. In contrast, the expression of the genes MKI67 and SOX2 was significantly downregulated in the treated MCF-7 cell line. The results of this study showed that the carotenoid extract isolated from *Haloarcula* sp. A15 could be a good candidate for the production of high-added-value bacterioruberin due to its possible anticancer properties [75]. The antiproliferative effect on breast cancer cell lines has been explored in other studies [15,75]. In particular, *Haloferax mediterranei* carotenoid extracts reduced cell adhesion, viability, diameter, and cell concentrations in cell lines representative of the four well-defined subtypes of breast cancer (Luminal A, Luminal B, HER2-enriched, and triple-negative) [15].

In conclusion, the observed antiproliferative effects of BR-rich extracts from various haloarchaeal strains, notably on hepatoma and breast cancer cell lines, suggest its potential as a valuable candidate for novel anticancer therapies. However, to translate these findings into clinically relevant interventions, further investigations are necessary to elucidate the underlying molecular mechanisms driving BR's anticancer properties. Additionally, comprehensive studies are needed to assess potential interactions between BR and current anticancer drugs, ensuring their compatibility and optimizing therapeutic outcomes. It is important to acknowledge the limitations associated with the use of carotenoids, including challenges in identifying optimal doses and potential variations in bioavailability. Moreover, while current preliminary studies may focus on treatment perspectives, clinical investigations with other carotenoids often adopt a preventive approach, which limits the accuracy of direct comparisons. Addressing these complexities will be essential for advancing our understanding of BR's therapeutic potential and developing effective strategies for cancer management.

6. Other Biological Activities of Interest for Biomedical and Pharmaceutical Applications

Aside from their antitumor activity, haloarchaeal carotenoids could have an impact on diabetes and obesity treatments. *Haloferax mediterranei* carotenoid extracts are capable of inhibiting α-glucosidase, α-amylase, and lipase enzymes which are involved in carbohydrate and lipid metabolism. The inhibition of these enzymes is the target of several drugs used to reduce blood glucose and lipid absorption, respectively [14]. Carotenoids from *Halorhabdus utahensis* reached 90% hyaluronidase inhibition with 1.5 μg, demonstrating great potential for applications in the skin care sector [17].

Halobacterium salinarum and *Haloarcula hispanica* carotenoid extracts can inhibit COX-2, acetylcholinesterase, and tyrosinase enzymes and, therefore, they could have potential applications as a treatment for inflammatory, neurological, and dermatological diseases [60]. In addition, haloarchaeal carotenoids exert antimicrobial activity against a wide range of species. For example, bacterioruberin from *Halorubrum tebenquichense* inhibited Staphylococcus aureus growth and biofilm formation [76]. Table 3 summaries more examples in which other biological activities have been described for BR.

Table 3. Other biological activities of BR and its precursors with potential uses in food, cosmetics, medicine, and pharmacy.

Species	Aim of the Research	Reference
Natronoccoccus sp. *Halorubrum tebenquichense*	Matrix metallopeptidase 9 (MMP-9) inhibition activities	[68]
Haloferax mediterranei	Characterisation of antiglycaemic and antilipidemic activities	[14]
Haloferax sp. ME16 *Halogeometricum* sp. ME3*Haloarcula* sp. BT9	Characterisation of the antibacterial activity of BR-rich extracts	[69]
Halorubrum sp. BS2	Isolation and characterization of total carotenoid extracts, and antibacterial activity quantification	[70]
Natrialba sp. M6	Isolation and characterisation of total carotenoid extracts, and antiviral activity quantification	[74]
Haloferax volcanii	Bioactive properties of BR on sperm cells (mainly in connection with antioxidant properties)	[62]
Halogeometricum rufum *Halogeometricum limi* *Haladaptatus litoreus* *Haloplanus vescus* *Halopelagius inordinatus* *Halogranum rubrum* *Haloferax volcanii*	Antihaemolytic activity apart from antitumoral and antioxidant activities	[61]

Finally, although synthetic colourants have been extensively used for numerous years in the cosmetics industry, their detrimental impacts on both the environment and health should not be disregarded. It is key to explore natural alternatives, with a particular focus on microbial colourants, to increase safety and reduce potential side effects [77–80]. Currently, there are multiple companies whose objective is to produce cosmetic and cosmeceutical products that are visually attractive as well as respectful of the environment and human health using ingredients of natural origin. In parallel, natural carotenoids are of interest and currently highly demanded by textile industries. Carotenoids from biological sources are increasingly used as ingredients in these kinds of formulations, due to both their colouring and biological properties [81]. β-carotene is one of the most frequently used carotenoids in this field and it can be obtained from the halophilic microalgae *Dunaliella salina* [82]. Other carotenoids that have been included in currently marketed cosmetic products are astaxanthin (*Haematococcus pluvialis*) and fucoxanthin (*Phaeodactylum tricornutum*) [81].

BR emerges as a promising candidate due to its intense pink-red hue and notable biological properties. As discussed earlier, BR possesses antioxidant, anti-inflammatory, and immunomodulatory characteristics, making it not only aesthetically appealing but also potentially beneficial for skin health. Its natural origin from halophilic archaea aligns with the growing consumer demand for eco-conscious and sustainable products. Despite its promising biological properties, its suitability for topical use on the skin is yet to be addressed. Investigating bacterioruberin's interactions with skin cells, its ability to penetrate the epidermal barrier, and its potential benefits in addressing dermatological conditions or enhancing cosmetic formulations would be invaluable.

BR's potential as a colouring agent also remains relatively unexplored. Given its intense pink-red hue, bacterioruberin holds promise as a natural and vibrant alternative to synthetic colorants in various applications. However, there is a notable gap in research regarding its efficacy, stability, and safety as a colouring agent, particularly in food, cosmetics, and textile industries. Understanding bacterioruberin's colour stability under different processing conditions, its compatibility with various matrices, and its potential allergenicity or toxicity is crucial for its widespread adoption as a colouring agent. Furthermore, exploring methods for extracting and purifying bacterioruberin on an industrial scale is essential for its commercial viability. By bridging these knowledge gaps, BR could be an alternative natural and sustainable colorant with diverse applications across industries.

7. Conclusions

Haloarchaeal carotenoids could have a diverse range of applications across the fields of biomedicine, food processing and conservation, pharmaceuticals, and textiles. These naturally occurring pigments have emerged as promising alternatives to synthetic colourants, addressing the growing demand for natural food colouring options worldwide as well as natural colourants as part of the formulations in cosmetics and pharmacology. Because of the antioxidant, anti-inflammatory, immunomodulatory, and antitumoral activities of BR, this C_{50} carotenoid offers new approaches and strategies for defining new drug formulations or drug immobilisation techniques as part of the treatments of pathologies related to the immune system and cancer, among others. By promoting research on haloarchaeal pigments, it is possible to uncover novel applications for these promising C_{50} carotenoids. Furthermore, the cultivation of haloarchaea and carotenoid extraction are more straightforward compared to other living beings, making them attractive subjects for the research and development of sustainable processes aiming at the production of natural pigments with a wider spectrum of applications, all following circular economy-based processes.

Author Contributions: R.M.M.-E. was involved in the conceptualization, supervision, project administration and funding acquisition. M.G., C.P. and R.M.M.-E. carried out formal analysis and investigation; M.G. and R.M.M.-E. wrote the original draft. All the authors were involved in writing the review. All authors have read and agreed to the published version of the manuscript.

Funding: This study has been funded by Universidad de Alicante (VIGROB-309) and Generalitat Valenciana, Spain (PROMETEO/2021/055).

Conflicts of Interest: The authors declare no conflicts of interest.

References

1. Oren, A. Halophilic Microbial Communities and Their Environments. *Curr. Opin. Biotechnol.* **2015**, *33*, 119–124. [CrossRef]
2. Abaramak, G.; Kırtel, O.; Toksoy Öner, E. Fructanogenic Halophiles: A New Perspective on Extremophiles. In *Physiological and Biotechnological Aspects of Extremophiles*; Elsevier: Amsterdam, The Netherlands, 2020; pp. 123–130, ISBN 978-0-12-818322-9.
3. Oren, A. The Microbiology of Red Brines. In *Advances in Applied Microbiology*; Elsevier: Amsterdam, The Netherlands, 2020; Volume 113, pp. 57–110. ISBN 978-0-12-820709-3.
4. Gupta, R.S.; Naushad, S.; Fabros, R.; Adeolu, M. A Phylogenomic Reappraisal of Family-Level Divisions within the Class *Halobacteria*: Proposal to Divide the Order *Halobacteriales* into the Families *Halobacteriaceae*, *Haloarculaceae* fam. nov., and *Halococcaceae* fam. nov., and the Order *Haloferacales* into the Families, *Haloferacaceae* and *Halorubraceae* fam nov. *Antonie Van Leeuwenhoek* **2016**, *109*, 565–587. [CrossRef]
5. Martínez, G.M.; Pire, C.; Martínez-Espinosa, R.M. Hypersaline Environments as Natural Sources of Microbes with Potential Applications in Biotechnology: The Case of Solar Evaporation Systems to Produce Salt in Alicante County (Spain). *Curr. Res. Microb. Sci.* **2022**, *3*, 100136. [CrossRef]
6. Torregrosa-Crespo, J.; Martínez-Espinosa, R.M.; Esclapez, J.; Bautista, V.; Pire, C.; Camacho, M.; Richardson, D.J.; Bonete, M.J. Anaerobic Metabolism in *Haloferax* Genus. In *Advances in Microbial Physiology*; Elsevier: Amsterdam, The Netherlands, 2016; Volume 68, pp. 41–85. ISBN 978-0-12-804823-8.
7. Oren, A. The Ecology of *Dunaliella* in High-Salt Environments. *J. Biol. Res.* **2014**, *21*, 23. [CrossRef]
8. Dutta, B.; Bandopadhyay, R. Biotechnological Potentials of Halophilic Microorganisms and Their Impact on Mankind. *Beni-Suef Univ. J. Basic Appl. Sci.* **2022**, *11*, 75. [CrossRef]
9. Torregrosa-Crespo, J.; Galiana, C.P.; Martínez-Espinosa, R.M. Biocompounds from Haloarchaea and Their Uses in Biotechnology. In *Archaea—New Biocatalysts, Novel Pharmaceuticals and Various Biotechnological Applications*; Sghaier, H., Najjari, A., Ghedira, K., Eds.; InTech: London, UK, 2017; ISBN 978-953-51-3569-2.
10. Thombre, R.S.; Shinde, V.; Thaiparambil, E.; Zende, S.; Mehta, S. Antimicrobial Activity and Mechanism of Inhibition of Silver Nanoparticles against Extreme Halophilic Archaea. *Front. Microbiol.* **2016**, *7*, 1424. [CrossRef]
11. Moopantakath, J.; Imchen, M.; Anju, V.T.; Busi, S.; Dyavaiah, M.; Martínez-Espinosa, R.M.; Kumavath, R. Bioactive Molecules from Haloarchaea: Scope and Prospects for Industrial and Therapeutic Applications. *Front. Microbiol.* **2023**, *14*, 1113540. [CrossRef]
12. Griffiths, B.S.; Philippot, L. Insights into the Resistance and Resilience of the Soil Microbial Community. *FEMS Microbiol. Rev.* **2013**, *37*, 112–129. [CrossRef]
13. Verma, D.K.; Vasudeva, G.; Sidhu, C.; Pinnaka, A.K.; Prasad, S.E.; Thakur, K.G. Biochemical and Taxonomic Characterization of Novel Haloarchaeal Strains and Purification of the Recombinant Halotolerant α-Amylase Discovered in the Isolate. *Front. Microbiol.* **2020**, *11*, 2082. [CrossRef]
14. Giani, M.; Gervasi, L.; Loizzo, M.R.; Martínez-Espinosa, R.M. Carbon Source Influences Antioxidant, Antiglycemic, and Antilipidemic Activities of *Haloferax mediterranei* Carotenoid Extracts. *Mar. Drugs* **2022**, *20*, 659. [CrossRef]
15. Giani, M.; Montoyo-Pujol, Y.G.; Peiró, G.; Martínez-Espinosa, R.M. Haloarchaeal Carotenoids Exert an in Vitro Antiproliferative Effect on Human Breast Cancer Cell Lines. *Sci. Rep.* **2023**, *13*, 7148. [CrossRef]
16. Squillaci, G.; Parrella, R.; Carbone, V.; Minasi, P.; La Cara, F.; Morana, A. Carotenoids from the Extreme Halophilic Archaeon *Haloterrigena turkmenica*: Identification and Antioxidant Activity. *Extremophiles* **2017**, *21*, 933–945. [CrossRef]
17. Serino, I.; Squillaci, G.; Errichiello, S.; Carbone, V.; Baraldi, L.; La Cara, F.; Morana, A. Antioxidant Capacity of Carotenoid Extracts from the Haloarchaeon *Halorhabdus utahensis*. *Antioxidants* **2023**, *12*, 1840. [CrossRef]
18. Mandelli, F.; Miranda, V.S.; Rodrigues, E.; Mercadante, A.Z. Identification of Carotenoids with High Antioxidant Capacity Produced by Extremophile Microorganisms. *World J. Microbiol. Biotechnol.* **2012**, *28*, 1781–1790. [CrossRef]
19. Kesbiç, F.I.; Gültepe, N. Carotenoid Characterization, Fatty Acid Profiles, and Antioxidant Activities of Haloarchaeal Extracts. *J. Basic Microbiol.* **2023**, *64*, e2300330. [CrossRef]
20. Kesbiç, F.I.; Gültepe, N. C_{50} Carotenoids Extracted from *Haloterrigena thermotolerans* strain K15: Antioxidant Potential and Identification. *Folia Microbiol.* **2022**, *67*, 71–79. [CrossRef]
21. Giani, M.; Martínez-Espinosa, R.M. Carotenoids as a Protection Mechanism against Oxidative Stress in *Haloferax mediterranei*. *Antioxidants* **2020**, *9*, 1060. [CrossRef]
22. Kesbiç, F.I.; Metin, H.; Fazio, F.; Parrino, V.; Kesbiç, O.S. Effects of Bacterioruberin-Rich Haloarchaeal Carotenoid Extract on the Thermal and Oxidative Stabilities of Fish Oil. *Molecules* **2023**, *28*, 8023. [CrossRef]
23. Hwang, C.Y.; Cho, E.-S.; Kim, S.; Kim, K.; Seo, M.-J. Optimization of Bacterioruberin Production from *Halorubrum ruber* and Assessment of Its Antioxidant Potential. *Microb. Cell Factories* **2024**, *23*, 2. [CrossRef]
24. Ávila-Román, J.; Gómez-Villegas, P.; De Carvalho, C.C.C.R.; Vigara, J.; Motilva, V.; León, R.; Talero, E. Up-Regulation of the Nrf2/HO-1 Antioxidant Pathway in Macrophages by an Extract from a New Halophilic Archaea Isolated in Odiel Saltworks. *Antioxidants* **2023**, *12*, 1080. [CrossRef]

25. Higa, L.H.; Schilrreff, P.; Briski, A.M.; Jerez, H.E.; De Farias, M.A.; Villares Portugal, R.; Romero, E.L.; Morilla, M.J. Bacterioruberin from Haloarchaea plus Dexamethasone in Ultra-Small Macrophage-Targeted Nanoparticles as Potential Intestinal Repairing Agent. *Colloids Surf. B Biointerfaces* **2020**, *191*, 110961. [CrossRef]
26. Serrano, S.; Mendo, S.; Caetano, T. Haloarchaea Have a High Genomic Diversity for the Biosynthesis of Carotenoids of Biotechnological Interest. *Res. Microbiol.* **2022**, *173*, 103919. [CrossRef]
27. Ren, Y.; Sun, H.; Deng, J.; Huang, J.; Chen, F. Carotenoid Production from Microalgae: Biosynthesis, Salinity Responses and Novel Biotechnologies. *Mar. Drugs* **2021**, *19*, 713. [CrossRef]
28. Sandmann, G. Carotenoids and Their Biosynthesis in Fungi. *Molecules* **2022**, *27*, 1431. [CrossRef]
29. Vargas-Sinisterra, A.F.; Ramírez-Castrillón, M. Yeast Carotenoids: Production and Activity as Antimicrobial Biomolecule. *Arch. Microbiol.* **2021**, *203*, 873–888. [CrossRef]
30. Maoka, T. Carotenoids as Natural Functional Pigments. *J. Nat. Med.* **2020**, *74*, 1–16. [CrossRef]
31. Nisar, N.; Li, L.; Lu, S.; Khin, N.C.; Pogson, B.J. Carotenoid Metabolism in Plants. *Mol. Plant* **2015**, *8*, 68–82. [CrossRef]
32. Alcaíno, J.; Baeza, M.; Cifuentes, V. Carotenoid Distribution in Nature. In *Carotenoids in Nature*; Stange, C., Ed.; Subcellular Biochemistry; Springer International Publishing: Cham, Switzerland, 2016; Volume 79, pp. 3–33. ISBN 978-3-319-39124-3.
33. Kushwaha, S.C.; Kramer, J.K.G.; Kates, M. Isolation and Characterization of C_{50}-Carotenoid Pigments and Other Polar Isoprenoids from Halobacterium Cutirubrum. *Biochim. Biophys. Acta* **1975**, *398*, 303–314. [CrossRef]
34. Kushwaha, S.C.; Kates, M. Studies of the Biosynthesis of C_{50} Carotenoids in *Halobacterium cutirubrum*. *Can. J. Microbiol.* **1979**, *25*, 1292–1297. [CrossRef]
35. Giani, M.; Garbayo, I.; Vílchez, C.; Martínez-Espinosa, R.M. Haloarchaeal Carotenoids: Healthy Novel Compounds from Extreme Environments. *Mar. Drugs* **2019**, *17*, 524. [CrossRef]
36. Asker, D.; Ohta, Y. Production of Canthaxanthin by Extremely Halophilic Bacteria. *J. Biosci. Bioeng.* **1999**, *88*, 617–621. [CrossRef]
37. Rodrigo-Baños, M.; Garbayo, I.; Vílchez, C.; Bonete, M.; Martínez-Espinosa, R. Carotenoids from Haloarchaea and Their Potential in Biotechnology. *Mar. Drugs* **2015**, *13*, 5508–5532. [CrossRef]
38. Chattopadhyay, M.K.; Jagannadham, M.V.; Vairamani, M.; Shivaji, S. Carotenoid Pigments of an Antarctic Psychrotrophic Bacterium *Micrococcus roseus*: Temperature Dependent Biosynthesis, Structure, and Interaction with Synthetic Membranes. *Biochem. Biophys. Res. Commun.* **1997**, *239*, 85–90. [CrossRef]
39. Flegler, A.; Lipski, A. The C_{50} Carotenoid Bacterioruberin Regulates Membrane Fluidity in Pink-Pigmented *Arthrobacter* Species. *Arch. Microbiol.* **2022**, *204*, 70. [CrossRef]
40. Silva, T.R.; Tavares, R.S.N.; Canela-Garayoa, R.; Eras, J.; Rodrigues, M.V.N.; Neri-Numa, I.A.; Pastore, G.M.; Rosa, L.H.; Schultz, J.A.A.; Debonsi, H.M.; et al. Chemical Characterization and Biotechnological Applicability of Pigments Isolated from Antarctic Bacteria. *Mar. Biotechnol.* **2019**, *21*, 416–429. [CrossRef]
41. Giani, M.; Miralles-Robledillo, J.M.; Peiró, G.; Pire, C.; Martínez-Espinosa, R.M. Deciphering Pathways for Carotenogenesis in Haloarchaea. *Molecules* **2020**, *25*, 1197. [CrossRef]
42. Yang, Y.; Yatsunami, R.; Ando, A.; Miyoko, N.; Fukui, T.; Takaichi, S.; Nakamura, S. Complete Biosynthetic Pathway of the C_{50} Carotenoid Bacterioruberin from Lycopene in the Extremely Halophilic Archaeon *Haloarcula japonica*. *J. Bacteriol.* **2015**, *197*, 1614–1623. [CrossRef]
43. Cerletti, M.; Rabino, A.; Paggi, R.A.; Ferrari, C.; Poetsch, A.; Savilahti, H.; Kiljunen, S.; De Castro, R.E. The C-Terminal Region of Phytoene Synthase Is a Key Element to Control Carotenoid Biosynthesis in the Haloarchaeon *Haloferax volcanii*. *Biochem. J.* **2022**, *479*, 2365–2377. [CrossRef]
44. Grivard, A.; Goubet, I.; Duarte Filho, L.M.D.S.; Thiéry, V.; Chevalier, S.; De Oliveira-Junior, R.G.; El Aouad, N.; Guedes Da Silva Almeida, J.R.; Sitarek, P.; Quintans-Junior, L.J.; et al. Archaea Carotenoids: Natural Pigments with Unexplored Innovative Potential. *Mar. Drugs* **2022**, *20*, 524. [CrossRef]
45. Sathasivam, R.; Radhakrishnan, R.; Kim, J.K.; Park, S.U. An Update on Biosynthesis and Regulation of Carotenoids in Plants. *S. Afr. J. Botany* **2021**, *140*, 290–302. [CrossRef]
46. Zhou, X.; Rao, S.; Wrightstone, E.; Sun, T.; Lui, A.C.W.; Welsch, R.; Li, L. Phytoene Synthase: The Key Rate-Limiting Enzyme of Carotenoid Biosynthesis in Plants. *Front. Plant Sci.* **2022**, *13*, 884720. [CrossRef]
47. Mata-Gómez, L.C.; Montañez, J.C.; Méndez-Zavala, A.; Aguilar, C.N. Biotechnological Production of Carotenoids by Yeasts: An Overview. *Microb. Cell Factories* **2014**, *13*, 12. [CrossRef]
48. Othman, R.; Mohd Zaifuddin, F.A.; Hassan, N.M. Carotenoid Biosynthesis Regulatory Mechanisms in Plants. *J. Oleo Sci.* **2014**, *63*, 753–760. [CrossRef]
49. Sandmann, G. Diversity and Evolution of Carotenoid Biosynthesis from Prokaryotes to Plants. In *Carotenoids. Biosynthetic and Biofunctional Approaches*; Misawa, N., Ed.; Advances in Experimental Medicine and Biology; Springer: Singapore, 2021; Volume 1261, pp. 79–94, ISBN 9789811573590.
50. Lu, S.; Li, L. Carotenoid Metabolism: Biosynthesis, Regulation, and Beyond. *J. Integr. Plant Biol.* **2008**, *50*, 778–785. [CrossRef]
51. Hirschberg, J. Carotenoid Biosynthesis in Flowering Plants. *Curr. Opin. Plant Biol.* **2001**, *4*, 210–218. [CrossRef]
52. Llorente, B.; Martinez-Garcia, J.F.; Stange, C.; Rodriguez-Concepcion, M. Illuminating Colors: Regulation of Carotenoid Biosynthesis and Accumulation by Light. *Curr. Opin. Plant Biol.* **2017**, *37*, 49–55. [CrossRef]
53. Mishra, S.; Singh Chanotiya, C.; Shanker, K.; Kumar Tripathi, A. Characterization of Carotenoids and Genes Encoding Their Biosynthetic Pathways in *Azospirillum brasilense*. *FEMS Microbiol. Lett.* **2021**, *368*, fnab025. [CrossRef]

54. Asker, D.; Ohta, Y. Haloferax Alexandrinus Sp. Nov., an Extremely Halophilic Canthaxanthin-Producing Archaeon from a Solar Saltern in Alexandria (Egypt). *Int. J. Syst. Evol. Microbiol.* **2002**, *52*, 729–738. [CrossRef]
55. Tao, L.; Cheng, Q. Novel β-Carotene Ketolases from Non-Photosynthetic Bacteria for Canthaxanthin Synthesis. *Mol. Genet. Genom.* **2004**, *272*, 530–537. [CrossRef]
56. Martín, J.F.; Gudiña, E.; Barredo, J.L. Conversion of β-Carotene into Astaxanthin: Two Separate Enzymes or a Bifunctional Hydroxylase-Ketolase Protein? *Microb. Cell Factories* **2008**, *7*, 3. [CrossRef]
57. Calegari-Santos, R.; Diogo, R.A.; Fontana, J.D.; Bonfim, T.M.B. Carotenoid Production by Halophilic Archaea Under Different Culture Conditions. *Curr. Microbiol.* **2016**, *72*, 641–651. [CrossRef] [PubMed]
58. Will Chen, C.; Hsu, S.; Lin, M.-T.; Hsu, Y. Mass Production of C_{50} Carotenoids by *Haloferax mediterranei* in Using Extruded Rice Bran and Starch under Optimal Conductivity of Brined Medium. *Bioprocess. Biosyst. Eng.* **2015**, *38*, 2361–2367. [CrossRef] [PubMed]
59. Abbes, M.; Baati, H.; Guermazi, S.; Messina, C.; Santulli, A.; Gharsallah, N.; Ammar, E. Biological Properties of Carotenoids Extracted from *Halobacterium halobium* Isolated from a Tunisian Solar Saltern. *BMC Complement. Altern. Med.* **2013**, *13*, 255. [CrossRef] [PubMed]
60. Gómez-Villegas, P.; Vigara, J.; Vila, M.; Varela, J.; Barreira, L.; Léon, R. Antioxidant, Antimicrobial, and Bioactive Potential of Two New Haloarchaeal Strains Isolated from Odiel Salterns (Southwest Spain). *Biology* **2020**, *9*, 298. [CrossRef] [PubMed]
61. Hou, J.; Cui, H.-L. In Vitro Antioxidant, Antihemolytic, and Anticancer Activity of the Carotenoids from Halophilic Archaea. *Curr. Microbiol.* **2018**, *75*, 266–271. [CrossRef] [PubMed]
62. Zalazar, L.; Pagola, P.; Miró, M.V.; Churio, M.S.; Cerletti, M.; Martínez, C.; Iniesta-Cuerda, M.; Soler, A.J.; Cesari, A.; De Castro, R. Bacterioruberin Extracts from a Genetically Modified Hyperpigmented *Haloferax volcanii* Strain: Antioxidant Activity and Bioactive Properties on Sperm Cells. *J. Appl. Microbiol.* **2019**, *126*, 796–810. [CrossRef]
63. Fang, C.-J.; Ku, K.-L.; Lee, M.-H.; Su, N.-W. Influence of Nutritive Factors on C_{50} Carotenoids Production by *Haloferax mediterranei* ATCC 33500 with Two-Stage Cultivation. *Bioresour. Technol.* **2010**, *101*, 6487–6493. [CrossRef]
64. Cao, Z.; Ding, X.; Peng, B.; Zhao, Y.; Ding, J.; Watts, A.; Zhao, X. Novel Expression and Characterization of a Light Driven Proton Pump Archaerhodopsin 4 in a *Halobacterium salinarum* Strain. *Biochim. Biophys. Acta–Bioenerg.* **2015**, *1847*, 390–398. [CrossRef] [PubMed]
65. Sun, C.; Ding, X.; Cui, H.; Yang, Y.; Chen, S.; Watts, A.; Zhao, X. In Situ Study of the Function of Bacterioruberin in the Dual-Chromophore Photoreceptor Archaerhodopsin-4. *Angew. Chem.* **2018**, *130*, 9075–9079. [CrossRef]
66. Yoshimura, K.; Kouyama, T. Structural Role of Bacterioruberin in the Trimeric Structure of Archaerhodopsin-2. *J. Mol. Biol.* **2008**, *375*, 1267–1281. [CrossRef]
67. Morilla, M.J.; Ghosal, K.; Romero, E.L. More Than Pigments: The Potential of Astaxanthin and Bacterioruberin-Based Nanomedicines. *Pharmaceutics* **2023**, *15*, 1828. [CrossRef] [PubMed]
68. Delgado-Garcia, M.; Gómez-Secundino, O.; Rodríguez, J.A.; Mateos-Díaz, J.C.; Muller-Santos, M.; Aguilar, C.N.; Camacho-Ruiz, R.M. Identification, Antioxidant Capacity, and Matrix Metallopeptidase 9 (MMP-9) In Silico Inhibition of Haloarchaeal Carotenoids from *Natronococcus* sp. and *Halorubrum tebenquichense*. *Microorganisms* **2023**, *11*, 2344. [CrossRef] [PubMed]
69. Sahli, K.; Gomri, M.A.; Esclapez, J.; Gómez-Villegas, P.; Bonete, M.-J.; León, R.; Kharroub, K. Characterization and Biological Activities of Carotenoids Produced by Three Haloarchaeal Strains Isolated from Algerian Salt Lakes. *Arch. Microbiol.* **2022**, *204*, 6. [CrossRef] [PubMed]
70. Sahli, K.; Gomri, M.A.; Esclapez, J.; Gómez-Villegas, P.; Ghennai, O.; Bonete, M.; León, R.; Kharroub, K. Bioprospecting and Characterization of Pigmented Halophilic Archaeal Strains from Algerian Hypersaline Environments with Analysis of Carotenoids Produced by *Halorubrum* sp. BS2. *J. Basic Microbiol.* **2020**, *60*, 624–638. [CrossRef] [PubMed]
71. Shahmohammadi, H.R.; Asgarani, E.; Terato, H.; Saito, T.; Ohyama, Y.; Gekko, K.; Yamamoto, O.; Ide, H. Protective Roles of Bacterioruberin and Intracellular KCl in the Resistance of *Halobacterium salinarium* against DNA-Damaging Agents. *J. Radiat. Res.* **1998**, *39*, 251–262. [CrossRef] [PubMed]
72. Kottemann, M.; Kish, A.; Iloanusi, C.; Bjork, S.; DiRuggiero, J. Physiological Responses of the Halophilic Archaeon *Halobacterium* sp. strain NRC1 to Desiccation and Gamma Irradiation. *Extremophiles* **2005**, *9*, 219–227. [CrossRef] [PubMed]
73. Alvares, J.J.; Furtado, I.J. Characterization of Multicomponent Antioxidants from *Haloferax alexandrinus* GUSF-1 (KF796625). *3 Biotech.* **2021**, *11*, 58. [CrossRef]
74. Hegazy, G.E.; Abu-Serie, M.M.; Abo-Elela, G.M.; Ghozlan, H.; Sabry, S.A.; Soliman, N.A.; Abdel-Fattah, Y.R. In Vitro Dual (Anticancer and Antiviral) Activity of the Carotenoids Produced by Haloalkaliphilic Archaeon *Natrialba* sp. M6. *Sci. Rep.* **2020**, *10*, 5986. [CrossRef]
75. Shahbazi, S.; Zargar, M.; Zolfaghari, M.R.; Amoozegar, M.A. Carotenoid Pigment of Halophilic Archaeon *Haloarcula* sp. A15 Induces Apoptosis of Breast Cancer Cells. *Cell Biochem. Funct.* **2023**, *41*, 344–354. [CrossRef]
76. Simioni, Y.R.; Perez, N.S.; Barbosa, L.R.S.; Perez, A.P.; Schilrreff, P.; Romero, E.L.; Morilla, M.J. Enhancing the Anti-Psoriatic Activity of Vitamin D3 Employing Nanostructured Archaeolipid Carriers. *J. Drug Del. Sci. Technol.* **2022**, *73*, 103455. [CrossRef]
77. Kumar, S.; Kumar, R.; Diksha; Kumari, A.; Panwar, A. Astaxanthin: A Super Antioxidant from Microalgae and Its Therapeutic Potential. *J. Basic Microbiol.* **2022**, *62*, 1064–1082. [CrossRef] [PubMed]
78. Kumar, A.; Vishwakarma, H.S.; Singh, J.; Kumar, M. Microbial pigments: Production and their applications in various industries. *Int. J. Pharm. Chem. Biol. Sci.* **2015**, *5*, 203–212.

79. Sharma, N.; Shekhar, P.; Kumar, V.; Kaur, H.; Jayasena, V. Microbial Pigments: Sources, Current Status, Future Challenges in Cosmetics and Therapeutic Applications. *J. Basic Microbiol.* **2024**, *64*, 4–21. [CrossRef] [PubMed]
80. Venil, C.K.; Dufossé, L.; Renuka Devi, P. Bacterial Pigments: Sustainable Compounds with Market Potential for Pharma and Food Industry. *Front. Sustain. Food Syst.* **2020**, *4*, 100. [CrossRef]
81. Morocho-Jácome, A.L.; Ruscinc, N.; Martinez, R.M.; De Carvalho, J.C.M.; Santos De Almeida, T.; Rosado, C.; Costa, J.G.; Velasco, M.V.R.; Baby, A.R. (Bio)Technological Aspects of Microalgae Pigments for Cosmetics. *Appl. Microbiol. Biotechnol.* **2020**, *104*, 9513–9522. [CrossRef]
82. Goyal, A.; Sharma, A.; Kaur, J.; Kumari, S.; Garg, M.; Sindhu, R.K.; Rahman, M.H.; Akhtar, M.F.; Tagde, P.; Najda, A.; et al. Bioactive-Based Cosmeceuticals: An Update on Emerging Trends. *Molecules* **2022**, *27*, 828. [CrossRef]

marine drugs

MDPI

Review

Marine-Derived Leads as Anticancer Candidates by Disrupting Hypoxic Signaling through Hypoxia-Inducible Factors Inhibition

Maria Rita Garcia [1,2,3], Paula B. Andrade [1], Florence Lefranc [4] and Nelson G. M. Gomes [1,*]

[1] REQUIMTE/LAQV, Laboratório de Farmacognosia, Departamento de Química, Faculdade de Farmácia, Universidade do Porto, 4050-313 Porto, Portugal; ritagarcia7@hotmail.com (M.R.G.); pandrade@ff.up.pt (P.B.A.)

[2] 1H-TOXRUN-Toxicology Research Unit, University Institute of Health Sciences, CESPU, CRL, 4585-116 Gandra, Portugal

[3] UCIBIO/REQUIMTE, Laboratory of Toxicology, Faculty of Pharmacy, University of Porto, 4050-313 Porto, Portugal

[4] Department of Neurosurgery, Hôpital Universitaire de Bruxelles (H.U.B), CUB Hôpital Erasme, Université Libre de Bruxelles (ULB), 1070 Brussels, Belgium; florence.lefranc@hubruxelles.be

* Correspondence: ngomes@ff.up.pt; Tel.: +351-122-042-8500

Abstract: The inadequate vascularization seen in fast-growing solid tumors gives rise to hypoxic areas, fostering specific changes in gene expression that bolster tumor cell survival and metastasis, ultimately leading to unfavorable clinical prognoses across different cancer types. Hypoxia-inducible factors (HIF 1 and HIF 2) emerge as druggable pivotal players orchestrating tumor metastasis and angiogenesis, thus positioning them as prime targets for cancer treatment. A range of HIF inhibitors, notably natural compounds originating from marine organisms, exhibit encouraging anticancer properties, underscoring their significance as promising therapeutic options. Bioprospection of the marine environment is now a well-settled approach to the discovery and development of anticancer agents that might have their medicinal chemistry developed into clinical candidates. However, despite the massive increase in the number of marine natural products classified as 'anticancer leads,' most of which correspond to general cytotoxic agents, and only a few have been characterized regarding their molecular targets and mechanisms of action. The current review presents a critical analysis of inhibitors of HIF-1 and HIF-2 and hypoxia-selective compounds that have been sourced from marine organisms and that might act as new chemotherapeutic candidates or serve as templates for the development of structurally similar derivatives with improved anticancer efficacy.

Keywords: caulerpin; discorhabdin; dolastatin-15; echinomycin; epolactaene; fascaplysin; kalkitoxin; latrunculin; plitidepsin; psammaplin

1. Introduction

1.1. Marine Natural Products in Cancer Therapy

Bioprospection of the marine environment has emerged as a new frontier in drug development due to the nearly unlimited potential of marine organisms as sources of lead structures that cover a wide range of pharmacological effects and biotechnological applications [1–3]. The vast repertoire of complex compounds with unconventional structural architectures, many possessing relevant and specific biological effects, turned the attention of organic chemists and pharmacologists to the depths of the oceans, leading to an exponential growth in the discovery of new marine natural products on the last 20 years [1,2,4–6].

Many of these compounds have been portrayed as 'chemical weapons' as they evolved to interact efficiently with biological targets, displaying an inherent degree of drug-likeness and frequently exerting relevant anticancer, antimicrobial, and immunosuppressive properties. For example, it is hypothesized that the decreased frequency of tumors in marine invertebrates may derive from an innate immune system [7]. Furthermore, there is also evidence that there is an inherent ability to overcome the sea dilution effect, which may partially explain the higher incidence of significant bioactivity compared with organisms from the terrestrial environment, with approximately half of the novel marine-derived natural products displaying biological activity [1,2,8,9].

It is clear that natural products have been the most successful source of anticancer agents ever [10–12]. Newman and Cragg have been updating the contribution of natural products to the development of drugs, with their latest review indicating that from all the chemotherapeutic drugs approved between 1946 and 2019, only 21% can be ascribed as truly synthetic, corroborating the major contribution of natural sources [13].

While most sources inspiring the development of anticancer agents have a terrestrial origin, marine-derived compounds are marking a milestone, providing new lead structures with unprecedented chemical diversity, striking anticancer properties and inspiring the design of several derivatives that keep feeding a constantly active marine pharmaceutical pipeline [1,13]. Cytarabine (Cytosar-U®) is traced back as the first marine-derived drug to receive market authorization from the Food and Drug Administration (FDA) in 1969. The development of cytarabine was inspired by the structural framework of two arabinose-containing nucleosides isolated from the sponge *Cryptotethya crypta* and completely transformed the approach to treating and handling hematological malignancies [14,15]. More than 50 years after cytarabine's approval, thirteen additional marine-derived drugs received market approval, with 38 candidates currently in clinical development [16]. As reviewed by us in 2019, the clinical pipeline of marine-derived drugs, consisting of approved drugs and clinical candidates, has been particularly fruitful in cancer therapy, not only enabling the broadening of the scope of action in cancer treatment but also the discovery of new mechanisms of action and molecular targets [17].

Despite the apparent and exciting richness of new potential anticancer agents from marine sources [17–21], it should be taken into account that the early research on the chemistry of marine natural products was mainly directed to the identification of novel chemical structures rather than in their potential biological properties [22,23]. Early anticancer screening has been mainly focused on the mere evaluation of the cytotoxic properties against cancer cell lines, with no emphasis on the effective anticancer activity against multidrug-resistant (MDR) cell lines, selectivity, or elucidation of their mechanisms of action [1,2]. Consequently, only a disappointing fraction of compounds, determined as cytotoxic against human cancer cell lines, ultimately displayed in vivo activity and, subsequently, clinical relevance [24,25]. Indeed, the complexity of a tumor derives from the continuous crosstalk between the tumor cells and the microenvironment over time, adding the complication of temporal heterogeneity on top of spatial heterogeneity, and by no means a purely cytotoxic or proapoptotic agent is likely to translate into an anticancer drug [26]. Conceivably, distinct environmental landscapes within a given tumor select for mutations that engender survival and expansion, thereby creating tumor cell heterogeneity and a complex regional difference in selective pressures, including hypoxia, that actively shapes tumor development [26,27].

1.2. Hypoxic Signaling in Cancer Development

Due to insufficient vascularization, hypoxic regions form within rapidly growing solid tumor masses, specific alterations of gene expression in these hypoxic tumor cells helping to facilitate the survival and metastatic spread of solid tumors, being therefore associated with poor clinical outcomes in many types of human cancers [28–30]. Hypoxic cancer cells are, in fact, resistant to radiotherapy, chemotherapy, and targeted therapy [28,31,32].

The hypoxic environment sparks cancer development by inducing an intricate cellular signaling network within cancer cells, encompassing the HIF, PI3K, MAPK, and NFκB pathways (Figure 1). These pathways interact with one another, leading to the formation of both positive and negative feedback loops, ultimately amplifying or reducing the impact of hypoxic conditions [33,34]. Hypoxia triggers the activation of HIFs, these factors consisting of hypoxia-regulated α and oxygen-insensitive β subunits, playing a crucial role in regulating gene expression during hypoxia, both in normal and solid tumor tissues (Figure 1) [28,35]. The HIF family comprises three members: HIF-1α, HIF-2α, and HIF-3α, each serving distinct functions. Unlike HIF-1α and HIF-2α, HIF-3α exhibits variations in protein structure and gene expression regulation. During hypoxia, HIF-3α exerts a transcriptional regulatory function that negatively impacts gene expression by competing with HIF-1α and HIF-2α for binding to transcriptional elements in target genes [35,36]. Additionally, HIF-1α plays a significant role in regulating mitochondrial homeostasis, as one of the essential adaptations to sustained hypoxia involves suppressing mitochondrial respiration and inducing glycolysis [37,38]. On the other hand, the activation of HIF-2α enhances peroxisome turnover through pexophagy, leading to changes in lipid composition akin to peroxisomal disorders [39–41].

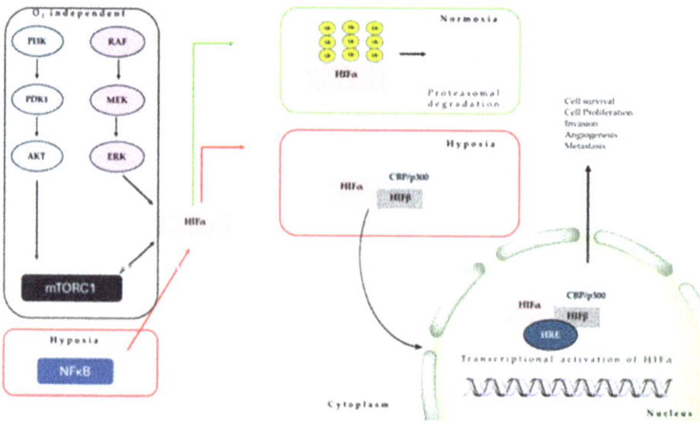

Figure 1. Pathways on hypoxia-inducible factor activation.

Activation of HIFs leads to a range of molecular effects, resulting in the transcription of numerous genes that play pivotal roles in processes such as angiogenesis, specification of cancer stem cells, cell motility, epithelial-mesenchymal transition, remodeling of the extracellular matrix, glucose and lipid metabolism, immune evasion, invasion, and metastasis (Figure 1) [42,43]. Such biochemical alterations evidence that the hypoxic tumor microenvironment influences the majority of hallmarks of aggressive cancer behavior, translating into clinical consequences that have been associated with increased patient mortality in several cancer types [42,44].

Considering such factors, inhibiting the activity of HIF-1 and HIF-2 in hypoxic regions of cancer could potentially increase the cancer's responsiveness to radiotherapy and/or chemotherapy [42,45], but despite the pivotal role of HIFs, only a reduced number of marine natural products have been investigated on their impact upon these heterodimeric transcription factors. Previous reviews covering natural products that impact the HIF pathway are worth mentioning, mostly covering plant-derived and synthetic inhibitors of HIF-1 with a brief mention of marine-sourced compounds [46–53]. Readers are also invited to take a glimpse at the structure–activity relationship (SAR) analysis of ten chemotypes reported to be HIF-1 inhibitors [54], as well as to the patent survey by Nakamura and colleagues, summarizing the information about patented HIF inhibitors over the time period from 2011 to 2015 [55].

As far as we are aware, there is only a descriptive review by Nagle and Zhou dealing with marine natural products that were identified as inhibitors of HIF-1 activation as of December 2008 [56], justifying the updated comprehensive analysis herein delivered. In the current analysis, we provide critical input as the marine natural products that are known to inhibit HIF-1 and HIF-2 are also highlighted, considering other effects that cooperate with the overall 'anticancer potential'. Our comprehensive literature search covers the period up to February 2024 without a start date restriction, with the keywords 'marine natural products', 'hypoxia-inducible factor', and 'cancer', as well as cross-referencing being used to expand the search criteria.

2. Marine Natural Products Acting as Inhibitors of HIF-1 and HIF-2

An expanding and motivating list of hundreds of additional lead structures produced by marine organisms currently feeds the preclinical pipeline, being expected that many new agents will step into clinical trials in the upcoming years. In the following sections, a comprehensive discussion will be presented on the most promising metabolites produced by marine organisms displaying anticancer properties via impact upon the HIF pathway.

2.1. Peptides

While originally discovered in terrestrial counterparts, actinomycin D (also known as dactinomycin) (**1**) (Figure 2) has also been reported from several marine strains of *Streptomycetes* [57,58]. The cyclic dipeptide antibiotic is a well-known chemotherapeutic and radiosensitizing agent (Cosmogen®) with anticancer effects mainly deriving from DNA intercalation and the subsequent impediment on the progression of RNA polymerases [59]. Actinomycin D (**1**) leads to an extremely fast action upon RNA polymerases but is a nonselective inhibitor of protein transcription, which determines some of the severe side effects [59]. Apart from the main anticancer mechanisms, **1** has been reported to inhibit HIF-1 binding activity to DNA in hepatocellular carcinoma Hep3B cells [60,61], but the effects in vascular smooth muscular cells demonstrated that actinomycin D (**1**) solely attenuated angiotensin II-mediated induction of HIF-1α protein expression levels and not the hypoxia-dependent induction [62].

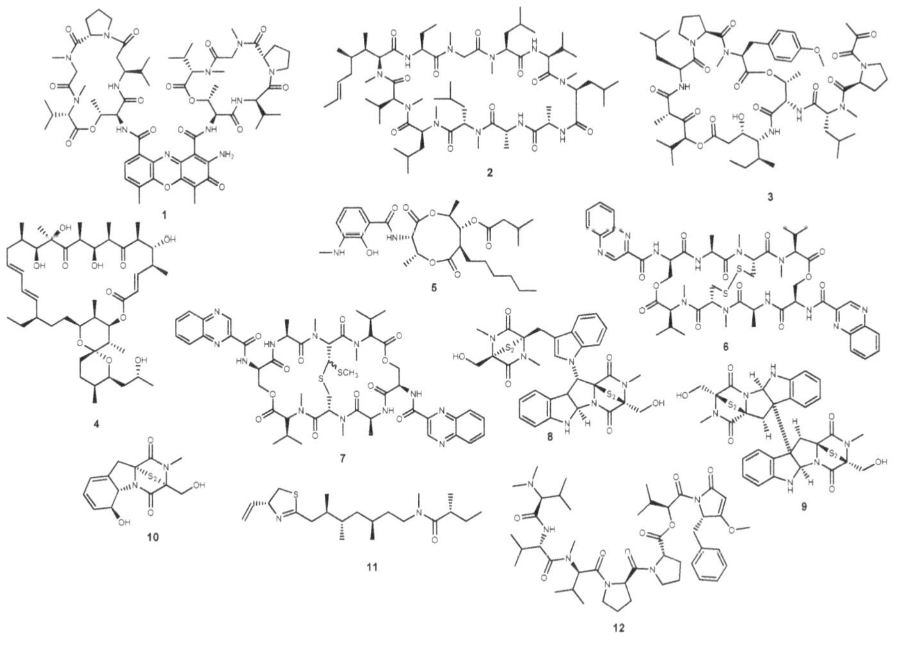

Figure 2. Structures of marine-derived peptides acting on the HIF pathway.

Also, the undecacyclopeptide cyclosporin A (**2**) (Figure 2) has been reported from marine-derived isolates of fungi [63]. The blockbuster immunosuppressant stimulates the activity of peptidylprolyl hydroxylases, ultimately modifying Pro-564 of the HIF-1α protein. The outcomes include the abolishment of hypoxic stabilization of HIF-1α and HIF-1α-mediated cellular responses in glioma C6 cells, being hypothesized that cyclosporin A (**2**) might limit adaptative responses to hypoxia [64].

Unlike actinomycin D (**1**) and cyclosporin A (**2**), the second-generation didemnin plitidepsin (**3**) (Figure 2), originally isolated from the Mediterranean tunicate *Aplidium albicans*, appears to be a strictly marine-derived metabolite [65]. Plitidepsin (**3**) received market approval under the trade name Aplidin® for the treatment of patients with relapsed and refractory multiple myeloma, acting as a pleiotropic chemotherapeutic agent [66]. While mainly acting as a disruptor of the translation elongation factor eEF1A2 protein complexes, leading to the induction of early oxidative stress and subsequent sustained activation of JNK in multiple myeloma cells, **3** was found to impact against angiogenic-related genes in anaplastic thyroid cancer xenografts [67]. Angiogenesis-related genes targeted by plitidepsin (**3**) include not only HIF-1 but also the transforming growth factor-β (TGFβ), TGFβR2, melanoma growth stimulating factor 1 (GRO1), cadherin and vasostatin, cumulatively inducing tumor starvation [67].

Reported from both terrestrial and marine *Streptomyces* spp., oligomycin A (**4**) (Figure 2) is mainly reputed as a mitochondrial F0F1-ATPase inhibitor [68,69]. Microbial antibiotics have been extensively used to elucidate the mechanistic aspects of ATP formation and energy requirements in tumor cell biology [70]. The effects of oligomycin A (**4**) on short-term hypoxia were investigated on the highly resistant human uveal melanoma Mum2B and U87 glioblastoma cells, results suggesting that the anticancer effects might be enhanced by preventing HIF-1α protein accumulation [71].

Described as a marine natural product [72], the microbial metabolite antimycin A (**5**) (Figure 2) also acts as an inhibitor of oxidative phosphorylation, specifically through the binding to the quinone reduction site of the cytochrome *bc1* complex [73]. Relevantly, the inhibitory effects of **5** upon the mitochondrial electron transport chain were followed by the inhibition of hypoxia-dependent HIF-1α protein induction by decreasing its half-life in osteosarcoma 143B cells [74]. Inhibition of HIF-1α protein induction was further suggested to occur independently of mitochondrial reactive oxygen species (ROS) production [74]. Together with the scientific outcomes delivered by Maeda and colleagues, antimycin A (**5**) is suggested to inhibit angiogenesis through the decreased production of the vascular endothelial growth factor (VEGF) caused by inhibition of HIF-1α activation [75].

While both triostin A (**6**) and echinomycin (**7**) (Figure 2) are labeled as competent HIF-1 inhibitors, the latter has been long into the spotlight as one of the most potent HIF-1 inhibitors, as well as impacting the coactivator/DNA interaction [76,77]. The anticancer effects of **6** and **7** derive from their DNA intercalating effects through the quinoxaline chromophores, preferentially binding at *CpG* steps in the minor groove of the double helix [77]. Echinomycin (**7**) was the first bifunctional intercalating agent proceeding to clinical development, but it was discontinued due to its poor effectiveness in patients with solid tumors [78,79]. While sharing the same structural backbone, **6** and **7** differ on the intrapeptide bridge between the two cysteine residues, determining a distinct HIF-1 inhibitory capacity [80]. Echinomycin (**7**) acts as a potent inhibitor of HIF-1α, blocking HIF-1 DNA binding of endogenous nuclear proteins but mainly the binding to the canonical hypoxia-responsive element (HRE) of VEGF promoter [80,81]. Triostatin (**6**), echinomycin (**7**), and a series of synthetic derivatives were evaluated for effects on the HIF-1 transcriptional activation under hypoxic conditions and cytotoxicity on MCF-7 cells, SAR analysis indicating that the cyclic depsipeptide architecture is as an attractive scaffold to develop selective anticancer agents targeting the hypoxic tumor microenvironment [80].

While both triostin A (**6**) and echinomycin (**7**) have been mainly reported from marine strains of bacterial isolates [82], epithiodiketopiperazines are almost exclusively reported from fungi, many of which obtained from marine sources and also impacting HIF-1 signaling [83]. The diketopiperazine dimers chetomin (**8**) and chaetocin (**9**) (Figure 2) occur both as terrestrial and marine-derived metabolites, being reported from marine strains of *Chaetomium cristatum* and *Nectria inventa*, respectively [84,85]. Both **8** and **9** are recognized for their ability to target the transcriptional coactivator p300 by displacing the zinc ion from its CH1 domain (C-TAD) [86,87]. This action disrupts the interactions with the C-terminal trans-activation domain of HIF-1, ultimately resulting in the attenuation of hypoxia-inducible transcription of downstream signaling components [88,89]. While chetomin (**8**) was identified as the first naturally occurring antagonist of the C-C chemokine receptor type 2 (CCR2) [90], it has played a significant role in uncovering the mechanisms that contribute to the invasiveness of specific cancer cell types, particularly highlighting the preponderant role of hypoxia in ovarian and triple-negative breast cancers [89,91]. Furthermore, the effective inhibition of HIF-1 by chetomin (**8**) leads to a reduction in CA9 and VEGF mRNA expression, enhancing the radiation response specifically under severely hypoxic conditions in HT 1080 human fibrosarcoma and U251MG and U343MG glioma cells [88,92]. Biological implications deriving from the disruption of the HIF-1/p300 complex include a direct antitumor effect but also antiangiogenic properties, with chaetocin (**9**) being more effective than chetomin (**8**) in this matter. The epithiodiketopiperazine dimer **9** is primarily acknowledged for its function as an epigenetic agent via the pharmacological inhibition of SUV39H, being the first histone lysine methyltransferase (HKMT) inhibitor [93–95], but several of its anticancer effects are also attributed to the disruption of the HIF-1α/p300 complex. For instance, chaetocin (**9**) exhibited a reduction in microvessel outgrowth in the low nM range, co-immunoprecipitation experiments providing additional evidence that these effects are, at least in part, a result of inhibiting the HIF-1/p300 interaction [96]. Downstream consequences include reduced levels of secreted VEGF and subsequent downregulation of glycolytic genes, namely *LDHA* and *ENO1*, suggesting a role in inhibiting cell survival under hypoxia and promoting cell death in hypoxic areas [96].

Described as the first member of epithiodiketopiperazines, gliotoxin (**10**) (Figure 2) has been progressively reported on its anticancer ability deriving from multiple targets, including the disruption of HIF-1 activity. The structurally simple epithiodiketopiperazine is commonly sourced from terrestrial and marine-derived strains of *Aspergillus* spp. [97–99]. Reece et al. (2014) also described the antiangiogenic effects of **10**, indicating similar mechanisms as those observed for the dimeric epipolythiodiketopiperazines chetomin (**8**) and chaetocin (**9**): (i) disruption of the C-TAD domain of HIF-1 and (ii) downregulation of the target genes *LDHA* and *ENO1*. In contrast, gliotoxin (**10**) did not impact VEGF expression in PC3 prostate cancer cells, pointing to cell-specific effects that differ from those of **8** and **9** [96].

First described by Gerwick and colleagues as a neurotoxic agent and originally sourced from the marine cyanobacterium *Lyngbya majuscula* [100], kalkitoxin (**11**) (Figure 2) was later found to be a competent disruptor of hypoxic signaling [101]. The lipopeptide inhibited hypoxia-induced activation of HIF-1 in T47D breast ductal carcinoma cells in the low nM range, acting through the suppression of mitochondrial oxygen consumption at electron transport chain (ETC) complex I (NADH-ubiquinone oxidoreductase). Kalkitoxin (**11**) efficiently inhibited the hypoxic induction of *VEGF* or glucose transporter-1 (*GLUT-1*) mRNA expression in a concentration-dependent manner, displaying also antiangiogenic effects via the suppression of hypoxia-induced secreted VEGF protein [101].

The discovery of the pentapeptides dolastatins from the sea hare *Dolabella auricularia* prompted the development of the CD30-targeted antibody-drug conjugate brentuximab vedotin (Adcetris®) that is currently available for the treatment of Hodgkin lymphoma [17,102]. Dolastatin-15 (**12**) (Figure 2) was also originally reported by Pettit and colleagues from the Indian Ocean sea hare *D. auricularia* [103] but has been progressively labeled as a cyanobacterial symbiont metabolite [104,105]. The pentapeptide is predominantly reputed as a potent cytostatic agent that, along with a series of synthetic analogs, proceeded to clinical development [106–111]. Despite mainly acting as a microtubule-destabilizer [112,113], **12** also displays HIF-mediated antiangiogenic activity, with inhibitory effects upon HIF-1α being recorded in vitro and in vivo [114]. Experiments in the single knockout cells HCT116$^{\text{HIF-1}\alpha-/-}$ and HCT116$^{\text{HIF-2}\alpha-/-}$ suggested that dolastatin 15 (**12**) preferentially targeted HIF-1α but not HIF-2α, showing decrease in potency against HCT116$^{\text{HIF-1}\alpha-/-\ \text{HIF-2}\alpha-/-}$ and

HCT116$^{HIF\text{-}1\alpha-/-}$ in contrast to the parental and HCT116$^{HIF\text{-}2\alpha-/-}$ cells [114]. Luesch's group further reported that **12** is able to suppress aberrant transcriptional upregulation of HIF-1α target genes in a zebrafish model, significantly diminishing pathological vascularization [114].

2.2. Alkaloids

During a screening on the ability of more than 170 200 crude natural product extracts to inhibit the HIF-1α/p300 interaction, a series of pyrroloiminoquinone alkaloids (**13**–**19**) (Figure 3) sourced from Australian and New Zealand collections of marine sponges, *Latrunculia* sp., were identified as inhibitors of HIF-1α transcriptional activity [115]. The peculiar structural features of pyrroloiminoquinone alkaloids include the azacarbocyclic spirocyclohexanone and pyrroloiminoquinone redox active core structures that frequently underlie the reported bioactive effects [116]. Pyrroloiminoquinone alkaloids were first screened through a cell-free protein–protein assay by measuring displacement of the HIF-1α binding domain of p300 (CH1) from the p300 binding domain of HIF-1α (C-TAD), with (−)-discorhabdin B dimer (**13**), (+)-discorhabdin B (**14**), (−)-discorhabdin H (**16**), and (−)-discorhabdin L (**17**) featuring as the most effective with IC_{50} values under 5 μM [115]. Results were also obtained in three cancer cell lines transfected with an HIF-1 reporter plasmid containing a hypoxia response element that mediates HIF-1-dependent gene transcription, with all the alkaloids (**13**–**19**) proving to significantly decrease the transcriptional activity of HIF-1α in human colorectal carcinoma HCT 116 cells, and (−)-discorhabdin B dimer (**13**) featuring as the most competent [115]. While most of the sponge-derived pyrroloiminoquinone alkaloids also led to a reduction in luciferase activity in human prostate adenocarcinoma LNCaP cells, there is a clear cell-type specificity on the HIF-1α transcriptional activity, as none proved to be active in COLO 205 colon cancer cells [115]. (−)-Discorhabdin H (**16**) also interfered with the secretion of the downstream target VEGF in LNCaP cells cultured under hypoxic conditions [115]. In addition to the significant inhibition of endothelial cell proliferation and tube formation recorded in HUVEC cells, ex vivo experiments demonstrated that the antiangiogenic effects of (−)-discorhabdin L (**17**) are also related to the decrease in microvessel outgrowth, as demonstrated in the aortic ring assay, at concentrations as low as 1 μM [117].

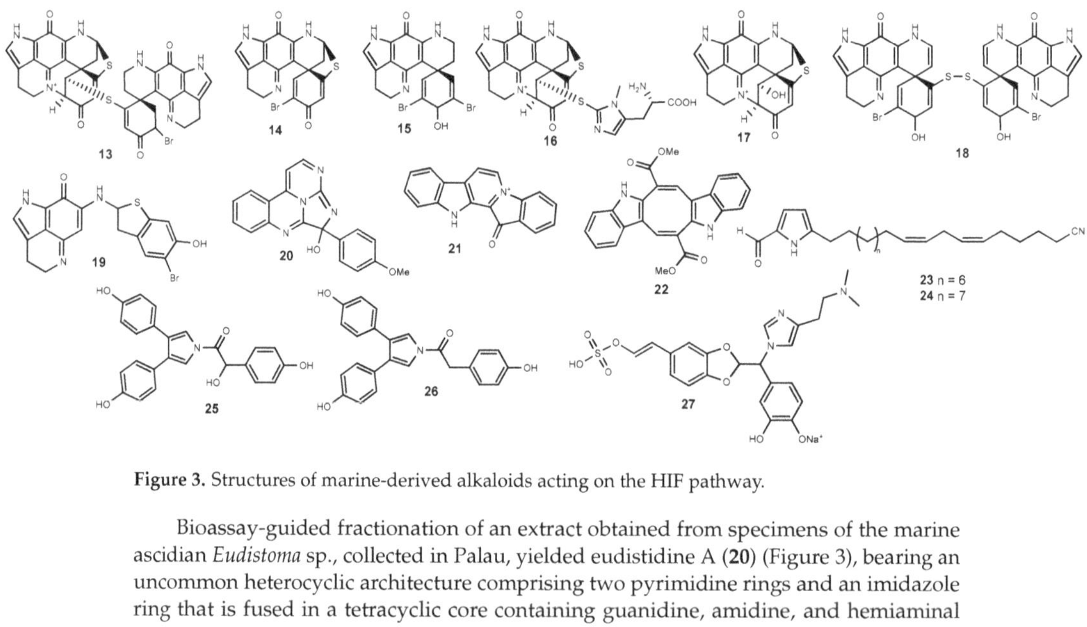

Figure 3. Structures of marine-derived alkaloids acting on the HIF pathway.

Bioassay-guided fractionation of an extract obtained from specimens of the marine ascidian *Eudistoma* sp., collected in Palau, yielded eudistidine A (**20**) (Figure 3), bearing an uncommon heterocyclic architecture comprising two pyrimidine rings and an imidazole ring that is fused in a tetracyclic core containing guanidine, amidine, and hemiaminal functionalities [118]. Eudistidine A (**20**) blocked the binding of soluble CH1 (p300) to immobilized C-TAD (HIF-1α) with concentration dependency, with an IC_{50} value of 75 μM being estimated [118].

Fascaplysin (**21**) (Figure 3), an indole alkaloid originally discovered from the marine sponge *Fascaplysinopsis reticulata* [119], has been reported as having a pleiotropic anticancer mechanism of action, including DNA intercalation [120], inhibition of angiogenesis [121], but mainly the selective inhibition of CDK4 [121–124]. The effects on tumor angiogenesis have been further elucidated in human melanoma A375 and colorectal carcinoma HCT116 cells, as well as in an A375 cell-injected xenograft model. Both in vitro and in vivo data suggested that the antiangiogenic effects of fascaplysin (**21**) derive from a strong suppression of VEGFR2 as well as of HIF-1α and its downstream genes [125].

The algal pigment caulerpin (**22**) (Figure 3), first reported in the 1970s from an ether extract of a *Caulerpa* sp. [126], was later identified as an inhibitor of HIF-1α activation in a human breast tumor T47D cell-based reporter assay [127]. Caulerpin (**22**) was able to inhibit both hypoxia (1% O_2)- and chemical hypoxia (10 μM 1,10-phenanthroline)-induced HIF-1α activation with comparable potency, and while being unable to inhibit the induction of VEGF and GLUT-1 mRNAs by 1,10-phenanthroline in human breast cancer T47D cells, there was a marked decrease on the hypoxia-derived induction of both target genes [127]. Liu et al. [127] further reported that **22** selectively suppresses mitochondrial respiration at complex I (NADH-ubiquinone oxidoreductase), suggesting that, as previously reported with other complex I inhibitors, the blockage of hypoxic induction of HIF-1α protein is mediated by the inhibition of complex III superoxide anion generation.

Chemical analysis of an extract obtained from a *Mycale* sp. sponge yielded 26 alkylpyrroles with variable HIF-1 inhibitory potency [128]. The most active lipophylic pyrroles, mycalenitrile-6 (**23**) and -7 (**24**) (Figure 3), displayed selective HIF-1 inhibitory effects using the T47D cell-based HIF-1 activation reporter assay, preferentially inhibiting hypoxia-induced HIF-1 activation in comparison to the effects on chemical hypoxia/iron chelator-induced activation [128]. Analogously to caulerpin (**22**), the inhibition of HIF-1 activation is mediated through the selective inhibition of mitochondrial respiration at complex I, and both **23** and **24** appear to prevent hypoxic mitochondria from releasing ROS signaling molecules, consequently avoiding the stabilization of HIF-1α protein [128].

Since the first report on the isolation of lamellarins from the Palauan mollusk *Lamellaria* sp. in 1985 [129], more than 50 lamellarins have been reported, mainly from *Didemnum* spp. ascidians [130–137], as well as from sponges [138,139]. Lacking the planar pentacyclic chromophore and consequently differing from the prototype structure of lamellarins, 7-hydroxyneolamellarin A (**25**) (Figure 3) was originally reported from the sponge *Dendrilla nigra* [140]. Unlike most congeners from the subfamily of neolamellarins isolated from the same source, 7-hydroxyneolamellarin A (**25**) effectively inhibited hypoxia-induced HIF-1 activation in a T47D human breast tumor cell-based reporter assay, suppressing also the activation of VEGF [140]. Effects were also demonstrated through in vivo experiments, **25** being able to suppress tumor growth of 4T1 cells in BALB/c mice by inhibiting the accumulation of HIF-1α in tumor tissue [141]. Li and colleagues further suggested that 7-hydroxyneolamellarin A (**25**) targets the protein with the ability to stabilize HIF-1α in hypoxia, as no impact on the degradation of synthesis of HIF-1α was observed [141]. While less effective than the 7-hydroxylated derivative, neolamellarin A (**26**) (Figure 3) also demonstrated HIF-1 inhibitory activity in the reporter gene assay based on T47D human breast tumor cells [140] and prompted the synthesis of a series of derivatives to identify the structural requirements underlying the effects towards HIF-1 [142]. Both naturally occurring constituents (**25** and **26**) proved to be more active than the synthetic derivatives, with SAR analysis indicating that the methoxylation of *p*-hydroxy groups diminished the HIF-1 inhibitory capacity and that a two-carbon aliphatic carbon chain linker was more favorable to the HIF-1 inhibitory activity than a single or triple carbon chain [142].

Displaying an unusual skeleton with a five-membered acetal ring, wondonin A (**27**) (Figure 3) was sourced from a two-sponge association (*Poecillastra wondoensis* and *Jaspis* sp.)

collected at Keomun Island, Korea [143]. Generally, wondonins are reputed for their strong ability to suppress the expression of HIF-1α and VEGF, but what sets them apart from most other antiangiogenic agents is their remarkable ability to inhibit angiogenesis without causing significant cytotoxicity [144]. Wondonin A (**27**) reduced the expression of HIF-1a and VEGF in endothelial cells and could suppress HIF-dependent transcription in HaCaT cells. Authors suggest that the enhancement of the assembly of pVHL and HIF-1α could be the underlying mechanism causing the proteasomal degradation of HIF-1 [144]. To optimize the antiangiogenic properties of wondonins, a series of synthetic analogs have been assayed on their effects towards VEGF-induced cell growth in HUVECs, replacement of benzodioxole and imidazole moieties by benzothiazole and 1,2,3-triazole rings, respectively, resulting in enhanced effects [145].

2.3. Polyketides

Psammaplin A (**28**) (Figure 4) is a spongean bromotyrosine derived dimer with intriguing anticancer properties that has been gaining increased attention since its discovery in 1987. It was originally isolated independently from three research groups, from a *Psammaplysilla sponge* [146], two unidentified sponges [147,148], and later from additional sponge species such as *Pseudoceratina purpurea* [149,150], *Aplysinella rhax* [151], and from the two-sponge association *Poecillastra wondoensis* and *Jaspis wondoensis* [152,153]. Displaying significant in vitro cytotoxicity against a wide panel of human cancer cells namely A549, SK-OV-3, SK-MEL-2, XF498, HCT15 [154], and leukemia cell lines [146,151], as well as in vivo growth inhibitory activity in an A549 lung xenograft mouse model [149], psammaplin A (**28**) has been mainly highlighted as an epigenetic modulator due to its dual inhibitory activity against the chromatin-modifying enzymes histone deacetylases (HDAC) and DNA methyltransferase (DNMT) [149]. Later, in 2015, Kim and coworkers reported psammaplin A (**28**) ability to induce autophagic cell death, markedly increasing the expression of damage-regulated autophagy modulator (DRAM), as well as causing the reduced expression of SIRT1, suggesting an association between SIRT1 expression and p53 acetylation in chemorresistant cancer cells [155]. A series of psammaplins obtained from a lipid extract sample of the sponge *Dendrilla lacunosa* were assayed on a cell-based reporter assay carried out in T47D cells transfected with pHRE-luc for HIF-1 activity. The results revealed intriguing effects with psammaplins being generally characterized by a biphasic pattern of activation, psammaplin A (**28**) strongly activating HIF-1 at 3 μM but displaying reduced effects at lower concentrations [156]. On the other hand, at concentrations ranging from 0.1 to 30 μM, the biphenylic dimer of **28**, bisaprasin (**29**) (Figure 4), inhibited HIF-1 in T47D cells [156].

Widely used in biological research, cycloheximide (**30**) (Figure 4) is mostly known as a transcription inhibitor that interferes with the translocation step and thus blocks translation elongation. Cycloheximide (**30**) was first reported as an antifungal agent by Whiffen-Barksdale of Upjohn Company in the mid-1940s from strains of *Streptomyces griseus* and remains commercially available as Actidione® [157]. Marine-derived strains of Actinomycetes are also reported to display the biosynthetic machinery to produce **30** [158,159]. Cycloheximide (**30**) was first reported to potently block HIF-1α protein expression and inhibit hypoxia- and iron chelator-induced HIF-1 activation in human liver adenocarcinoma Hep3B cells [160]. Semenza et al. (1994) later demonstrated that the induction of erythropoietin, a hormone encoded by a gene whose transcription is regulated by O_2 tension, was also attenuated in Hep3B and HeLa cells [161].

Bioassay-guided fractionation of an extract obtained from cultures of a marine isolate of *Penicillium* sp. led to the isolation of the neuritogenic compound epolactaene (**31**) (Figure 4) [162]. Epolactaene (**31**) was later found to bind human heat shock protein (HSP) 60 Cys^{442}, both in in vitro and in situ settings, inhibiting its chaperone activity [163] and supporting the identification of HSP60 as a regulator of the hypoxia-inducible factor subunit HIF-1α [163,164].

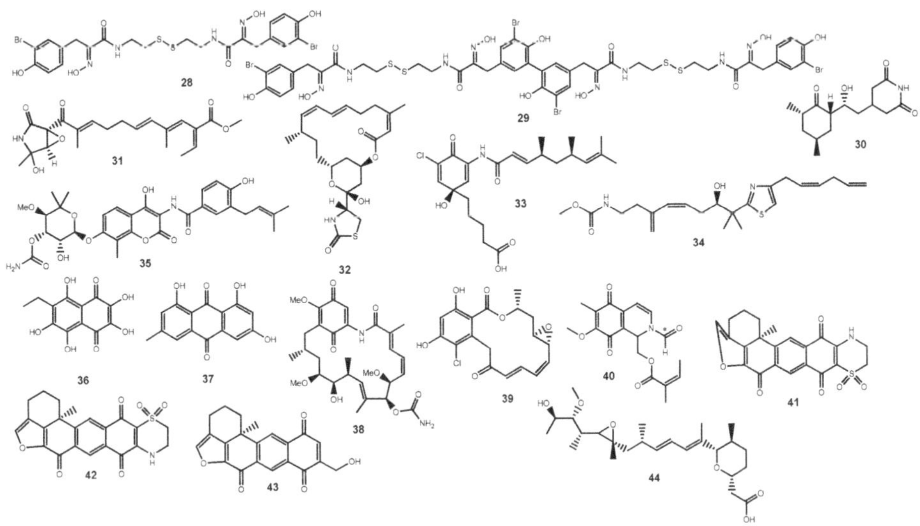

Figure 4. Structures of marine-derived polyketides acting on the HIF pathway.

First described 50 years ago, the 16-membered macrolide toxin latrunculin A (**32**) (Figure 4) was early reported as a microfilament disruptor [165]. Originally isolated from the sponge *Latruncula magnifica* [166,167], the toxin was also reported from *Spongia mycofijiensis* [168] and curiously from associated nudibranchs [168,169]. Latrunculin A (**32**) forms reversible complexes with G-actin, preventing its polymerization, ultimately leading to the disruption of microfilament organization, with no effect on the organization of the microtubular system [165,170]. A potent anti-invasive activity was also observed in prostate cancer PC-3M cells treated with **32**, attenuating their invasiveness and cell migration and selectively suppressing hypoxia-induced HIF-1 activation in T47D breast tumor cells [171]. Relevantly, the blockage of actin dynamics by latrunculin A (**32**), through the inhibition of either polymerization or depolymerization, appears to underlie the attenuation of HIF-1α protein expression via the mTOR/p70^{S6K}/Mdm2 signaling pathway in a p53-independent manner [171,172].

Chemical analyses of an extract and fractions obtained from a saltern-derived halophilic *Streptomyces* strain collected on Shinui Island in the Republic of Korea yielded a series of cytotoxic salternamides [173,174]. Reported as the first chlorinated compound in the manumycin family, salternamide A (**33**) (Figure 4) displayed strong cytotoxicity towards a panel of cancer cell lines, being particularly active towards human colorectal carcinoma HCT-116 cells and human gastric carcinoma SNU638 cells, with IC_{50} values below 1 μM [173]. The anticancer activity of **33** towards HCT116 cells appears to derive from two distinct mechanisms involving G2/M cell cycle arrest and subsequent apoptotic cell death, but also via suppression of HIF-1α translation through the modulation of the mTOR signaling and the downregulation of the axis of the PI3K/ STAT3 signaling pathways [175].

Originally reported by Crews's group in the sponge *Spongia mycofijiensis* [176] and later from the sponge *Dactylospongia* sp. [177], the thiazolo-polyene mycothiazole (**34**) (Figure 4) was initially described as an anthelminthic agent. NCI 60 tumor cell panel screening revealed a potent cytotoxic effect against several cancer cell lines with selective nM potency toward lung cancer cells, namely SCLC and NSCLC cancer lines [178]. Analogously to other HIF-1 inhibitors, **34** selectively disrupts the mitochondrial electron transport chain by suppressing mitochondrial respiration at complex I (NADH-ubiquinone oxidoreductase) and potently blocking hypoxia-induced HIF-1 activation (IC_{50} = 1 nM) [179]. Additionally, mycothiazole (**34**) was found not only to cause a decrease in ROS levels but also to suppress the hypoxic induction of the HIF-1 target genes, VEGF and GLUT-1 [179].

While its nM cytostatic effect in sensitive cells showing a hypoxic response is explained through the disruption of mitochondrial function and inhibition of mitochondrial electron transport complex I, a biphasic response was observed in some sensitive cells, suggesting an additional target. Furthermore, the mycothiazole (**34**) effect in mitochondrial genome-knock out ρo insensitive HL-60, LN18, and Jurkat cells, not affected by mitochondrial electron transport chain suppression, leads to a cytotoxic effect rather than cytostatic at μM concentrations, suggesting the involvement of a distinct nonmitochondrial mechanism of action [178].

Previously used in clinical settings as an antistaphylococcal agent [180], the clinical utility of novobiocin (**35**) (Figure 4) continues to be repurposed, particularly as a chemotherapeutic agent [181,182]. Novobiocin (**35**) was first obtained from cultures of the actinomycete *Streptomyces niveus* [183–185] but is also known to occur in marine counterparts [186]. The antibiotic has been in the spotlight as a first-in-class polymerase theta (Polθ) inhibitor, acting as a noncompetitive inhibitor of ATP hydrolysis, and it is currently under clinical development in patients with tumors that harbor aberrant DNA repair genes [182,187]. However, the anticancer mechanism of **35** has long been recognized as being pleiotropic and also includes the inhibition of HSP90 autophosphorylation by interacting with a C-terminal ATP-binding pocket, consequently hampering hypoxia-induced HIF-1α accumulation [188–190]. Antiproliferative effects of novobiocin (**35**) in A549 and MCF-7 cells appear to derive from the disruptions between the HIF1α CTAD and p300 CH1 complex, which downregulates the transcriptional activation of HIF-responsive genes such as CA9, being also able to downregulate the mRNA expression of Akt1 and mTOR in both cell lines [191].

Currently available in Russia, echinochrome A (**36**) (Figure 4) is used as an active substance of the drug Histochrome®, clinically used on the prophylaxis of reperfusion damages after myocardial infarction for treating ischemia and infarction in acute forms and also as retinoprotector for dystrophic damages of the retina and diabetic retinopathy, for cataract, keratitis, and uveitis [192–195]. The polyhydroxylated 1,4-naphthoquinone was first described as a bactericidal agent by Mac Munn in 1885 from the coelomocytes of the sea urchin *Echinus esculentus* [196,197] but was recently reported to act as a SOD3 mimetic, controlling the expression of cell enzymes through the interference with HIFs, but also enhancing the transcription of PPAR-α and the coactivator1 PPAR-γ (PCG-1 α) [198].

While emodin (**37**) (Figure 4) is mainly reported from several plant genera [199,200], it is also commonly documented as a fungal natural product [201]. The anthraquinone has been isolated from several marine-derived strains of fungi [202,203], with Gomes and colleagues reporting its isolation from cultures of a marine-sponge-associated strain of *Eurotium cristatum* [204]. Emodin (**37**) is widely reputed for its anticancer effects and the interference with a series of molecular events underlying cancer development and progression [205]. The interference with the HIF-1 pathway emerges as a common mechanism underlying an array of potential therapeutic effects of **37**, ranging from neuroprotection and anti-inflammatory effects to the preservation of intestinal barrier function and amelioration of pulmonary inflammation [206–210]. Similarly, the response to the hypoxic environment in the cancer microenvironment has also been commonly reported. Emodin (**37**) inhibited HIF-1α expression in five human pancreatic cancer cell lines, as well as attenuating cancer cachexia in in vivo models. Treatment of athymic mice xenografted with MiaPaCa2 cells resulted in diminishing cancer cell growth and enhancing energy homeostasis through the improvement of cancer-induced hepatic gluconeogenesis and skeletal muscle wasting [211]. Emodin (**37**) also demonstrated in vitro and in vivo suppressive effects against anaplastic thyroid cancer by affecting TRAF6-mediated pathways. Besides blocking angiogenesis by inhibiting the TRAF6/HIF-1α/VEGF pathway in 8505c and SW1736 cells, **37** also suppressed anaplastic thyroid cancer metastasis by inhibiting the TRAF6/CD147/MMP9 pathway [212]. Relevant effects were also noted in hypoxia-induced radioresistance in HepG2 cells, with emodin (**37**) synergistically improving irradiation effects through the inhibition of hypoxia-induced signaling factors such as HIF-1α and histone demethylase

(JMJD1A), but mainly via increased PARP1 cleavage, activation of caspase-9, and inhibition of JMJD2B [213].

Labeled as the first naturally occurring HSP90 inhibitor and originally reported in the culture filtrates of *Streptomyces hygroscopicus* var. *geldanus* var. *nova* [214], the ansamycin antibiotic geldanamycin (**38**) (Figure 4) is commonly described in marine strains of *Streptomyces* [215–218]. The pivotal work of Whitesell and Neckers demonstrated that **38** inhibited the formation of a *v*-Src–HSP90 complex through binding to the ATP-binding site in the N-terminal domain of HSP90 [219,220]. Geldanamycin (**38**), the inaugural HSP90 inhibitor to undergo clinical trials, was unable to progress further clinical development due to its marked hepatotoxicity, likely linked to the electrophilic methoxybenzoquinone group [221]. As observed in prostate cancer PC-3 and LNCaP cells, the interaction of **38** with the N-terminal ATP binding domain of HSP90 induces destabilization and degradation of numerous HSP90 client proteins by the ubiquitin–proteasome pathway, among them HIF-1α [222,223]. Both in vitro studies and xenograft animal models employing various human tumor cell lines have demonstrated the therapeutic promise of geldanamycin (**38**) in cancer treatment, particularly in solid cancer types, not only due to potent cytotoxicity but also due to a significant decrease in cell invasion deriving from HIF-1α-mediated effects [224–227].

Despite bearing a dissimilar structural architecture, radicicol (**39**) (Figure 4) shares a close mechanistic similarity with geldanamycin (**38**), disrupting the folding of protein kinases dependent on HSP90, and implying the degradation of the client protein HIF-1α [220]. While less commonly reported from marine sources, Crews' group described the isolation of **39** from an EtOAc extract obtained from cultures of the fungus *Humicola fuscoatra* isolated from sediments collected in Tutuila, American Samoa [228].

Convergent with the late identification of HIF-2 as a potential target for the development of alternative chemotherapeutic agents, only a limited number of marine-derived candidates have been identified as inhibitors. McKee and collaborators screened over 146,000 extracts of plants, microorganisms, and marine invertebrates on their effects upon HIF-2, and only three extracts from soft corals scored positively [229], ten sponge extracts being also selected for further studies [230]. The inseparable mixture of isomers *N*-formyl-1,2-dihydrorenierone (**40a/40b**) (Figure 4), isolated from *Haliclona velinea*, displayed selectivity for the HIF-2α induced transcription of mRNAs [230].

The potential of adociaquinones A (**41**) and B (**42**) (Figure 4) as lead structures for the development of chemotherapeutic agents dates back to 1988 with their discovery from an unspecified sponge from the genus *Adocia* and the first report on their in vitro cytotoxic effect against cancer cell lines [231]. Later, and being isolated from a *Xestospongia* sp. MeOH extract, both xestoquinones were found to inhibit topoisomerase II [232]. In a recent report, the bioassay-guided isolation of an extract of the sponge *Petrosia alfiani* yielded a new structurally related quinone, 14-hydroxymethylxestoquinone (**43**) (Figure 4), along with **41** and **42** [233]. Adociaquinones A (**41**) and B (**42**) selectively suppressed iron chelator-induced HIF-1 activation in T47D cells, each with IC_{50} values of 0.2 μM, and led to the suppression of secreted VEGF protein by 1,10-phenanthroline, causing a moderate increase in secreted VEGF under hypoxic condition. While both **41** and **42** promoted oxygen consumption without affecting mitochondrial membrane potential, 14-hydroxymethylxestoquinone (**43**) acted as a protonophoric uncoupler of oxidative phosphorylation and decreased mitochondrial membrane potential [233]. Furthermore, while the majority of the Cdc25B inhibitors are quinones, adociaquinone B (**42**) attracted special and increased attention due to its potent and remarkable selectivity, being identified as the most potent known Cdc25B inhibitor [234].

Herboxidiene (**44**) (Figure 4) was originally described as a metabolite of *Streptomyces chromofuscus* by researchers in Monsanto Company [235], being later rediscovered in cultures of the *Streptomyces* sp. GMY01 strain isolated from a marine sediment sample collected from Krakal beach in Yogyakarta, Indonesia [236]. On the initial reports, herboxidiene (**44**) displayed cytotoxicity in the low nM range against several human tumor cell lines, with the main mode of action being attributed to the targeted effects upon SF3B and interference with spliceosome assembly [237,238]. Cooperating with the effects towards SF3B1, **44** also causes a dual impact of the signaling mediated by VEGFR2 and the expression of HIF-1α, inhibiting the transcription and splicing of *HIF-1α* mRNA in HUVECs [239]. Furthermore, the antiangiogenic effects of herboxidiene (**44**) are also suggested based on the inhibition of neovascularization of the chorioallantoic membrane in developing chick embryos [239].

2.4. Phenolics

Bioassay-guided fractionation of a CH_2Cl_2/MeOH extract obtained from samples of the marine crinoid *Comantheria rotula* afforded a series of benzochromenones that were assayed on their inhibitory effects upon HIF-1α in cell-based reporter assay [240]. The benzochromenones **45–52** (Figure 5) significantly inhibited HIF-1 activation in T47D breast tumor cells with IC_{50} values ranging from 1.7 to 7.3 μM and from 0.6 to 3.0 μM for hypoxia-induced and 1,10-phenanthroline-induced activation, respectively [240]. However, solely comaparvin (**52**) led to a decrease in the hypoxic induction of secreted VEGF proteins. When assayed on the NCI 60-cell line panel, the dimeric neocomantherin derivative **45** decreased tumor cell growth with a low level of selectivity, but TMC-256A1 (**51**) was characterized by a unique pattern of anticancer activity as indicated by the COMPARE analysis [240].

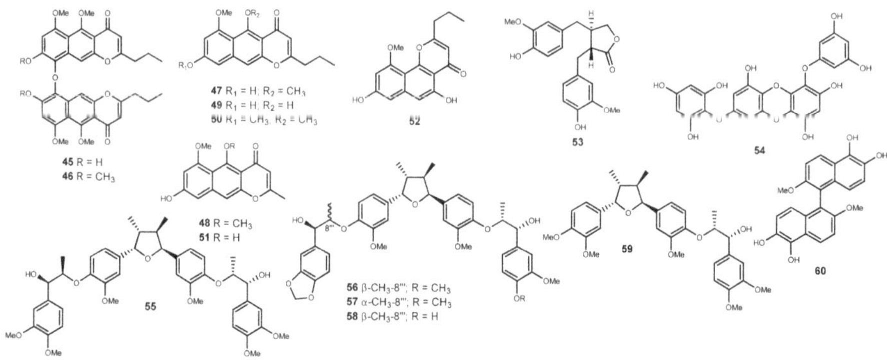

Figure 5. Structures of marine-derived phenolics acting on the HIF pathway.

While matairesinol (**53**) (Figure 5) has been restrictively described as a plant lignan, Urbatzka's group reported the dibenzylbutyrolactone lignan in hexane extracts obtained from the leaves and stems of the marine seagrass *Halophila stipulacea* [241]. Now also labeled as a marine natural product, **53** reduced hypoxia-induced accumulation of HIF-1α protein with concentration dependency, with no effects upon the synthesis of cytoskeletal (tubulin) or cell cycle (cyclin D1) proteins in HeLa cells, inhibiting also tumor-conditioned media-induced angiogenesis via the diminished expression of VEGF [242]. Matairesinol (**53**) demonstrated efficient suppression of hypoxia and VEGF-induced angiogenesis at concentrations lower than those required to hinder HUVEC growth, suggesting that it might selectively disrupt angiogenic signaling pathways by suppressing mitochondrial ROS generation [242].

The phlorotannin 7-phloroeckol (**54**) (Figure 5) is a common metabolite of *Ecklonia* kelps and has been progressively reported as being active towards a series of biologically relevant targets [243–246]. 7-Phloroeckol (**54**) is acknowledged to inhibit tumor angiogenesis in HepG2 cells and HUVECs via inhibition of HIF-1α protein expression and the secretion of VEGF protein by blocking PI3K/AKT/mTOR/P70S6K and RAS/MEK/ERK/MNK mediated signal transduction pathways [247].

Chemical analysis of the aquatic plant *Saururus cernuus* led to the isolation of a series of neolignans with nM potency towards HIF-1α [248,249]. Manassantins A (**55**), B (**56**), and B_1 (**57**) (Figure 5) potently inhibited hypoxia-activated HIF-1 with IC_{50} values of 3 nM, while 4-O-demethylmanassantin B (**58**) and 4-O-methylsaucerneol (**59**) (Figure 5) were weaker on their inhibitory capacity (IC_{50} values of 30 and 20 nM, respectively) [248,249]. The SAR analysis by Nagle and colleagues evidenced that the absence of both hydroxylated side chain segments is an essential structural requirement for the HIF-1 inhibitory activity by this series of lignans, absence of one side chain phenylpropyl unit, as in the sesquilignan **59**, reducing also the inhibitory potency [249]. Additionally, the replacement of the methylenedioxyl moiety by O-methyl groups and the difference in relative configuration of at least one of the two side chains in **56** and **57** have only a slight influence on the potency of HIF-1 inhibition [249]. Hypoxic induction of VEGF was attenuated by the manassantins **55**–**58**, with manassantin A (**55**) and B_1 (**57**) also blocking the hypoxia-induced increase in *CDKN1A* and *GLUT-1* mRNA levels [249].

In an attempt to elucidate the constituents underlying the effects of an extract obtained from a *Lendenfeldia* sp. sponge on hypoxia-induced HIF-1 activation in T47D breast tumor cells, Dai and colleagues carried out the isolation of a series of structurally dissimilar constituents [250]. In addition to a series of active constituents, the naphthalene dimer **60** (Figure 5) also significantly inhibited both hypoxia- and 1,10-phenanthrolin-induced HIF-1 activation in T47D breast tumor cells, with an IC_{50} value of 4.3 μM [250].

2.5. Terpenes

The trichothecene-type mycotoxin diacetoxyscirpenol (**61**) (Figure 6) is a well-known metabolite from phytopathogenic *Fusarium* spp. [251,252]. However, it was also reported from a marine bacterial parasite *Bacillus licheniformis* isolated from the red alga *Gelidium pacificum* [253]. While several mycotoxins are able to upregulate the HIF pathway [254], diacetoxyscirpenol (**61**) dampened the activation of hypoxic genes by HIF, thereby reducing anchorage-independent colony formation, endothelial tube formation, and tumor growth in mice [253]. The impact of **61** upon HIF-1 is suggested to occur either through the inhibition of HIF-1α translation or its dimerization with ARNT, as well as by hampering the hypoxia-induced production of VEGF [253].

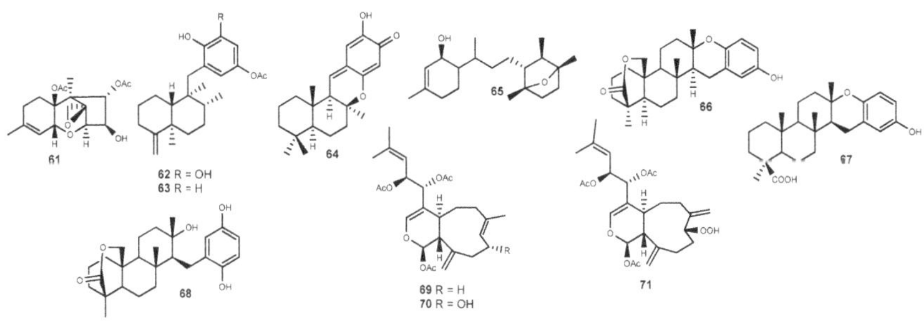

Figure 6. Structures of marine-derived sesquiterpenes (**61**–**64**) and diterpenes (**65**–**71**) acting on the HIF pathway.

Kobayashi's group reported the isolation of several sesquiterpene phenols, namely dictyoceratins A (also known as smenospondiol) (**62**) and C (**63**) (Figure 6) from the sponge *Dactylospongia elegans* [255]. While **62** was originally described from an Okinawan *Hippospongia* sp. [256], its congener dictyoceratin C (**63**) was initially reported from a *Dactylospongia* sp. [257], both being reported later from the sponges *Polyfibrospongia australis* [258] and *Spongia* sp. [259]. Both **62** and **63** were originally described as antimicrobial agents; however, they were found later to display hypoxia-selective antiproliferative effects, inhibiting the proliferation of human prostate cancer DU145 cells under hypoxic conditions in low μM concentrations [255] and also showing a strong antitumor effect in mice xenografted with sarcoma S180 cells upon oral administration [260,261]. Molecular studies performed with dictyoceratins A (**62**) and C (**63**) revealed that their selective antiproliferative activity was derived from their inhibitory effects toward HIF-1α, inhibiting the accumulation of

HIF-1α in hypoxia-adapted DU145 cells [255]. Kawachi and coauthors further detailed the mode of action of dictyoceratins A (**62**) and C (**63**), demonstrating that both HIF inhibitors bind to RNA polymerase II-associated protein 3 (RPAP3) in the vicinity of the TRP1 domain and disturbed the R2TP/PEDL/HSP90 complex, consequently leading to dysfunction of mTOR and the reduced accumulation of HIF-1 [262].

The bioassay-guided screening on HIF-2 inhibitors by McKee and coworkers also led to the isolation of the meroterpene puupehenone (**64**) (Figure 6) from the sponge *Hyrtios reticulatus* [230]. However, analogously to the remaining HIF-2 inhibitors isolated from the active sponge extracts, puupehenone's (**64**) effect on VEGF secretion was coupled with a decrease in total protein, suggesting that it was related to cellular toxicity [230]. The sesquiterpene quinone and several analogs have been repeatedly described in various sponges from distinct genera such as *Heteronema* [263], *Hyrtios* [264–267], *Stronglyphora* [268], *Xestospongia* [269], *Dysidea* [270,271] and from *Dactylospongia* [272]. Concomitantly, **64** has also been documented to have a wide range of biological properties, namely as a potent and selective human 5-lipoxygenase inhibitor [267,273]. Puupehenone (**64**) was further assayed as a potential antiangiogenic agent, inhibiting the endothelial cell differentiation in bovine aortic endothelial (BAE) cells in vitro with an IC_{50} value of 10 ± 2 μM, but without apparent selectivity since, at the same range of concentrations, it was also cytotoxic against a panel of human cancer cell lines [274]. Interestingly, puupehenone (**64**) was also reported as useful in tumor immunotherapy, being attached to a modified antigenic peptide derived from Melan-A/MART-1 protein, frequently recognized by MHC class I-restricted CD8+ cytotoxic T-lymphocytes (CTL). Despite the low affinity for HLA-A2 molecules, the resulting adduct fitted on the TCR/HLA-A2 interface, leading to the stimulation of CTL [275].

Displaying an uncommon 7-oxabicyclo[2.2.1]heptane ring system, lauranditerpenol (**65**) (Figure 6) was reported from an extract of samples of the red alga *Laurencia intricata* collected in Discovery Bay, Jamaica [276]. The algal metabolite enhanced the degradation of HIF-1α in breast cancer T47D cells, with an IC_{50} value as low as 0.4 μM, exhibiting selective anticancer effects under hypoxic conditions without affecting normoxic cell growth [276]. Lauranditerpenol (**65**) also inhibited the mitochondrial electron transport pathway as a complex I inhibitor, evidencing that the inhibitory effects on hypoxia-induced HIF-1 activation were dependent on the increase in cellular O_2 availability under hypoxia [276].

The chemical family strongylophorines has been gaining attention since the first report on the isolation of the first members from the sponge *Strongylophora durissima* in the late 1970s [277]. Several strongylophorines have been into the spotlight due to the reports on their versatile modes of action towards cancer cells, acting as Rho-dependent inhibitors of tumor cell invasion [278], proteasome inhibitors [279], and as inhibitors of the HIF-1 transcriptional pathway [280]. The bioassay-oriented isolation of strongylophorine-2, -3, and -8 (**66–68**) (Figure 6) from the MeOH extract obtained from the sponge *Petrosia (Strongylophora) strongylata* enabled their identification as inhibitors of the HIF-1-dependent luciferase expression in U251-HRE glioblastoma cells without interference with luciferase expression in U251-pGL3 control cells [280]. While the study was limited to strongylophorine-2, -3, and -8 (**66–68**) and chromanol, a preliminary SAR analysis suggests that the presence of the A-ring lactone is a structural requirement that enhances the HIF-1 inhibitory activity of strongylophorines [280]. Besides their HIF-1 selectivity, the strongylophorines **66–68** also effectively decreased the expression of VEGF [280].

Chemical analysis of an extract obtained from the soft coral *Asteropicularia laurae*, collected from a large reef west of Mabul in Malaysia, yielded a series of cembrane diterpenes [229]. While most proved to be inactive, 13-*epi*-9-deacetylxenicin (**69**), 13-*epi*-9-deacetoxyxenicin (**70**) and its hydroperoxide (**71**) (Figure 6) effectively suppressed HIF-2α activity in renal carcinoma 786-0 cells with IC_{50} values of 6.2, 3.4, and 11.8 μM, without exhibiting significant cytotoxicity [229].

Diacarnoxide B (**72**) (Figure 7), a norsesterterpene peroxide isolated from the Papua New Guinea sponge *Diacarnus levii*, was found to inhibit hypoxia-induced HIF-1 activation in T47D cells with an IC_{50} value of 12.7 μM [281]. Interestingly, while diacarnoxide B

(**72**) inhibited prostate DU145 and PC-3 cells and breast MCF-7 and MDA-MB-231 cell proliferation, both under normoxic and hypoxic conditions, it caused an unusual enhanced and selective inhibitory effect at low concentration in MCF-7 and MDA-MB-231 cells under hypoxic conditions [281].

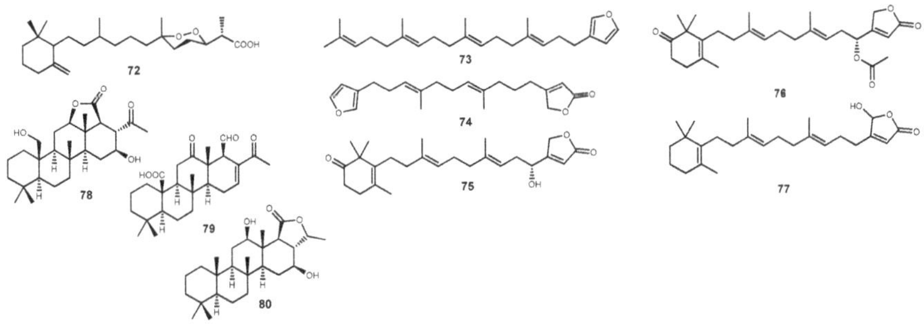

Figure 7. Structures of marine-derived sesterterpenes acting on the HIF pathway.

In addition to its potent and selective inhibitory effect toward Cdc25A [282] and in vitro cytotoxicity against a set of isogenic HCT-116 colon cancer cell lines [283], the spongean metabolite furospinosulin-1 (**73**) (Figure 7) has been claiming much attention for its hypoxia-selective growth inhibitory effect. Furospinosulin-1 (**73**) is a furanosesterterpene originally described from an *Ircinia* sp. sponge more than 50 years ago [284] but has also been widely reported from other spongean genera such as *Hippospongia* [256], *Fasciospongia* [285], *Spongia* [282,286], and *Smenospongia* [283,287]. In 2010, on the report on its isolation from the Indonesian sponge *Dactylospongia elegans*, **73** was found to lead to concentration-dependent and selective suppression of human prostate cancer DU145 cells under hypoxic conditions, as well as displaying in vivo antitumor effects in mice xenografted with mouse sarcoma S180 cells, with no side effects being recorded upon oral administration [288]. Curiously, despite its hypoxia-selective growth inhibitory effect, furospinosulin-1 (**73**) did not inhibit the accumulation of HIF-1 or VEGF, instead modulating the activation of several genes involved in the hypoxia signaling pathway. The selective growth inhibitory effect of **73** against hypoxia-adaptable cancer cells was initially attributed to the suppression of the insulin-like growth factor-2 (IGF-2) gene transcription, selectively induced under hypoxic conditions [288]. Recently, the same group further detailed the mechanism of action of furospinosulin-1 (**73**), reporting an effective and selective effect against hypoxic regions of tumors, stemming from the direct binding to the transcriptional regulators p54^{nrb} and LEDGF/p75, both known as mediators of hypoxia adaptation in cancer cells [289].

Discovered more than 35 years ago as a metabolic product of the Red Sea sponge *Dysidea herbacea* [290] and later from the sponges *Lendenfeldia* sp. [291] and *Spongia officinalis* [292], furospongolide (**74**) (Figure 7) was reported as the first marine-derived furanolipid able to inhibit hypoxia-induced HIF-1 activation [291]. During a screening on extracts from natural sources with the ability to inhibit HIF-1 activation, the lipid extract of *Lendenfeldia* sp. was found to be active, and the subsequent bioassay-guided isolation afforded three scalarene-type sesterterpenes with similar activity and selectivity profile as HIF-1 inhibitors along with furospongolide (**74**) [291]. Unlike the co-isolated sesterterpenes displaying significant cytotoxicity, only **74** preferentially inhibited HIF-1 activation with a 10-fold selectivity compared to its antiproliferative/cytotoxic effect against T47D cells, as well as blocking VEGF induction. The HIF-1 inhibitory activity of furospongolide (**74**) is mediated through the suppression of tumor cell respiration via the blockade of NADH-ubiquinone oxidoreductase (complex I)-mediated mitochondrial electron transfer, consequently blocking the HIF-1 transcription regulator protein HIF-1α [291].

Bioassay-guided isolation of the Palau sponge *Hyrtios communis* afforded several sesterterpenes with HIF-1 inhibitory activity [293]. Among them, the new sesterterpenes thorectidaeolide A (**75**), 4-acetoxythorectidaeolide A (**76**), and the previously reported luffariellolide (**77**) (Figure 7) were found to be the most potent inhibitors of hypoxia-induced HIF-1 activation with IC_{50} values of 3.2, 3.5, and 3.6 μM, respectively [293]. Unlike the other sesterterpenes, **77** displayed a significant antiproliferative effect in T47D and MDA-MR-231 breast cancer cells [293]. Luffariellolide (**77**) has been previously reported in several sponge species from the genera *Luffariella* [294], *Cacospongia* [295], *Acanthodendrilla* [296], and *Thorectandra* [297], being initially reported as a reversible phospholipase A2 inhibitor [294] and later as a weak inhibitor of the protein tyrosine phosphatase Cdc25 [298]. More relevant, its in vitro cytotoxicity against human cancer cell lines was attributed to its agonistic effect on retinoic acid receptors (RARs) [299]. Unlike other RAR ligands, luffariellolide (**77**) adopts a distinct binding mode in RARα through a covalent modification with its unusual i-hydroxybutenolide ring terminus, stabilizing the interaction of RARs with its ligands. It displayed significant cytotoxic effects against monocytic leukemia and promyeloid leukemic cell lines, as well as against MCF-7 breast cancer cells [299]. Furthermore, **77** was also effective against the retinoic acid-resistant colon cancer HCT-116 cell line, inducing the expression of the tumor suppressors RARβ and CRABPII [299].

In addition to the naphthalene dimer **60** (Figure 5), the homoscalarane sesterterpenes **78–80** (Figure 7) were obtained from the lipid extract of Indonesian samples of *Lendenfeldia* sp. [250]. While the three homoscalarane sesterterpenes proved to be efficient inhibitors of hypoxia-induced HIF-1 activation in T47D cells, **79** featured as the most active, with an IC_{50} value as low as 0.64 μM [250], evidencing that the free C-25 aldehyde moiety is essential for HIF-1 inhibition and that its lactonization markedly decreases the inhibitory potency [250].

Mainly reported from the red algae *Laurencia* spp. [300–305], thyrsiferol (**81**) (Figure 8) selectively suppresses mitochondrial respiration at complex I, inhibiting also the hypoxia-induced HIF-1 activation in T47D human breast tumor cells at the same concentration (3 μM) [306]. Roussis and colleagues further described the ability to counteract the hypoxic induction of the HIF-1 target genes *VEGF* and *GLUT-1* in a concentration-dependent manner [306]. The variance in cytotoxicity observed between the sensitive breast cancer T47D cells, which heavily depend on mitochondrial oxidative phosphorylation, and the relatively unresponsive breast cancer MDA-MB-231 cells, which primarily utilize glycolysis, can be explained by the impact of thyrsiferol (**81**) on mitochondrial function [306].

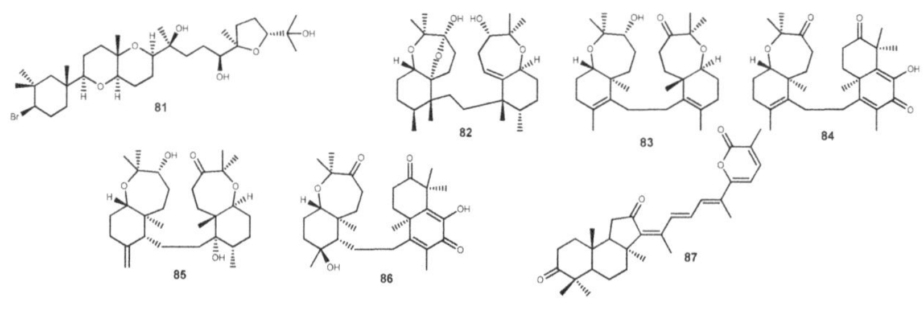

Figure 8. Structures of marine-derived triterpenoids acting on the HIF pathway.

A series of cytotoxic triterpenoids bearing an uncommon condensed oxepane-cyclohexane scaffold have been widely reported in sponges from the genera *Axinella* [307–314] and *Ptilocaulis* [311,315], with several members from this series of spongean terpenoids being reported as HIF-1 inhibitors. Sodwanone V (**82**) (Figure 8) is featured as the most active, inhibiting both hypoxia- and phenanthroline-induced HIF-1 activation in T47D breast tumor cells and being the only sodwanone derivative suppressing hypoxia-induced HIF-1 activation in PC-3 prostate tumor cells [314]. Displaying weaker inhibitory effects, with IC_{50} values in the range 20–25 μM, sodwanone T (**83**) and 10,11-dihydrosodwanone B (**84**) (Figure 8) inhibited both hypoxia- and phenanthroline-induced HIF-1 activation in T47D cells, while 3-*epi*-sodwanone K (**85**) and sodwanone A (**86**) (Figure 8) could only inhibit the hypoxia-induced activation [314].

There is an increasing number of reports describing the anticancer effects of stellettin B (**87**) (Figure 8), an isomalabaricane-type triterpene commonly reported from sponges of the genera *Geodia* [316,317], *Jaspis* [318,319], *Rhabdastrella* [320,321], and *Stelletta* [322,323]. Stellettin B (**87**) appears to act mainly due to the induction of autophagy and apoptosis by interfering with the PI3K/Akt, Stat3, and mTOR signaling pathways in glioblastoma [324,325] and chronic myeloid leukemia cells [319]. The antiproliferative effects upon the oral squamous cell carcinoma cells OC2 and SCC4 derive from autophagic cell death, dropping the expression levels of p62 and increasing Beclin-1 and LC3-II levels [326]. In addition to the modes of action mentioned above, **87** treatment led to antiangiogenic effects in human glioblastoma U87MG and GBM8401 cells, being observed to significantly downregulate p-Stat3 and HIF-1α and culminating in the diminished expression and secretion of VEGF [325]. The antiangiogenic effects of stellettin B (**87**) were confirmed in two in vivo models, with VEGF mRNA expression being decreased in zebrafish embryos and reduction in angiogenesis also being recorded in murine Matrigel Plug models [325].

3. Discussion

As demonstrated above, a considerable number of marine natural products prove to be effective in interfering with HIFs and might have potential utility in treating various types of tumors (Table S1), particularly those with a negative prognosis due to hypoxia-induced resistance and metastasis. However, as already demonstrated, some are accompanied by severe toxicity that limits their translation to clinical use, while others are in the preliminary phase of characterizing their mechanisms of action and validation in disease models more indicative of therapeutic utility.

For example, the clinical development of diacetoxyscirpenol (**61**) ceased after a phase II clinical trial for cancer treatment demonstrated severe side effects [327,328]. However, it should be noted that **61** proved to inhibit HIF-1 at concentrations 20-fold lower than those displaying cytotoxicity [253,329]. The clinical development of echinomycin (**7**) was also discontinued due to the lack of anticancer efficacy in patients with solid tumors [330–332], but its incorporation in liposomes has been recently suggested as a safe and effective therapeutic option, profiting from the HIF-1α inhibition in metastatic cancers [333]. The same applies to gliotoxin (**10**), whose clinical use has been precluded despite its discovery more than 80 years ago. Its clinical use has been revisited in recent years, with a particular focus on investigating the possible strategies to reduce toxicity, such as the targeted delivery of **10** through nanoparticles [334] or the use of lower doses in combination with other anticancer drugs [335]. In other instances, as in the case of kalkitoxin (**11**), it is possible to anticipate toxicity even in the absence of clinical data, as the sodium channel and mitochondria-associated neurotoxicity may limit the therapeutic potential [101]. It is also unlikely that radicicol (**39**) might become a chemotherapeutic agent despite the HSP90 inhibitory ability and anticancer effects observed in vitro, as it was found to be devoid of any in vivo activity in animal models [336].

Certainly, there will be other limitations, particularly those inherent in obtaining active constituents from marine natural sources that are scarce or produced in limited quantities. The inhibitory mode of action of strongylophorine-2 (**66**) for the HIF-1 oriented transcription pathway has not been properly elucidated because of the scarcity of isolating the same from natural sources, prompting its total synthesis [337]. However, there will still be cases where the synthesis of synthetic analogs may not overcome limitations inherent to the structural architecture itself. For example, wondonin (**27**) and derivatives are highly unstable in acidic environments due to the five-membered acetal ring and the vinyl sulfate moieties [145].

However, in analogy to the numerous successful cases associated with the development of drugs inspired by natural molecules, particularly those obtained from marine sources, many of the HIF inhibitors presented here are *bona fide* leads for the translation into therapy. This could occur either in their original structural form or, more likely, through the synthesis of synthetic derivatives optimized for efficacy, toxicity, and pharmacokinetic parameters.

Supplementary Materials: The following supporting information can be downloaded at: https://www.mdpi.com/article/10.3390/md22040143/s1, Table S1: Marine derived HIF inhibitors.

Author Contributions: Conceptualization, N.G.M.G.; validation, N.G.M.G., P.B.A. and F.L.; formal analysis, M.R.G.; writing—original draft preparation, M.R.G.; writing—review and editing, N.G.M.G., P.B.A. and F.L.; supervision, N.G.M.G. All authors have read and agreed to the published version of the manuscript.

Funding: This work received financial support from PT national funds (FCT/MCTES, Fundação para a Ciência e Tecnologia and Ministério da Ciência, Tecnologia e Ensino Superior) through the project UIDB/50006/2020 of REQUIMTE/LAQV.

Institutional Review Board Statement: Not applicable.

Data Availability Statement: Not applicable.

Acknowledgments: Nelson G. M. Gomes thanks FCT (Fundação para a Ciência e Tecnologia) for funding through the Scientific Employment Stimulus Individual Call (Ref. 2022.07375.CEECIND); https://doi.org/10.54499/2022.07375.CEECIND/CP1724/CT0013 accessed on 20 January 2024.

Conflicts of Interest: The authors declare no conflicts of interest.

References

1. Mayer, A.M.S.; Pierce, M.L.; Howe, K.; Rodríguez, A.D.; Taglialatela-Scafati, O.; Nakamura, F.; Fusetani, N. Marine Pharmacology in 2018: Marine Compounds with Antibacterial, Antidiabetic, Antifungal, Anti-Inflammatory, Antiprotozoal, Antituberculosis and Antiviral Activities; Affecting the Immune and Nervous Systems, and Other Miscellaneous Mechanisms of Action. *Pharmacol. Res.* **2022**, *183*, 106391. [CrossRef]
2. Carroll, A.R.; Copp, B.R.; Davis, R.A.; Keyzers, R.A.; Prinsep, M.R. Marine Natural Products. *Nat. Prod. Rep.* **2023**, *40*, 275–325. [CrossRef]
3. Kijjoa, A.; Sawangwong, P. Drugs and Cosmetics from the Sea. *Mar. Drugs* **2004**, *2*, 73–82. [CrossRef]
4. Pecoraro, C.; Terrana, F.; Panzeca, G.; Parrino, B.; Cascioferro, S.; Diana, P.; Giovannetti, E.; Carbone, D. Nortopsentins as Leads from Marine Organisms for Anticancer and Anti-Inflammatory Agent Development. *Molecules* **2023**, *28*, 6450. [CrossRef]
5. Molinski, T.F.; Dalisay, D.S.; Lievens, S.L.; Saludes, J.P. Drug Development from Marine Natural Products. *Nat. Rev. Drug Discov.* **2009**, *8*, 69–85. [CrossRef] [PubMed]
6. Gomes, N.G.M.; Madureira-Carvalho, Á.; Dias-da-Silva, D.; Valentão, P.; Andrade, P.B. Biosynthetic Versatility of Marine-Derived Fungi on the Delivery of Novel Antibacterial Agents against Priority Pathogens. *Biomed. Pharmacother.* **2021**, *140*, 111756. [CrossRef] [PubMed]
7. Robert, J. Comparative Study of Tumorigenesis and Tumor Immunity in Invertebrates and Nonmammalian Vertebrates. *Dev. Comp. Immunol.* **2010**, *34*, 915–925. [CrossRef]
8. Montaser, R.; Luesch, H. Marine Natural Products: A New Wave of Drugs? *Future Med. Chem.* **2011**, *3*, 1475–1489. [CrossRef]
9. Munro, M.H.G.; Blunt, J.W.; Dumdei, E.J.; Hickford, S.J.H.; Lill, R.E.; Li, S.; Battershill, C.N.; Duckworth, A.R. The Discovery and Development of Marine Compounds with Pharmaceutical Potential. *J. Biotechnol.* **1999**, *70*, 15–25. [CrossRef]
10. Atanasov, A.G.; Zotchev, S.B.; Dirsch, V.M.; Orhan, I.E.; Banach, M.; Rollinger, J.M.; Barreca, D.; Weckwerth, W.; Bauer, R.; Bayer, E.A.; et al. Natural Products in Drug Discovery: Advances and Opportunities. *Nat. Rev. Drug Discov.* **2021**, *20*, 200–216. [CrossRef]
11. Cech, N.B.; Oberlies, N.H. From Plant to Cancer Drug: Lessons Learned from the Discovery of Taxol. *Nat. Prod. Rep.* **2023**, *40*, 1153–1157. [CrossRef]
12. Newman, D.J. Natural Products and Drug Discovery. *Natl. Sci. Rev.* **2022**, *9*, nwac206. [CrossRef]
13. Newman, D.J.; Cragg, G.M. Natural Products as Sources of New Drugs over the Nearly Four Decades from 01/1981 to 09/2019. *J. Nat. Prod.* **2020**, *83*, 770–803. [CrossRef] [PubMed]
14. Bergmann, W.; Burke, D.C. Contributions to the Study of Marine Products. XXXIX. The Nucleosides of Sponges. III.1 Spongothymidine and Spongouridine. *J. Org. Chem.* **1955**, *20*, 1501–1507. [CrossRef]
15. Lichtman, M.A. A Historical Perspective on the Development of the Cytarabine (7days) and Daunorubicin (3 days) Treatment Regimen for Acute Myelogenous Leukemia: 2013 the 40th Anniversary of 7+3. *Blood Cells Mol. Dis.* **2013**, *50*, 119–130. [CrossRef]
16. Mayer, A.M.S. The Global Marine Pharmaceuticals Pipeline. Available online: https://www.marinepharmacology.org/ (accessed on 24 July 2023).

17. Pereira, R.B.; Evdokimov, N.M.; Lefranc, F.; Valentaõ, P.; Kornienko, A.; Pereira, D.M.; Andrade, P.B.; Gomes, N.G.M. Marine-Derived Anticancer Agents: Clinical Benefits, Innovative Mechanisms, and New Targets. *Mar. Drugs* **2019**, *17*, 329. [CrossRef] [PubMed]
18. Gomes, N.; Lefranc, F.; Kijjoa, A.; Kiss, R. Can Some Marine-Derived Fungal Metabolites Become Actual Anticancer Agents? *Mar. Drugs* **2015**, *13*, 3950–3991. [CrossRef] [PubMed]
19. Barreca, M.; Spanò, V.; Montalbano, A.; Cueto, M.; Díaz Marrero, A.R.; Deniz, I.; Erdoğan, A.; Lukić Bilela, L.; Moulin, C.; Taffin-de-Givenchy, E.; et al. Marine Anticancer Agents: An Overview with a Particular Focus on Their Chemical Classes. *Mar. Drugs* **2020**, *18*, 619. [CrossRef] [PubMed]
20. Jimenez, P.C.; Wilke, D.V.; Branco, P.C.; Bauermeister, A.; Rezende-Teixeira, P.; Gaudêncio, S.P.; Costa-Lotufo, L. V Enriching Cancer Pharmacology with Drugs of Marine Origin. *Br. J. Pharmacol.* **2020**, *177*, 3–27. [CrossRef]
21. Lefranc, F.; Koutsaviti, A.; Ioannou, E.; Kornienko, A.; Roussis, V.; Kiss, R.; Newman, D. Algae Metabolites: From: In Vitro Growth Inhibitory Effects to Promising Anticancer Activity. *Nat. Prod. Rep.* **2019**, *36*, 810–841. [CrossRef]
22. Faulkner, D.J. Marine Natural Products. *Nat. Prod. Rep.* **1997**, *14*, 259–302. [CrossRef]
23. John Faulkner, D. Highlights of Marine Natural Products Chemistry (1972–1999). *Nat. Prod. Rep.* **2000**, *17*, 1–6. [CrossRef]
24. Blunden, G. Biologically Active Compounds from Marine Organisms. *Phyther. Res.* **2001**, *15*, 89–94. [CrossRef]
25. Kinghorn, A.D.; Chin, Y.-W.; Swanson, S.M. Discovery of Natural Product Anticancer Agents from Biodiverse Organisms. *Curr. Opin. Drug Discov. Devel.* **2009**, *12*, 189–196.
26. Junttila, M.R.; de Sauvage, F.J. Influence of Tumour Micro-Environment Heterogeneity on Therapeutic Response. *Nature* **2013**, *501*, 346–354. [CrossRef]
27. Dagogo-Jack, I.; Shaw, A.T. Tumour Heterogeneity and Resistance to Cancer Therapies. *Nat. Rev. Clin. Oncol.* **2018**, *15*, 81–94. [CrossRef]
28. Karakashev, S.V.; Reginato, M.J. Progress toward Overcoming Hypoxia-Induced Resistance to Solid Tumor Therapy. *Cancer Manag. Res.* **2015**, *7*, 253–264. [CrossRef]
29. Matuszewska, K.; Pereira, M.; Petrik, D.; Lawler, J.; Petrik, J. Normalizing Tumor Vasculature to Reduce Hypoxia, Enhance Perfusion, and Optimize Therapy Uptake. *Cancers* **2021**, *13*, 4444. [CrossRef]
30. Chen, Z.; Han, F.; Du, Y.; Shi, H.; Zhou, W. Hypoxic Microenvironment in Cancer: Molecular Mechanisms and Therapeutic Interventions. *Signal Transduct. Target. Ther.* **2023**, *8*, 70. [CrossRef]
31. Bouleftour, W.; Rowinski, E.; Louati, S.; Sotton, S.; Wozny, A.-S.; Moreno-Acosta, P.; Mery, B.; Rodriguez-Lafrasse, C.; Magne, N. A Review of the Role of Hypoxia in Radioresistance in Cancer Therapy. *Med. Sci. Monit. Int. Med. J. Exp. Clin. Res.* **2021**, *27*, e934116. [CrossRef]
32. Codony, V.L.; Tavassoli, M. Hypoxia-Induced Therapy Resistance: Available Hypoxia-Targeting Strategies and Current Advances in Head and Neck Cancer. *Transl. Oncol.* **2021**, *14*, 101017. [CrossRef] [PubMed]
33. Muz, B.; de la Puente, P.; Azab, F.; Azab, A.K. The Role of Hypoxia in Cancer Progression, Angiogenesis, Metastasis, and Resistance to Therapy. *Hypoxia* **2015**, *3*, 83–92. [CrossRef]
34. Tímár, J.; Sebestyén, A.; Kopper, L.; Dankó, T. Hypoxia Signaling in Cancer: From Basics to Clinical Practice. *Pathol. Oncol. Res.* **2021**, *27*, 1609802. [CrossRef]
35. Koh, M.Y.; Powis, G. Passing the Baton: The HIF Switch. *Trends Biochem. Sci.* **2012**, *37*, 364–372. [CrossRef] [PubMed]
36. Yang, S.-L.; Wu, C.; Xiong, Z.-F.; Fang, X. Progress on Hypoxia-Inducible Factor-3: Its Structure, Gene Regulation and Biological Function (Review). *Mol. Med. Rep.* **2015**, *12*, 2411–2416. [CrossRef] [PubMed]
37. Schönenberger, M.; Kovacs, W. Hypoxia Signaling Pathways: Modulators of Oxygen-Related Organelles. *Front. Cell Dev. Biol.* **2015**, *3*, 42. [CrossRef] [PubMed]
38. Bao, X.; Zhang, J.; Huang, G.; Yan, J.; Xu, C.; Dou, Z.; Sun, C.; Zhang, H. The Crosstalk between HIFs and Mitochondrial Dysfunctions in Cancer Development. *Cell Death Dis.* **2021**, *12*, 215. [CrossRef]
39. Germain, K.; Kim, P.K. Pexophagy: A Model for Selective Autophagy. *Int. J. Mol. Sci.* **2020**, *21*, 578. [CrossRef]
40. Kim, J.-A. Peroxisome Metabolism in Cancer. *Cells* **2020**, *9*, 1692. [CrossRef]
41. Tiburcio, P.D.; Choi, H.; Huang, L.E. Complex Role of HIF in Cancer: The Known, the Unknown, and the Unexpected. *Hypoxia* **2014**, *2*, 59–70. [CrossRef]
42. Wicks, E.E.; Semenza, G.L. Hypoxia-Inducible Factors: Cancer Progression and Clinical Translation. *J. Clin. Investig.* **2022**, *132*, e159839. [CrossRef]
43. Sharma, A.; Sinha, S.; Shrivastava, N. Therapeutic Targeting Hypoxia-Inducible Factor (HIF-1) in Cancer: Cutting Gordian Knot of Cancer Cell Metabolism. *Front. Genet.* **2022**, *13*, 849040. [CrossRef]
44. Semenza, G.L. Targeting HIF-1 for Cancer Therapy. *Nat. Rev. Cancer* **2003**, *3*, 721–732. [CrossRef]
45. Infantino, V.; Santarsiero, A.; Convertini, P.; Todisco, S.; Iacobazzi, V. Cancer Cell Metabolism in Hypoxia: Role of HIF-1 as Key Regulator and Therapeutic Target. *Int. J. Mol. Sci.* **2021**, *22*, 5703. [CrossRef]
46. Nagle, D.G.; Zhou, Y.-D. Natural Product-Based Inhibitors of Hypoxia-Inducible Factor-1 (HIF-1). *Curr. Drug Targets* **2006**, *7*, 355–369. [CrossRef]
47. Nagle, D.G.; Zhou, Y.-D. Natural Product-Derived Small Molecule Activators of Hypoxia-Inducible Factor-1 (HIF-1). *Curr. Pharm. Des.* **2006**, *12*, 2673–2688. [CrossRef]

48. Ikeda, H.; Kakeya, H. Targeting Hypoxia-Inducible Factor 1 (HIF-1) Signaling with Natural Products toward Cancer Chemotherapy. *J. Antibiot.* **2021**, *74*, 687–695. [CrossRef]
49. Zhong, J.-C.; Li, X.-B.; Lyu, W.-Y.; Ye, W.-C.; Zhang, D.-M. Natural Products as Potent Inhibitors of Hypoxia-Inducible Factor-1α in Cancer Therapy. *Chin. J. Nat. Med.* **2020**, *18*, 696–703. [CrossRef]
50. Manolescu, B.; Oprea, E.; Busu, C.; Cercasov, C. Natural Compounds and the Hypoxia-Inducible Factor (HIF) Signalling Pathway. *Biochimie* **2009**, *91*, 1347–1358. [CrossRef]
51. Ma, Z.; Xiang, X.; Li, S.; Xie, P.; Gong, Q.; Goh, B.-C.; Wang, L. Targeting Hypoxia-Inducible Factor-1, for Cancer Treatment: Recent Advances in Developing Small-Molecule Inhibitors from Natural Compounds. *Semin. Cancer Biol.* **2022**, *80*, 379–390. [CrossRef]
52. Jones, D.T.; Harris, A.L. Small-Molecule Inhibitors of the HIF Pathway and Synthetic Lethal Interactions. *Expert Opin. Ther. Targets* **2012**, *16*, 463–480. [CrossRef] [PubMed]
53. Ghosh, R.; Samanta, P.; Sarkar, R.; Biswas, S.; Saha, P.; Hajra, S.; Bhowmik, A. Targeting HIF-1α by Natural and Synthetic Compounds: A Promising Approach for Anti-Cancer Therapeutics Development. *Molecules* **2022**, *27*, 5192. [CrossRef]
54. Bhattarai, D.; Xu, X.; Lee, K. Hypoxia-Inducible Factor-1 (HIF-1) Inhibitors from the Last Decade (2007 to 2016): A "Structure–Activity Relationship" Perspective. *Med. Res. Rev.* **2018**, *38*, 1404–1442. [CrossRef] [PubMed]
55. Ban, H.S.; Uto, Y.; Won, M.; Nakamura, H. Hypoxia-Inducible Factor (HIF) Inhibitors: A Patent Survey (2011–2015). *Expert Opin. Ther. Pat.* **2016**, *26*, 309–322. [CrossRef] [PubMed]
56. Nagle, D.G.; Zhou, Y.-D. Marine Natural Products as Inhibitors of Hypoxic Signaling in Tumors. *Phytochem. Rev.* **2009**, *8*, 415–429. [CrossRef]
57. Govindarajan, G.; Yao, Z.; Zhou, Z.; Zheng, X.; Ma, J.; Kumar, P.S.; Ju, J.; Sun, C. Genome Sequencing of *Streptomyces griseus* SCSIO PteL053, the Producer of 2,2′-Bipyridine and Actinomycin Analogs, and Associated Biosynthetic Gene Cluster Analysis. *J. Mar. Sci. Eng.* **2023**, *11*, 396. [CrossRef]
58. Liu, M.; Jia, Y.; Xie, Y.; Zhang, C.; Ma, J.; Sun, C.; Ju, J. Identification of the Actinomycin D Biosynthetic Pathway from Marine-Derived *Streptomyces costaricanus* SCSIO ZS0073. *Mar. Drugs* **2019**, *17*, 240. [CrossRef] [PubMed]
59. Bensaude, O. Inhibiting Eukaryotic Transcription: Which Compound to Choose? How to Evaluate Its Activity? *Transcription* **2011**, *2*, 103–108. [CrossRef]
60. Berra, E.; Richard, D.E.; Gothié, E.; Pouysségur, J. HIF-1-Dependent Transcriptional Activity Is Required for Oxygen-Mediated HIF-1α Degradation. *FEBS Lett.* **2001**, *491*, 85–90. [CrossRef]
61. Wang, G.L.; Semenza, G.L. Characterization of Hypoxia-Inducible Factor 1 and Regulation of DNA Binding Activity by Hypoxia. *J. Biol. Chem.* **1993**, *268*, 21513–21518. [CrossRef]
62. Pagé, E.L.; Robitaille, G.A.; Pouysségur, J.; Richard, D.E. Induction of Hypoxia-Inducible Factor-1α by Transcriptional and Translational Mechanisms *J. Biol. Chem.* **2002**, *277*, 48403–48409. [CrossRef] [PubMed]
63. Bhosale, S.H.; Patil, K.B.; Parameswaran, P.S.; Naik, C.G.; Jagtap, T.G. Active Pharmaceutical Ingredient (Api) from an Estuarine Fungus, *Microdochium nivale* (Fr.). *J. Environ. Biol.* **2011**, *32*, 653–658. [PubMed]
64. D'Angelo, G.; Duplan, E.; Vigne, P.; Frelin, C. Cyclosporin A Prevents the Hypoxic Adaptation by Activating Hypoxia-Inducible Factor-1α Pro-564 Hydroxylation. *J. Biol. Chem.* **2003**, *278*, 15406–15411. [CrossRef] [PubMed]
65. Rinehart, K.L.J.; Gloer, J.B.; Cook, J.C.J.; Mizsak, S.A.; Scahill, T.A. Structures of the Didemnins, Antiviral and Cytotoxic Depsipeptides from a Caribbean Tunicate. *J. Am. Chem. Soc.* **1981**, *103*, 1857–1859. [CrossRef]
66. Gomes, N.G.M.; Valentaõ, P.; Andrade, P.B.; Pereira, R.B. Plitidepsin to Treat Multiple Myeloma. *Drugs Today* **2020**, *56*, 337–347. [CrossRef]
67. Straight, A.M.; Oakley, K.; Moores, R.; Bauer, A.J.; Patel, A.; Tuttle, R.M.; Jimeno, J.; Francis, G.L. Aplidin Reduces Growth of Anaplastic Thyroid Cancer Xenografts and the Expression of Several Angiogenic Genes. *Cancer Chemother. Pharmacol.* **2006**, *57*, 7–14. [CrossRef]
68. Symersky, J.; Osowski, D.; Walters, D.E.; Mueller, D.M. Oligomycin Frames a Common Drug-Binding Site in the ATP Synthase. *Proc. Natl. Acad. Sci. USA* **2012**, *109*, 13961–13965. [CrossRef]
69. Dame, Z.T.; Islam, M.T.; Helmke, E.; von Tiedemann, A.; Laatsch, H. Oligomycins and Pamamycin Homologs Impair Motility and Induce Lysis of Zoospores of the Grapevine Downy Mildew Pathogen, Plasmopara Viticola. *FEMS Microbiol. Lett.* **2016**, *363*, fnw167. [CrossRef]
70. Nagle, D.G.; Zhou, Y.-D. 2.20—Natural Products as Probes of Selected Targets in Tumor Cell Biology and Hypoxic Signaling. In *Comprehensive Natural Products II*; Liu, H.-W., Mander, L., Eds.; Elsevier: Oxford, UK, 2010; pp. 651–683, ISBN 978-0-08-045382-8.
71. Gong, Y.; Agani, F.H. Oligomycin Inhibits HIF-1α Expression in Hypoxic Tumor Cells. *Am. J. Physiol. Physiol.* **2005**, *288*, C1023–C1029. [CrossRef] [PubMed]
72. Paul, S.K.; Chakraborty, M.; Rahman, M.; Gupta, D.R.; Mahmud, N.U.; Rahat, A.A.M.; Sarker, A.; Hannan, M.A.; Rahman, M.M.; Akanda, A.M.; et al. Marine Natural Product Antimycin A Suppresses Wheat Blast Disease Caused by Magnaporthe Oryzae Triticum. *J. Fungi* **2022**, *8*, 618. [CrossRef] [PubMed]
73. Huang, L.-S.; Cobessi, D.; Tung, E.Y.; Berry, E.A. Binding of the Respiratory Chain Inhibitor Antimycin to the Mitochondrial Bc1 Complex: A New Crystal Structure Reveals an Altered Intramolecular Hydrogen-Bonding Pattern. *J. Mol. Biol.* **2005**, *351*, 573–597. [CrossRef]

74. Chua, Y.L.; Dufour, E.; Dassa, E.P.; Rustin, P.; Jacobs, H.T.; Taylor, C.T.; Hagen, T. Stabilization of Hypoxia-Inducible Factor-1alpha Protein in Hypoxia Occurs Independently of Mitochondrial Reactive Oxygen Species Production. *J. Biol. Chem.* **2010**, *285*, 31277–31284. [CrossRef]
75. Maeda, M.; Hasebe, Y.; Egawa, K.; Shibanuma, M.; Nose, K. Inhibition of Angiogenesis and HIF-1alpha Activity by Antimycin A1. *Biol. Pharm. Bull.* **2006**, *29*, 1344–1348. [CrossRef]
76. Vlaminck, B.; Toffoli, S.; Ghislain, B.; Demazy, C.; Raes, M.; Michiels, C. Dual effect of echinomycin on hypoxia-inducible factor-1 activity under normoxic and hypoxic conditions. *FEBS J.* **2007**, *274*, 5533–5542. [CrossRef] [PubMed]
77. Waring, M.J. Echinomycin, Triostin, and Related Antibiotics. In *Mechanism of Action of Antieukaryotic and Antiviral Compounds*; Hahn, F.E., Ed.; Springer: Berlin/Heidelberg, Germany, 1979; pp. 173–194, ISBN 978-3-642-46407-2.
78. Park, Y.-S.; Shin, W.-S.; Kim, C.-S.; Ahn, C.M.; Qi, X.-F.; Kim, S.-K. Molecular and Cellular Toxicological Profiling of DNA Bis-Intercalator, Quinoxaline Compounds: Echinomycin as the Versatile Lead. *Mol. Cell. Toxicol.* **2018**, *14*, 9–18. [CrossRef]
79. Foster, B.J.; Clagett-Carr, K.; Shoemaker, D.D.; Suffness, M.; Plowman, J.; Trissel, L.A.; Grieshaber, C.K.; Leyland-Jones, B. Echinomycin: The First Bifunctional Intercalating Agent in Clinical Trials. *Investig. New Drugs* **1985**, *3*, 403–410. [CrossRef] [PubMed]
80. Hattori, K.; Koike, K.; Okuda, K.; Hirayama, T.; Ebihara, M.; Takenaka, M.; Nagasawa, H. Solution-Phase Synthesis and Biological Evaluation of Triostin A and Its Analogues. *Org. Biomol. Chem.* **2016**, *14*, 2090–2111. [CrossRef] [PubMed]
81. Kong, D.; Park, E.J.; Stephen, A.G.; Calvani, M.; Cardellina, J.H.; Monks, A.; Fisher, R.J.; Shoemaker, R.H.; Melillo, G. Echinomycin, a Small-Molecule Inhibitor of Hypoxia-Inducible Factor-1 DNA-Binding Activity. *Cancer Res.* **2005**, *65*, 9047–9055. [CrossRef] [PubMed]
82. Fernández, J.; Marín, L.; Álvarez-Alonso, R.; Redondo, S.; Carvajal, J.; Villamizar, G.; Villar, C.J.; Lombó, F. Biosynthetic Modularity Rules in the Bisintercalator Family of Antitumor Compounds. *Mar. Drugs* **2014**, *12*, 2668–2699. [CrossRef] [PubMed]
83. Gomes, N.G.M.; Pereira, R.B.; Andrade, P.B.; Valentão, P. Double the Chemistry, Double the Fun: Structural Diversity and Biological Activity of Marine-Derived Diketopiperazine Dimers. *Mar. Drugs* **2019**, *17*, 551. [CrossRef]
84. Watts, K.R.; Ratnam, J.; Ang, K.-H.; Tenney, K.; Compton, J.E.; McKerrow, J.; Crews, P. Assessing the Trypanocidal Potential of Natural and Semi-Synthetic Diketopiperazines from Two Deep Water Marine-Derived Fungi. *Bioorg. Med. Chem.* **2010**, *18*, 2566–2574. [CrossRef]
85. Yun, K.; Khong, T.T.; Leutou, A.S.; Kim, G.-D.; Hong, J.; Lee, C.-H.; Son, B.W. Cristazine, a New Cytotoxic Dioxopiperazine Alkaloid from the Mudflat-Sediment-Derived Fungus *Chaetomium cristatum*. *Chem. Pharm. Bull.* **2016**, *64*, 59–62. [CrossRef] [PubMed]
86. Cook, K.M.; Hilton, S.T.; Mecinović, J.; Motherwell, W.B.; Figg, W.D.; Schofield, C.J. Epidithiodiketopiperazines Block the Interaction between Hypoxia-Inducible Factor-1α (HIF-1α) and P300 by a Zinc Ejection Mechanism. *J. Biol. Chem.* **2009**, *284*, 26831–26838. [CrossRef] [PubMed]
87. Kung, A.L.; Zabludoff, S.D.; France, D.S.; Freedman, S.J.; Tanner, E.A.; Vieira, A.; Cornell-Kennon, S.; Lee, J.; Wang, B.; Wang, J.; et al. Small Molecule Blockade of Transcriptional Coactivation of the Hypoxia-Inducible Factor Pathway. *Cancer Cell* **2004**, *6*, 33–43. [CrossRef] [PubMed]
88. Kessler, J.; Hahnel, A.; Wichmann, H.; Rot, S.; Kappler, M.; Bache, M.; Vordermark, D. HIF-1α Inhibition by SiRNA or Chetomin in Human Malignant Glioma Cells: Effects on Hypoxic Radioresistance and Monitoring via CA9 Expression. *BMC Cancer* **2010**, *10*, 605. [CrossRef] [PubMed]
89. Horiuchi, A.; Hayashi, T.; Kikuchi, N.; Hayashi, A.; Fuseya, C.; Shiozawa, T.; Konishi, I. Hypoxia Upregulates Ovarian Cancer Invasiveness via the Binding of HIF-1α to a Hypoxia-Induced, Methylation-Free Hypoxia Response Element of S100A4 Gene. *Int. J. Cancer* **2012**, *131*, 1755–1767. [CrossRef] [PubMed]
90. Herath, K.B.; Jayasuriya, H.; Ondeyka, J.G.; Polishook, J.D.; Bills, G.F.; Dombrowski, A.W.; Cabello, A.; Vicario, P.P.; Zweerink, H.; Guan, Z.; et al. Isolation and Structures of Novel Fungal Metabolites as Chemokine Receptor (CCR2) Antagonists. *J. Antibiot.* **2005**, *58*, 686–694. [CrossRef]
91. Indelicato, M.; Pucci, B.; Schito, L.; Reali, V.; Aventaggiato, M.; Mazzarino, M.C.; Stivala, F.; Fini, M.; Russo, M.A.; Tafani, M. Role of Hypoxia and Autophagy in MDA-MB-231 Invasiveness. *J. Cell. Physiol.* **2010**, *223*, 359–368. [CrossRef]
92. Staab, A.; Loeffler, J.; Said, H.M.; Diehlmann, D.; Katzer, A.; Beyer, M.; Fleischer, M.; Schwab, F.; Baier, K.; Einsele, H.; et al. Effects of HIF-1 Inhibition by Chetomin on Hypoxia-Related Transcription and Radiosensitivity in HT 1080 Human Fibrosarcoma Cells. *BMC Cancer* **2007**, *7*, 213. [CrossRef]
93. Greiner, D.; Bonaldi, T.; Eskeland, R.; Roemer, E.; Imhof, A. Reply to "Chaetocin Is a Nonspecific Inhibitor of Histone Lysine Methyltransferases". *Nat. Chem. Biol.* **2013**, *9*, 137. [CrossRef]
94. Greiner, D.; Bonaldi, T.; Eskeland, R.; Roemer, E.; Imhof, A. Identification of a Specific Inhibitor of the Histone Methyltransferase SU(VAR)3-9. *Nat. Chem. Biol.* **2005**, *1*, 143–145. [CrossRef] [PubMed]
95. Han, L.; Lee, J.B.; Indermaur, E.W.; Keung, A.J. Chaetocin Disrupts the SUV39H1–HP1 Interaction Independent of SUV39H1 Methyltransferase Activity. *Biochem. J.* **2023**, *480*, 421–432. [CrossRef] [PubMed]
96. Reece, K.M.; Richardson, E.D.; Cook, K.M.; Campbell, T.J.; Pisle, S.T.; Holly, A.J.; Venzon, D.J.; Liewehr, D.J.; Chau, C.H.; Price, D.K.; et al. Epidithiodiketopiperazines (ETPs) Exhibit in Vitro Antiangiogenic and in Vivo Antitumor Activity by Disrupting the HIF-1α/P300 Complex in a Preclinical Model of Prostate Cancer. *Mol. Cancer* **2014**, *13*, 91. [CrossRef] [PubMed]

97. Fu, J.; Luo, X.; Lin, M.; Xiao, Z.; Huang, L.; Wang, J.; Zhu, Y.; Liu, Y.; Tao, H. Marine-Fungi-Derived Gliotoxin Promotes Autophagy to Suppress *Mycobacteria tuberculosis* Infection in Macrophage. *Mar. Drugs* **2023**, *21*, 616. [CrossRef]
98. Zhang, S.; Guo, J.; Zhang, H.; Tong, L.; Zhang, L. Gliotoxin Induced Ferroptosis by Downregulating SUV39H1 Expression in Esophageal Cancer Cells. *Recent Pat. Anticancer. Drug Discov.* **2023**, *18*, 397–407. [CrossRef]
99. Mohamed, A.F.; Abuamara, T.M.M.; Amer, M.E.; El-Moselhy, L.E.; Gomah, T.A.; Matar, E.R.; Shebl, R.I.; Desouky, S.E.; Abu-Elghait, M. Genetic and Histopathological Alterations in Caco-2 and HuH-7 Cells Treated with Secondary Metabolites of Marine Fungi. *J. Gastrointest. Cancer* **2022**, *53*, 480–495. [CrossRef]
100. Berman, F.W.; Gerwick, W.H.; Murray, T.F. Antillatoxin and Kalkitoxin, Ichthyotoxins from the Tropical Cyanobacterium Lyngbya Majuscula, Induce Distinct Temporal Patterns of NMDA Receptor-Mediated Neurotoxicity. *Toxicon* **1999**, *37*, 1645–1648. [CrossRef]
101. Morgan, J.B.; Liu, Y.; Coothankandaswamy, V.; Mahdi, F.; Jekabsons, M.B.; Gerwick, W.H.; Valeriote, F.A.; Zhou, Y.D.; Nagle, D.G. Kalkitoxin Inhibits Angiogenesis, Disrupts Cellular Hypoxic Signaling, and Blocks Mitochondrial Electron Transport in Tumor Cells. *Mar. Drugs* **2015**, *13*, 1552–1568. [CrossRef]
102. Senter, P.D.; Sievers, E.L. The Discovery and Development of Brentuximab Vedotin for Use in Relapsed Hodgkin Lymphoma and Systemic Anaplastic Large Cell Lymphoma. *Nat. Biotechnol.* **2012**, *30*, 631–637. [CrossRef]
103. Pettit, G.R.; Kamano, Y.; Dufresne, C.; Cerny, R.L.; Herald, C.L.; Schmidt, J.M. Isolation and Structure of the Cytostatic Linear Depsipeptide Dolastatin 15. *J. Org. Chem.* **1989**, *54*, 6005–6006. [CrossRef]
104. Gomes, N.G.M.; Dasari, R.; Chandra, S.; Kiss, R.; Kornienko, A. Marine Invertebrate Metabolites with Anticancer Activities: Solutions to the "Supply Problem". *Mar. Drugs* **2016**, *14*, 98. [CrossRef]
105. Swain, S.S.; Padhy, R.N.; Singh, P.K. Anticancer Compounds from Cyanobacterium Lyngbya Species: A Review. *Antonie Leeuwenhoek Int. J. Gen. Mol. Microbiol.* **2015**, *108*, 223–265. [CrossRef]
106. Kerbrat, P.; Dieras, V.; Pavlidis, N.; Ravaud, A.; Wanders, J.; Fumoleau, P. Phase II Study of LU 103793 (Dolastatin Analogue) in Patients with Metastatic Breast Cancer. *Eur. J. Cancer* **2003**, *39*, 317–320. [CrossRef]
107. Marks, R.S.; Graham, D.L.; Sloan, J.A.; Hillman, S.; Fishkoff, S.; Krook, J.E.; Okuno, S.H.; Mailliard, J.A.; Fitch, T.R.; Addo, F. A Phase II Study of the Dolastatin 15 Analogue LU 103793 in the Treatment of Advanced Non-Small-Cell Lung Cancer. *Am. J. Clin. Oncol. Cancer Clin. Trials* **2003**, *26*, 336–337. [CrossRef] [PubMed]
108. Mross, K. Clinical and Pharmacologic Phase I Study of Cemadotin-HCl (LU103793), a Novel Antimitotic Peptide, given as 24-Hour Infusion in Patients with Advanced Cancer. *Ann. Oncol.* **1998**, *9*, 1323–1330. [CrossRef] [PubMed]
109. Villalona-Calero, M.A.; Baker, S.D.; Hammond, L.; Aylesworth, C.; Eckhardt, S.G.; Kraynak, M.; Fram, R.; Fischkoff, S.; Velagapudi, R.; Toppmeyer, D.; et al. Phase I and Pharmacokinetic Study of the Water-Soluble Dolastatin 15 Analog LU103793 in Patients with Advanced Solid Malignancies. *J. Clin. Oncol.* **1998**, *16*, 2770–2779. [CrossRef] [PubMed]
110. Cunningham, C.; Appleman, L.J.; Kirvan-Visovatti, M.; Ryan, D.P.; Regan, E.; Vukelja, S.; Bonate, P.L.; Ruvuna, F.; Fram, R.J.; Jekunen, A.; et al. Phase I and Pharmacokinetic Study of the Dolastatin-15 Analogue Tasidotin (ILX651) Administered Intravenously on Days 1, 3, and 5 Every 3 Weeks in Patients with Advanced Solid Tumors. *Clin. Cancer Res.* **2005**, *11*, 7825–7833. [CrossRef] [PubMed]
111. Ebbinghaus, S.; Rubin, E.; Hersh, E.; Cranmer, L.D.; Bonate, P.L.; Fram, R.J.; Jekunen, A.; Weitman, S.; Hammond, L.A. A Phase I Study of the Dolastatin-15 Analogue Tasidotin (ILX651) Administered Intravenously Daily for 5 Consecutive Days Every 3 Weeks in Patients with Advanced Solid Tumors. *Clin. Cancer Res.* **2005**, *11*, 7807–7816. [CrossRef] [PubMed]
112. Bai, R.; Friedman, S.J.; Pettit, G.R.; Hamel, E. Dolastatin 15, a Potent Antimitotic Depsipeptide Derived from Dolabella Auricularia. Interaction with Tubulin and Effects on Cellular Microtubules. *Biochem. Pharmacol.* **1992**, *43*, 2637–2645. [CrossRef] [PubMed]
113. Lopus, M. Mechanism of Mitotic Arrest Induced by Dolastatin 15 Involves Loss of Tension across Kinetochore Pairs. *Mol. Cell. Biochem.* **2013**, *382*, 93–102. [CrossRef] [PubMed]
114. Ratnayake, R.; Gunasekera, S.P.; Ma, J.J.; Dang, L.H.; Carney, T.J.; Paul, V.J.; Luesch, H. Dolastatin 15 from a Marine Cyanobacterium Suppresses HIF-1α Mediated Cancer Cell Viability and Vascularization. *ChemBioChem* **2020**, *21*, 2356–2366. [CrossRef]
115. Goey, A.K.L.; Chau, C.H.; Sissung, T.M.; Cook, K.M.; Venzon, D.J.; Castro, A.; Ransom, T.R.; Henrich, C.J.; McKee, T.C.; McMahon, J.B.; et al. Screening and Biological Effects of Marine Pyrroloiminoquinone Alkaloids: Potential Inhibitors of the HIF-1α/P300 Interaction. *J. Nat. Prod.* **2016**, *79*, 1267–1275. [CrossRef] [PubMed]
116. Hu, J.-F.; Fan, H.; Xiong, J.; Wu, S.-B. Discorhabdins and Pyrroloiminoquinone-Related Alkaloids. *Chem. Rev.* **2011**, *111*, 5465–5491. [CrossRef]
117. Harris, E.M.; Strope, J.D.; Beedie, S.L.; Huang, P.A.; Goey, A.K.L.; Cook, K.M.; Schofield, C.J.; Chau, C.H.; Cadelis, M.M.; Copp, B.R.; et al. Preclinical Evaluation of Discorhabdins in Antiangiogenic and Antitumor Models. *Mar. Drugs* **2018**, *16*, 241. [CrossRef] [PubMed]
118. Chan, S.T.S.; Patel, P.R.; Ransom, T.R.; Henrich, C.J.; Mckee, T.C.; Goey, A.K.L.; Cook, K.M.; Figg, W.D.; Mcmahon, J.B.; Schnermann, M.J.; et al. Structural Elucidation and Synthesis of Eudistidine A: An Unusual Polycyclic Marine Alkaloid That Blocks Interaction of the Protein Binding Domains of P300 and HIF-1α. *J. Am. Chem. Soc.* **2015**, *137*, 5569–5575. [CrossRef]
119. Roll, D.M.; Ireland, C.M.; Lu, H.S.M.; Clardy, J. Fascaplysin, an Unusual Antimicrobial Pigment from the Marine Sponge *Fascaplysinopsis* Sp. *J. Org. Chem.* **1988**, *53*, 3276–3278. [CrossRef]
120. Hörmann, A.; Chaudhuri, B.; Fretz, H. DNA Binding Properties of the Marine Sponge *Pigment fascaplysin*. *Bioorg. Med. Chem.* **2001**, *9*, 917–921. [CrossRef]

121. Lin, J.; Yan, X.-J.; Chen, H.-M. Fascaplysin, a Selective CDK4 Inhibitor, Exhibit Anti-Angiogenic Activity in Vitro and in Vivo. *Cancer Chemother. Pharmacol.* **2007**, *59*, 439–445. [CrossRef] [PubMed]
122. Soni, R.; Muller, L.; Furet, P.; Schoepfer, J.; Stephan, C.; Zumstein-Mecker, S.; Fretz, H.; Chaudhuri, B. Inhibition of Cyclin-Dependent Kinase 4 (Cdk4) by Fascaplysin, a Marine Natural Product. *Biochem. Biophys. Res. Commun.* **2000**, *275*, 877–884. [CrossRef]
123. Bharate, S.B.; Manda, S.; Mupparapu, N.; Battini, N.; Vishwakarma, R.A. Chemistry and Biology of Fascaplysin, a Potent Marine-Derived CDK-4 Inhibitor. *Mini Rev. Med. Chem.* **2012**, *12*, 650–664. [CrossRef]
124. Shafiq, M.I.; Steinbrecher, T.; Schmid, R. Fascaplysin as a Specific Inhibitor for CDK4: Insights from Molecular Modelling. *PLoS ONE* **2012**, *7*, e42612. [CrossRef]
125. Oh, T.-I.; Lee, Y.-M.; Nam, T.-J.; Ko, Y.-S.; Mah, S.; Kim, J.; Kim, Y.; Reddy, R.H.; Kim, Y.J.; Hong, S.; et al. Fascaplysin Exerts Anti-Cancer Effects through the Downregulation of Survivin and HIF-1α and Inhibition of VEGFR2 and TRKA. *Int. J. Mol. Sci.* **2017**, *18*, 2074. [CrossRef]
126. Aguilar-Santos, G. Caulerpin, a New Red Pigment from Green Algae of the Genus Caulerpa. *J. Chem. Soc. C* **1970**, *6*, 842–843. [CrossRef] [PubMed]
127. Liu, Y.; Morgan, J.B.; Coothankandaswamy, V.; Liu, R.; Jekabsons, M.B.; Mahdi, F.; Nagle, D.G. The Caulerpa Pigment Caulerpin Inhibits HIF-1 Activation and Mitochondrial Respiration. *J. Nat. Prod.* **2009**, *1*, 2104–2109. [CrossRef] [PubMed]
128. Mao, S.; Liu, Y.; Morgan, J.B.; Jekabsons, M.B.; Zhou, Y.; Nagle, D.G. Lipophilic 2,5-Disubstituted Pyrroles from the Marine Sponge *Mycale* Sp. Inhibit Mitochondrial Respiration and HIF-1 Activation. *J. Nat. Prod.* **2009**, *72*, 1927–1936. [CrossRef] [PubMed]
129. Andersen, R.J.; Faulkner, D.J.; He, C.H.; Van Duyne, G.D.; Clardy, J. Metabolites of the Marine Prosobranch Mollusk *Lamellaria* Sp. *J. Am. Chem. Soc.* **1985**, *107*, 5492–5495. [CrossRef]
130. Lindquist, N.; Fenical, W.; Van Duyne, G.D.; Clardy, J. New Alkaloids of the Lamellarin Class from the Marine Ascidian *Didemnum chartaceum* (Sluiter, 1909). *J. Org. Chem.* **1988**, *53*, 4570–4574. [CrossRef]
131. Urban, S.; Capon, R.J. Lamellarin-S: A New Aromatic Metabolite From an Australian Tunicate, *Didemnum* Sp. *Aust. J. Chem.* **1996**, *49*, 711–713. [CrossRef]
132. Reddy, M.V.R.; Faulkner, D.J.; Venkateswarlu, Y.; Rao, M.R. New Lamellarin Alkaloids from an Unidentified Ascidian from the Arabian Sea. *Tetrahedron* **1997**, *53*, 3457–3466. [CrossRef]
133. Davis, R.A.; Carroll, A.R.; Pierens, G.K.; Quinn, R.J. New Lamellarin Alkaloids from the Australian Ascidian, *Didemnum chartaceum*. *J. Nat. Prod.* **1999**, *62*, 419–424. [CrossRef]
134. Ham, J.-Y.; Kang, H.-J. A Novel Cytotoxic Alkaloid of Lamellarin Class from a Marine Ascidian *Didemnum* Sp. *Bull. Korean Chem. Soc.* **2002**, *23*, 163–166. [CrossRef]
135. Krishnaiah, P.; Reddy, V.L.N.; Venkataramana, G.; Ravinder, K.; Srinivasulu, M.; Raju, T.V.; Ravikumar, K.; Chandrasekar, D.; Ramakrishna, S.; Venkateswarlu, Y. New Lamellarin Alkaloids from the Indian Ascidian *Didemnum obscurum* and Their Antioxidant Properties. *J. Nat. Prod.* **2004**, *67*, 1168–1171. [CrossRef] [PubMed]
136. Malla Reddy, S.; Srinivasulu, M.; Satyanarayana, N.; Kondapi, A.K.; Venkateswarlu, Y. New Potent Cytotoxic Lamellarin Alkaloids from Indian Ascidian *Didemnum obscurum*. *Tetrahedron* **2005**, *61*, 9242–9247. [CrossRef]
137. Plisson, F.; Huang, X.-C.; Zhang, H.; Khalil, Z.; Capon, R.J. Lamellarins as Inhibitors of P-Glycoprotein-Mediated Multidrug Resistance in a Human Colon Cancer Cell Line. *Chem. Asian J.* **2012**, *7*, 1616–1623. [CrossRef]
138. Urban, S.; Butler, M.S.; Capon, R.J. Lamellarins O and P. New Aromatic Metabolites from the Australian Marine Sponge *Dendrilla cactos*. *Aust. J. Chem.* **1994**, *47*, 1919–1924. [CrossRef]
139. Huang, X.-C.; Xiao, X.; Zhang, Y.-K.; Talele, T.T.; Salim, A.A.; Chen, Z.-S.; Capon, R.J. Lamellarin O, a Pyrrole Alkaloid from an Australian Marine Sponge, *Ianthella* Sp., Reverses BCRP Mediated Drug Resistance in Cancer Cells. *Mar. Drugs* **2014**, *12*, 3818–3837. [CrossRef]
140. Liu, R.; Liu, Y.; Zhou, Y.-D.; Nagle, D.G. Molecular-Targeted Antitumor Agents. 15. Neolamellarins from the Marine Sponge *Dendrilla nigra* Inhibit Hypoxia-Inducible Factor-1 Activation and Secreted Vascular Endothelial Growth Factor Production in Breast Tumor Cells. *J. Nat. Prod.* **2007**, *70*, 1741–1745. [CrossRef]
141. Li, G.; Shao, Y.; Pan, Y.; Li, Y.; Wang, Y.; Wang, L.; Wang, X.; Shao, K.; Wang, S.; Liu, N.; et al. Total Synthesis and Biological Evaluation of 7-Hydroxyneolamellarin A as Hypoxia-Inducible Factor-1α Inhibitor for Cancer Therapy. *Bioorg. Med. Chem. Lett.* **2021**, *50*, 128338. [CrossRef]
142. Li, G.; Dong, H.; Ma, Y.; Shao, K.; Li, Y.; Wu, X.; Wang, S.; Shao, Y.; Zhao, W. Structure-Activity Relationships Study of Neolamellarin A and Its Analogues as Hypoxia Inducible Factor-1 (HIF-1) Inhibitors. *Bioorg. Med. Chem. Lett.* **2019**, *29*, 2327–2331. [CrossRef]
143. Shin, J.; Rho, J.-R.; Seo, Y.; Lee, H.-S.; Cho, K.W.; Kwon, H.J.; Sim, C.J. Wondonins A and B, New Bis(Dihydroxystyryl)Imidazoles from a Two-Sponge Association. *Tetrahedron Lett.* **2001**, *42*, 1965–1968. [CrossRef]
144. Jun, H.-O.; Kim, Y.; Kwon, Y.-W.; Hong, S.-S.; Kim, K.-W.; Shin, J.; Kim, T.-Y. Wondonin, a Novel Compound, Inhibits Hypoxia-Induced Angiogenesis through Hypoxia-Inducible Factor 1 Alpha. *FEBS Lett.* **2007**, *581*, 4977–4982. [CrossRef] [PubMed]
145. Yu, S.; Oh, J.; Li, F.; Kwon, Y.; Cho, H.; Shin, J.; Lee, S.K.; Kim, S. New Scaffold for Angiogenesis Inhibitors Discovered by Targeted Chemical Transformations of Wondonin Natural Products. *ACS Med. Chem. Lett.* **2017**, *8*, 1066–1071. [CrossRef] [PubMed]
146. Quiñoà, E.; Crews, P. Phenolic Constituents of Psammaplysilla. *Tetrahedron Lett.* **1987**, *28*, 3229–3232. [CrossRef]

147. Arabshahi, L.; Schmitz, F.J. Brominated Tyrosine Metabolites from an Unidentified Sponge. *J. Org. Chem.* **1987**, *52*, 3584–3586. [CrossRef]
148. Rodriguez, A.D.; Akee, R.K.; Scheuer, P.J. Two Bromotyrosine-Cysteine Derived Metabolites from a Sponge. *Tetrahedron Lett.* **1987**, *28*, 4989–4992. [CrossRef]
149. Piña, I.C.; Gautschi, J.T.; Wang, G.-Y.-S.; Sanders, M.L.; Schmitz, F.J.; France, D.; Cornell-Kennon, S.; Sambucetti, L.C.; Remiszewski, S.W.; Perez, L.B.; et al. Psammaplins from the Sponge *Pseudoceratina purpurea*: Inhibition of Both Histone Deacetylase and DNA Methyltransferase. *J. Org. Chem.* **2003**, *68*, 3866–3873. [CrossRef]
150. McCulloch, M.W.B.; Coombs, G.S.; Banerjee, N.; Bugni, T.S.; Cannon, K.M.; Harper, M.K.; Veltri, C.A.; Virshup, D.M.; Ireland, C.M. Psammaplin A as a General Activator of Cell-Based Signaling Assays via HDAC Inhibition and Studies on Some Bromotyrosine Derivatives. *Bioorg. Med. Chem.* **2009**, *17*, 2189–2198. [CrossRef]
151. Shin, J.; Lee, H.-S.; Seo, Y.; Rho, J.-R.; Cho, K.W.; Paul, V.J. New Bromotyrosine Metabolites from the Sponge *Aplysinella rhax*. *Tetrahedron* **2000**, *56*, 9071–9077. [CrossRef]
152. Jung, J.H.; Sim, C.J.; Lee, C.-O. Cytotoxic Compounds from a Two-Sponge Association. *J. Nat. Prod.* **1995**, *58*, 1722–1726. [CrossRef]
153. Li, C.J.; Schmitz, F.J.; Kelly Borges, M. A New Lysine Derivative and New 3-Bromopyrrole Carboxylic Acid Derivative from Two Marine Sponges. *J. Nat. Prod.* **1998**, *61*, 387–389. [CrossRef] [PubMed]
154. Park, Y.; Liu, Y.; Hong, J.; Lee, C.-O.; Cho, H.; Kim, D.-K.; Im, K.S.; Jung, J.H. New Bromotyrosine Derivatives from an Association of Two Sponges, *Jaspis wondoensis* and *Poecillastra wondoensis*. *J. Nat. Prod.* **2003**, *66*, 1495–1498. [CrossRef] [PubMed]
155. Kim, T.H.; Kim, H.S.; Kang, Y.J.; Yoon, S.; Lee, J.; Choi, W.S.; Jung, J.H.; Kim, H.S. Psammaplin A Induces Sirtuin 1-Dependent Autophagic Cell Death in Doxorubicin-Resistant MCF-7/Adr Human Breast Cancer Cells and Xenografts. *Biochim. Biophys. Acta* **2015**, *1850*, 401–410. [CrossRef] [PubMed]
156. Zhou, Y.D.; Li, J.; Du, L.; Mahdi, F.; Le, T.P.; Chen, W.L.; Swanson, S.M.; Watabe, K.; Nagle, D.G. Biochemical and Anti-Triple Negative Metastatic Breast Tumor Cell Properties of Psammaplins. *Mar. Drugs* **2018**, *16*, 442. [CrossRef] [PubMed]
157. Leach, B.E.; Ford, J.H.; Whiffen, A.J. Actidione, an Antibiotic from *Streptomyces griseus*. *J. Am. Chem. Soc.* **1947**, *69*, 474. [CrossRef] [PubMed]
158. Xu, X.; Yin, L.; Wang, S.; Liu, H.; Gao, J.; Zhao, S. Cycloheximide Acid A, a New Cycloheximide Derivative from Marine Derived *Streptomyces* Sp. from East China Sea. *Rec. Nat. Prod.* **2013**, *7*, 292–295.
159. Flora, D.O.; Adeyemi, A.I.; George, W.P. Himalomycin A and Cycloheximide-Producing Marine Actinomycete from Lagos Lagoon Soil Sediment. *J. Coast. Life Med.* **2015**, *3*, 361–365. [CrossRef]
160. Semenza, G.L.; Wang, G.L. A Nuclear Factor Induced by Hypoxia via de Novo Protein Synthesis Binds to the Human Erythropoietin Gene Enhancer at a Site Required for Transcriptional Activation. *Mol. Cell. Biol.* **1992**, *12*, 5447–5454. [CrossRef]
161. Semenza, G.L.; Roth, P.H.; Fang, H.M.; Wang, G.L. Transcriptional Regulation of Genes Encoding Glycolytic Enzymes by Hypoxia-Inducible Factor 1. *J. Biol. Chem.* **1994**, *269*, 23757–23763. [CrossRef]
162. Kakeya, H.; Takahashi, I.; Okada, G.; Isono, K.; Osada, H. Epolactaene, a Novel Neuritogenic Compound in Human Neuroblastoma Cells, Produced by a Marine Fungus. *J. Antibiot.* **1995**, *48*, 733–735. [CrossRef]
163. Nagumo, Y.; Kakeya, H.; Shoji, M.; Hayashi, Y.; Dohmae, N.; Osada, H. Epolactaene Binds Human Hsp60 Cys442 Resulting in the Inhibition of Chaperone Activity. *Biochem. J.* **2005**, *387*, 835–840. [CrossRef]
164. Ban, H.S.; Shimizu, K.; Minegishi, H.; Nakamura, H. Identification of Heat Shock Protein 60 as the Regulator of the Hypoxia-Inducible Factor Subunit HIF-1α. *Pure Appl. Chem.* **2012**, *84*, 2325–2337. [CrossRef]
165. Spector, I.; Shochet, N.R.; Blasberger, D.; Kashman, Y. Latrunculins--Novel Marine Macrolides That Disrupt Microfilament Organization and Affect Cell Growth: I. Comparison with Cytochalasin D. *Cell Motil. Cytoskelet.* **1989**, *13*, 127–144. [CrossRef]
166. Nèeman, I.; Fishelson, L.; Kashman, T. Isolation of a New Toxin from the Sponge *Latrunculia magnifica* in the Gulf of Aqaba (Red Sea). *Mar. Biol.* **1975**, *30*, 293–296. [CrossRef]
167. Kashman, Y.; Groweiss, A.; Shmueli, U. Latrunculin, a New 2-Thiazolidinone Macrolide from the Marine Sponge *Latrunculia magnifica*. *Tetrahedron Lett.* **1980**, *21*, 3629–3632. [CrossRef]
168. Kakou, Y.; Crews, P.; Bakus, G.J. Dendrolasin and Latrunculin A from the Fijian Sponge *Spongia mycofijiensis* and an Associated Nudibranch Chromodoris Lochi. *J. Nat. Prod.* **1987**, *50*, 482–484. [CrossRef]
169. Okuda, R.K.; Scheuer, P.J. Latrunculin-A, Ichthyotoxic Constituent of the Nudibranch *Chromodoris elisabethina*. *Experientia* **1985**, *41*, 1355–1356. [CrossRef]
170. Khanfar, M.A.; Youssef, D.T.A.; El Sayed, K.A. 3D-QSAR Studies of Latrunculin-Based Actin Polymerization Inhibitors Using CoMFA and CoMSIA Approaches. *Eur. J. Med. Chem.* **2010**, *45*, 3662–3668. [CrossRef]
171. El Sayed, K.A.; Khanfar, M.A.; Shallal, H.M.; Muralidharan, A.; Awate, B.; Youssef, D.T.A.; Liu, Y.; Zhou, Y.D.; Nagle, D.G.; Shah, G. Latrunculin A and Its C-17-O-Carbamates Inhibit Prostate Tumor Cell Invasion and HIF-1 Activation in Breast Tumor Cells. *J. Nat. Prod.* **2008**, *71*, 396–402. [CrossRef]
172. Shin, I.J.; Park, B.K.; Ahn, Y.T.; Kim, Y.; An, W.G. Actin Disruption Inhibits Hypoxia Inducible Factor-1α Expression via Inactivity of Mdm2-Mediated P70S6K. *Mol. Med. Rep.* **2010**, *3*, 815–819. [CrossRef] [PubMed]
173. Kim, S.-H.; Shin, Y.; Lee, S.-H.; Oh, K.-B.; Lee, S.K.; Shin, J.; Oh, D.-C. Salternamides A-D from a Halophilic *Streptomyces* Sp. Actinobacterium. *J. Nat. Prod.* **2015**, *78*, 836–843. [CrossRef]

174. Kim, S.-H.; Shin, Y.; Lee, S.K.; Shin, J.; Oh, D.-C. Salternamide E from a Saltern-Derived Marine Actinomycete *Streptomyces* Sp. *Nat. Prod. Sci.* **2015**, *21*, 273–277. [CrossRef]
175. Bach, D.H.; Kim, S.H.; Hong, J.Y.; Park, H.J.; Oh, D.C.; Lee, S.K. Salternamide a Suppresses Hypoxia-Induced Accumulation of HIF-1α and Induces Apoptosis in Human Colorectal Cancer Cells. *Mar. Drugs* **2015**, *13*, 6962–6976. [CrossRef] [PubMed]
176. Crews, P.; Kakou, Y.; Quinoa, E. Mycothiazole, a Polyketide Heterocycle from a Marine Sponge. *J. Am. Chem. Soc.* **1988**, *110*, 4365–4368. [CrossRef]
177. Cutignano, A.; Bruno, I.; Bifulco, G.; Casapullo, A.; Debitus, C.; Gomez-Paloma, L.; Riccio, R. Dactylolide, a New Cytotoxic Macrolide from the Vanuatu Sponge *Dactylospongia* Sp. *Eur. J. Org. Chem.* **2001**, *2001*, 775–778. [CrossRef]
178. Meyer, K.J.; Singh, A.J.; Cameron, A.; Tan, A.S.; Leahy, D.C.; O'Sullivan, D.; Joshi, P.; La Flamme, A.C.; Northcote, P.T.; Berridge, M.V.; et al. Mitochondrial Genome-Knockout Cells Demonstrate a Dual Mechanism of Action for the Electron Transport Complex I Inhibitor Mycothiazole. *Mar. Drugs* **2012**, *10*, 900–917. [CrossRef]
179. Morgan, J.B.; Mahdi, F.; Liu, Y.; Coothankandaswamy, V.; Jekabsons, M.B.; Johnson, T.A.; Sashidhara, K.V.; Crews, P.; Nagle, D.G.; Zhou, Y.-D. The Marine Sponge Metabolite Mycothiazole: A Novel Prototype Mitochondrial Complex I Inhibitor. *Bioorg. Med. Chem.* **2010**, *18*, 5988–5994. [CrossRef]
180. Walsh, T.J.; Standiford, H.C.; Reboli, A.C.; John, J.F.; Mulligan, M.E.; Ribner, B.S.; Montgomerie, J.Z.; Goetz, M.B.; Mayhall, C.G.; Rimland, D. Randomized Double-Blinded Trial of Rifampin with Either Novobiocin or Trimethoprim-Sulfamethoxazole against Methicillin-Resistant Staphylococcus Aureus Colonization: Prevention of Antimicrobial Resistance and Effect of Host Factors on Outcome. *Antimicrob. Agents Chemother.* **1993**, *37*, 1334–1342. [CrossRef]
181. Eder, J.P.; Wheeler, C.A.; Teicher, B.A.; Schnipper, L.E. A Phase I Clinical Trial of Novobiocin, a Modulator of Alkylating Agent Cytotoxicity. *Cancer Res.* **1991**, *51*, 510–513.
182. Zhou, J.; Gelot, C.; Pantelidou, C.; Li, A.; Yücel, H.; Davis, R.E.; Färkkilä, A.; Kochupurakkal, B.; Syed, A.; Shapiro, G.I.; et al. A First-in-Class Polymerase Theta Inhibitor Selectively Targets Homologous-Recombination-Deficient Tumors. *Nat. Cancer* **2021**, *2*, 598–610. [CrossRef]
183. Hoeksema, H.; Johnson, J.L.; Hinman, J.W. Structural Studies on Streptonivicin,1 a New Antibiotic. *J. Am. Chem. Soc.* **1955**, *77*, 6710–6711. [CrossRef]
184. Smith, C.G.; Dietz, A.; Sokolski, W.T.; Savage, G.M. Streptonivicin, a New Antibiotic. I. Discovery and Biologic Studies. *Antibiot. Chemother.* **1956**, *6*, 135–142.
185. Hoeksema, H.; Bergy, M.E.; Jackson, W.G.; Shell, J.W.; Hinman, J.W.; Fonken, A.E.; Boyack, G.A.; Caron, E.L.; Ford, J.H.; Devries, W.H.; et al. Streptonivicin, a New Antibiotic. II. Isolation and Characterization. *Antibiot. Chemother.* **1956**, *6*, 143–148.
186. Dalisay, D.S.; Williams, D.E.; Wang, X.L.; Centko, R.; Chen, J.; Andersen, R.J. Marine Sediment-Derived Streptomyces Bacteria from British Columbia, Canada Are a Promising Microbiota Resource for the Discovery of Antimicrobial Natural Products. *PLoS ONE* **2013**, *8*, e77078. [CrossRef]
187. Syed, A.; Filandr, F.; Patterson-Fortin, J.; Bacolla, A.; Ravindranathan, R.; Zhou, J.; McDonald, D.T.; Albuhluli, M.E.; Verway-Cohen, A.; Newman, J.A.; et al. Novobiocin Blocks Nucleic Acid Binding to Polθ and Inhibits Stimulation of Its ATPase Activity. *Nucleic Acids Res.* **2023**, *51*, 9920–9937. [CrossRef]
188. Conde, R.; Belak, Z.R.; Nair, M.; O'Carroll, R.F.; Ovsenek, N. Modulation of Hsf1 Activity by Novobiocin and Geldanamycin. *Biochem. Cell Biol.* **2009**, *87*, 845–851. [CrossRef] [PubMed]
189. Katschinski, D.M.; Le, L.; Heinrich, D.; Wagner, K.F.; Hofer, T.; Schindler, S.G.; Wenger, R.H. Heat Induction of the Unphosphorylated Form of Hypoxia-Inducible Factor-1α Is Dependent on Heat Shock Protein-90 Activity. *J. Biol. Chem.* **2002**, *277*, 9262–9267. [CrossRef] [PubMed]
190. Lupescu, A.; Bissinger, R.; Herrmann, T.; Oswald, G.; Jilani, K.; Lang, F. Induction of Suicidal Erythrocyte Death by Novobiocin. *Cell. Physiol. Biochem. Int. J. Exp. Cell. Physiol. Biochem. Pharmacol.* **2014**, *33*, 670–680. [CrossRef] [PubMed]
191. Wu, D.; Zhang, R.; Zhao, R.; Chen, G.; Cai, Y.; Jin, J. A Novel Function of Novobiocin: Disrupting the Interaction of HIF 1α and P300/CBP through Direct Binding to the HIF1α C-Terminal Activation Domain. *PLoS ONE* **2013**, *8*, e62014. [CrossRef] [PubMed]
192. Egorov, E.A.; Alekhina, V.A.; Volobueva, T.M.; Fedoreev, S.A.; Mishchenko, N.P.; Kol'tsova, E.A. Histochrome, a new antioxidant, in the treatment of ocular diseases. *Vestn. Oftalmol.* **1999**, *115*, 34–35.
193. Mishchenko, N.P.; Fedoreev, S.A.; Bagirova, V.L. Histochrome: A New Original Domestic Drug. *Pharm. Chem. J.* **2003**, *37*, 48–52. [CrossRef]
194. Hwang, J.-W.; Park, J.-H.; Park, B.-W.; Kim, H.; Kim, J.-J.; Sim, W.-S.; Mishchenko, N.P.; Fedoreyev, S.A.; Vasileva, E.A.; Ban, K.; et al. Histochrome Attenuates Myocardial Ischemia-Reperfusion Injury by Inhibiting Ferroptosis-Induced Cardiomyocyte Death. *Antioxidants* **2021**, *10*, 1624. [CrossRef]
195. Artyukov, A.A.; Popov, A.M.; Tsybulsky, A.V.; Krivoshapko, O.N.; Polyakova, N.V. Pharmacological Activity of Echinochrome a Alone and in the Biologically Active Additive Timarin. *Biochem. Suppl. Ser. B Biomed. Chem.* **2013**, *7*, 237–242. [CrossRef]
196. Munn, C.A. Mac On the Chromatology of the Blood of Some Invertebrates. *J. Cell Sci.* **1885**, *s2-25*, 469–490. [CrossRef]
197. Service, M.; Wardlaw, A.C. Echinochrome-A as a Bactericidal Substance in the Coelomic Fluid of *Echinus esculentus* (L.). *Comp. Biochem. Physiol. Part B Comp. Biochem.* **1984**, *79*, 161–165. [CrossRef]
198. Artyukov, A.A.; Zelepuga, E.A.; Bogdanovich, L.N.; Lupach, N.M.; Novikov, V.L.; Rutckova, T.A.; Kozlovskaya, E.P. Marine Polyhydroxynaphthoquinone, Echinochrome A: Prevention of Atherosclerotic Inflammation and Probable Molecular Targets. *J. Clin. Med.* **2020**, *9*, 1494. [CrossRef] [PubMed]

199. Dong, X.; Fu, J.; Yin, X.; Cao, S.; Li, X.; Lin, L.; Ni, J. Emodin: A Review of Its Pharmacology, Toxicity and Pharmacokinetics. *Phytother. Res.* **2016**, *30*, 1207–1218. [CrossRef]
200. Stompor-Gorący, M. The Health Benefits of Emodin, a Natural Anthraquinone Derived from Rhubarb-A Summary Update. *Int. J. Mol. Sci.* **2021**, *22*, 9522. [CrossRef]
201. de Mattos-Shipley, K.M.J.; Simpson, T.J. The "emodin Family" of Fungal Natural Products-Amalgamating a Century of Research with Recent Genomics-Based Advances. *Nat. Prod. Rep.* **2023**, *40*, 174–201. [CrossRef]
202. Greco, G.; Turrini, E.; Catanzaro, E.; Fimognari, C. Marine Anthraquinones: Pharmacological and Toxicological Issues. *Mar. Drugs* **2021**, *19*, 272. [CrossRef]
203. Hafez Ghoran, S.; Taktaz, F.; Ayatollahi, S.A.; Kijjoa, A. Anthraquinones and Their Analogues from Marine-Derived Fungi: Chemistry and Biological Activities. *Mar. Drugs* **2022**, *20*, 474. [CrossRef] [PubMed]
204. Gomes, N.M.; Dethoup, T.; Singburaudom, N.; Gales, L.; Silva, A.M.S.; Kijjoa, A. Eurocristatine, a New Diketopiperazine Dimer from the Marine Sponge-Associated Fungus *Eurotium cristatum*. *Phytochem. Lett.* **2012**, *5*, 717–720. [CrossRef]
205. Tuli, H.S.; Aggarwal, V.; Tuorkey, M.; Aggarwal, D.; Parashar, N.C.; Varol, M.; Savla, R.; Kaur, G.; Mittal, S.; Sak, K. Emodin: A Metabolite That Exhibits Anti-Neoplastic Activities by Modulating Multiple Oncogenic Targets. *Toxicol. Vitr.* **2021**, *73*, 105142. [CrossRef] [PubMed]
206. Cao, M.; Fang, Y.; Jia, W.; Wang, Y.; Sun, J.; Tao, D. Emodin Relieves Hypoxia-Triggered Injury via Elevation of MicroRNA-25 in PC-12 Cells. *Artif. Cells Nanomed. Biotechnol.* **2019**, *47*, 2678–2687. [CrossRef] [PubMed]
207. Ha, M.K.; Song, Y.H.; Jeong, S.J.; Lee, H.J.; Jung, J.H.; Kim, B.; Song, H.S.; Huh, J.E.; Kim, S.H. Emodin Inhibits Proinflammatory Responses and Inactivates Histone Deacetylase 1 in Hypoxic Rheumatoid Synoviocytes. *Biol. Pharm. Bull.* **2011**, *34*, 1432–1437. [CrossRef] [PubMed]
208. Li, X.; Shan, C.; Wu, Z.; Yu, H.; Yang, A.; Tan, B. Emodin Alleviated Pulmonary Inflammation in Rats with LPS-Induced Acute Lung Injury through Inhibiting the MTOR/HIF-1α/VEGF Signaling Pathway. *Inflamm. Res.* **2020**, *69*, 365–373. [CrossRef]
209. Qi, L.; Fu, Q.; Du, C.; Wu, D.; Zhang, G.; Yuan, B.; Yan, L. Amelioration of Hypoxia and LPS-Induced Intestinal Epithelial Barrier Dysfunction by Emodin through the Suppression of the NF-KB and HIF-1α Signaling Pathways. *Int. J. Mol. Med.* **2014**, *34*, 1629–1639. [CrossRef]
210. Lv, B.; Zheng, K.; Sun, Y.; Wu, L.; Qiao, L.; Wu, Z.; Zhao, Y.; Zheng, Z. Network Pharmacology Experiments Show That Emodin Can Exert a Protective Effect on MCAO Rats by Regulating Hif-1α/VEGF-A Signaling. *ACS Omega* **2022**, *7*, 22577–22593. [CrossRef]
211. Hu, L.; Cui, R.; Liu, H.; Wang, F. Emodin and Rhein Decrease Levels of Hypoxia-Inducible Factor-1a in Human Pancreatic Cancer Cells and Attenuate Cancer Cachexia in Athymic Mice Carrying These Cells. *Oncotarget* **2017**, *8*, 88008–88020. [CrossRef]
212. Shi, G.H.; Zhou, L. Emodin Suppresses Angiogenesis and Metastasis in Anaplastic Thyroid Cancer by Affecting TRAF6-Mediated Pathways in Vivo and in Vitro. *Mol. Med. Rep.* **2018**, *18*, 5191–5197. [CrossRef]
213. Hwang, S.Y.; Heo, K.; Kim, J.S.; Im, J.W.; Lee, S.M.; Cho, M.; Kang, D.H.; Heo, J.; Lee, J.W.; Choi, C.W.; et al. Emodin Attenuates Radioresistance Induced by Hypoxia in HepG2 Cells via the Enhancement of PARP1 Cleavage and Inhibition of JMJD2B. *Oncol. Rep.* **2015**, *33*, 1691–1698. [CrossRef]
214. Deboer, C.; Meulman, P.A.; Wnuk, R.J.; Peterson, D.H. Geldanamycin, a New Antibiotic. *J. Antibiot.* **1970**, *23*, 442–447. [CrossRef]
215. Yi, K.-X.; Xie, Q.-Y.; Ma, Q.-Y.; Yang, L.; Dai, H.-F.; Zhao, Y.-X.; Hao, Y.-E. Diverse Ansamycin Derivatives from the Marine-Derived *Streptomyces* Sp. ZYX-F-97 and Their Antibacterial Activities. *Fitoterapia* **2024**, *173*, 105814. [CrossRef]
216. Lu, X.; Zhang, M.; Qiu, Y.; Liu, X.; Wang, C.; Chen, J.; Zhang, H.; Wei, B.; Yu, Y.; Ying, Y.; et al. α-Glucosidase Inhibitors from Two Mangrove-Derived Actinomycetes. *Molecules* **2023**, *28*, 3822. [CrossRef] [PubMed]
217. Yi, W.; Lian, X.-Y.; Zhang, Z. Cytotoxic Metabolites from the Marine-Associated *Streptomyces* Sp. ZZ1944. *Phytochemistry* **2022**, *201*, 113292. [CrossRef] [PubMed]
218. Nong, X.-H.; Tu, Z.-C.; Qi, S.-H. Ansamycin Derivatives from the Marine-Derived *Streptomyces* Sp. SCSGAA 0027 and Their Cytotoxic and Antiviral Activities. *Bioorg. Med. Chem. Lett.* **2020**, *30*, 127168. [CrossRef]
219. Whitesell, L.; Mimnaugh, E.G.; De Costa, B.; Myers, C.E.; Neckers, L.M. Inhibition of Heat Shock Protein HSP90-Pp60v-Src Heteroprotein Complex Formation by Benzoquinone Ansamycins: Essential Role for Stress Proteins in Oncogenic Transformation. *Proc. Natl. Acad. Sci. USA* **1994**, *91*, 8324–8328. [CrossRef] [PubMed]
220. Roe, S.M.; Prodromou, C.; O'Brien, R.; Ladbury, J.E.; Piper, P.W.; Pearl, L.H. Structural Basis for Inhibition of the Hsp90 Molecular Chaperone by the Antitumor Antibiotics Radicicol and Geldanamycin. *J. Med. Chem.* **1999**, *42*, 260–266. [CrossRef] [PubMed]
221. Avendaño, C.; Menéndez, J.C. Chapter 14—Miscellaneous Small- Molecule and Biological Approaches to Targeted Cancer Therapy. In *Medicinal Chemistry of Anticancer Drugs*, 3rd ed.; Avendaño, C., Menéndez, J.C., Eds.; Elsevier: Boston, MA, USA, 2023; pp. 743–822, ISBN 978-0-12-818549-0.
222. Mabjeesh, N.J.; Post, D.E.; Willard, M.T.; Kaur, B.; Van Meir, E.G.; Simons, J.W.; Zhong, H. Geldanamycin Induces Degradation of Hypoxia-Inducible Factor 1alpha Protein via the Proteosome Pathway in Prostate Cancer Cells. *Cancer Res.* **2002**, *62*, 2478–2482. [PubMed]
223. Suzuki, Y.; Kondo, Y.; Hara, S.; Kimata, R.; Nishimura, T. Effect of the Hsp90 Inhibitor Geldanamycin on Androgen Response of Prostate Cancer under Hypoxic Conditions. *Int. J. Urol.* **2010**, *17*, 281–285. [CrossRef]
224. Alqawi, O.; Moghaddas, M.; Singh, G. Effects of Geldanamycin on HIF-1alpha Mediated Angiogenesis and Invasion in Prostate Cancer Cells. *Prostate Cancer Prostatic Dis.* **2006**, *9*, 126–135. [CrossRef]

225. van der Bilt, J.D.W.; Soeters, M.E.; Duyverman, A.M.M.J.; Nijkamp, M.W.; Witteveen, P.O.; van Diest, P.J.; Kranenburg, O.; Borel Rinkes, I.H.M. Perinecrotic Hypoxia Contributes to Ischemia/Reperfusion-Accelerated Outgrowth of Colorectal Micrometastases. *Am. J. Pathol.* **2007**, *170*, 1379–1388. [CrossRef] [PubMed]
226. Koga, F.; Tsutsumi, S.; Neckers, L.M. Low Dose Geldanamycin Inhibits Hepatocyte Growth Factor and Hypoxia-Stimulated Invasion of Cancer Cells. *Cell Cycle* **2007**, *6*, 1393–1402. [CrossRef] [PubMed]
227. Liu, Y.V.; Baek, J.H.; Zhang, H.; Diez, R.; Cole, R.N.; Semenza, G.L. RACK1 Competes with HSP90 for Binding to HIF-1alpha and Is Required for O(2)-Independent and HSP90 Inhibitor-Induced Degradation of HIF-1alpha. *Mol. Cell* **2007**, *25*, 207–217. [CrossRef] [PubMed]
228. Mejia, E.J.; Loveridge, S.T.; Stepan, G.; Tsai, A.; Jones, G.S.; Barnes, T.; White, K.N.; Drašković, M.; Tenney, K.; Tsiang, M.; et al. Study of Marine Natural Products Including Resorcyclic Acid Lactones from *Humicola fuscoatra* That Reactivate Latent HIV-1 Expression in an in Vitro Model of Central Memory CD4+ T Cells. *J. Nat. Prod.* **2014**, *77*, 618–624. [CrossRef] [PubMed]
229. Grkovic, T.; Whitson, E.L.; Rabe, D.C.; Gardella, R.S.; Bottaro, D.P.; Linehan, W.M.; McMahon, J.B.; Gustafson, K.R.; McKee, T.C. Identification and Evaluation of Soft Coral Diterpenes as Inhibitors of HIF-2α Induced Gene Expression. *Bioorg. Med. Chem. Lett.* **2011**, *21*, 2113–2115. [CrossRef]
230. McKee, T.C.; Rabe, D.; Bokesch, H.R.; Grkovic, T.; Whitson, E.L.; Diyabalanage, T.; Van Wyk, A.W.W.; Marcum, S.R.; Gardella, R.S.; Gustafson, K.R.; et al. Inhibition of Hypoxia Inducible Factor-2 Transcription: Isolation of Active Modulators from Marine Sponges. *J. Nat. Prod.* **2012**, *75*, 1632–1636. [CrossRef]
231. Schmitz, F.J.; Bloor, S.J. Xesto- and Halenaquinone Derivatives from a Sponge, *Adocia* Sp., from *Truk lagoon*. *J. Org. Chem.* **1988**, *53*, 3922–3925. [CrossRef]
232. Concepción, G.P.; Foderaro, T.A.; Eldredge, G.S.; Lobkovsky, E.; Clardy, J.; Barrows, L.R.; Ireland, C.M. Topoisomerase II-Mediated DNA Cleavage by Adocia- and Xestoquinones from the Philippine Sponge *Xestospongia* Sp. *J. Med. Chem.* **1995**, *38*, 4503–4507. [CrossRef]
233. Du, L.; Mahdi, F.; Datta, S.; Jekabsons, M.B.; Zhou, Y.-D.; Nagle, D.G. Structures and Mechanisms of Antitumor Agents: Xestoquinones Uncouple Cellular Respiration and Disrupt HIF Signaling in Human Breast Tumor Cells. *J. Nat. Prod.* **2012**, *75*, 1553–1559. [CrossRef]
234. Cao, S.; Foster, C.; Brisson, M.; Lazo, J.S.; Kingston, D.G.I. Halenaquinone and Xestoquinone Derivatives, Inhibitors of Cdc25B Phosphatase from a *Xestospongia* Sp. *Bioorg. Med. Chem.* **2005**, *13*, 999–1003. [CrossRef]
235. Isaac, B.G.; Ayer, S.W.; Elliott, R.C.; Stonard, R.J. Herboxidiene: A Potent Phytotoxic Polyketide from *Streptomyces* Sp. A7847. *J. Org. Chem.* **1992**, *57*, 7220–7226. [CrossRef]
236. Damayanti, E.; Nisa, K.; Handayani, S.; Dewi, R.T.; Mustofa, M.; Dinoto, A.; Dinoto, A.; Widada, J. Cytotoxicity and Molecular Mechanism of Marine-Derived *Streptomyces* Sp. Gmy01 on Human Lung Cancer Cell Line A549. *J. Appl. Pharm. Sci.* **2021**, *11*, 46–55. [CrossRef]
237. Hasegawa, M.; Miura, T.; Kuzuya, K.; Inoue, A.; Won Ki, S.; Horinouchi, S.; Yoshida, T.; Kunoh, T.; Koseki, K.; Mino, K.; et al. Identification of SAP155 as the Target of GEX1A (Herboxidiene), an Antitumor Natural Product. *ACS Chem. Biol.* **2011**, *6*, 229–233. [CrossRef] [PubMed]
238. Kaida, D.; Motoyoshi, H.; Tashiro, E.; Nojima, T.; Hagiwara, M.; Ishigami, K.; Watanabe, H.; Kitahara, T.; Yoshida, T.; Nakajima, H.; et al. Spliceostatin A Targets SF3b and Inhibits Both Splicing and Nuclear Retention of Pre-MRNA. *Nat. Chem. Biol.* **2007**, *3*, 576–583. [CrossRef]
239. Jung, H.J.; Kim, Y.; Shin, J.Y.; Sohng, J.K.; Kwon, H.J. Antiangiogenic Activity of Herboxidiene via Downregulation of Vascular Endothelial Growth Factor Receptor-2 and Hypoxia-Inducible Factor-1α. *Arch. Pharm. Res.* **2015**, *38*, 1728–1735. [CrossRef] [PubMed]
240. Dai, J.; Liu, Y.; Jia, H.; Zhou, Y.D.; Nagle, D.G. Benzochromenones from the Marine Crinoid Comantheria Rotula Inhibit Hypoxia-Inducible Factor-1 (HIF-1) in Cell-Based Reporter Assays and Differentially Suppress the Growth of Certain Tumor Cell Lines. *J. Nat. Prod.* **2007**, *70*, 1462–1466. [CrossRef] [PubMed]
241. Mabrouk, S.B.; Reis, M.; Sousa, M.L.; Ribeiro, T.; Almeida, J.R.; Pereira, S.; Antunes, J.; Rosa, F.; Vasconcelos, V.; Achour, L.; et al. The Marine Seagrass *Halophila stipulacea* as a Source of Bioactive Metabolites against Obesity and Biofouling. *Mar. Drugs* **2020**, *18*, 88. [CrossRef] [PubMed]
242. Lee, B.; Kim, K.H.; Jung, H.J.; Kwon, H.J. Matairesinol Inhibits Angiogenesis via Suppression of Mitochondrial Reactive Oxygen Species. *Biochem. Biophys. Res. Commun.* **2012**, *421*, 76–80. [CrossRef] [PubMed]
243. Hannan, M.A.; Dash, R.; Haque, M.N.; Mohibbullah, M.; Sohag, A.A.; Rahman, M.A.; Uddin, M.J.; Alam, M.; Moon, I.S. Neuroprotective Potentials of Marine Algae and Their Bioactive Metabolites: Pharmacological Insights and Therapeutic Advances. *Mar. Drugs* **2020**, *18*, 347. [CrossRef] [PubMed]
244. Ferreres, F.; Lopes, G.; Gil-Izquierdo, A.; Andrade, P.B.; Sousa, C.; Mouga, T.; Valentão, P. Phlorotannin Extracts from Fucales Characterized by HPLC-DAD-ESI-MSn: Approaches to Hyaluronidase Inhibitory Capacity and Antioxidant Properties. *Mar. Drugs* **2012**, *10*, 2766–2781. [CrossRef]
245. Wijesekara, I.; Yoon, N.Y.; Kim, S.-K. Phlorotannins from *Ecklonia cava* (Phaeophyceae): Biological Activities and Potential Health Benefits. *BioFactors* **2010**, *36*, 408–414. [CrossRef]
246. Lopes, G.; Andrade, P.B.; Valentão, P. Phlorotannins: Towards New Pharmacological Interventions for Diabetes Mellitus Type 2. *Molecules* **2017**, *22*, 56. [CrossRef]

247. Yang, S.; Liu, Y.; Xiao, Z.; Tang, Y.; Hong, P.; Sun, S.; Zhou, C.; Qian, Z.J. Inhibition Effects of 7-Phloro-Eckol from *Ecklonia cava* on Metastasis and Angiogenesis Induced by Hypoxia through Regulation of AKT/MTOR and ERK Signaling Pathways. *Arab. J. Chem.* **2021**, *14*, 103187. [CrossRef]
248. Hodges, T.W.; Hossain, C.F.; Kim, Y.P.; Zhou, Y.D.; Nagle, D.G. Molecular-Targeted Antitumor Agents: The *Saururus cernuus* Dineolignans Manassantin B and 4-O-Demethylmanassantin B Are Potent Inhibitors of Hypoxia-Activated HIF-1. *J. Nat. Prod.* **2004**, *67*, 767–771. [CrossRef] [PubMed]
249. Hossain, C.F.; Kim, Y.P.; Baerson, S.R.; Zhang, L.; Bruick, R.K.; Mohammed, K.A.; Agarwal, A.K.; Nagle, D.G.; Zhou, Y.D. *Saururus cernuus* Lignans—Potent Small Molecule Inhibitors of Hypoxia-Inducible Factor-1. *Biochem. Biophys. Res. Commun.* **2005**, *333*, 1026–1033. [CrossRef]
250. Dai, J.; Liu, Y.; Zhou, Y.D.; Nagle, D.G. Cytotoxic Metabolites from an Indonesian Sponge *Lendenfeldia* Sp. *J. Nat. Prod.* **2007**, *70*, 1824–1826. [CrossRef]
251. Wang, J.; Zhang, M.; Yang, J.; Yang, X.; Zhang, J.; Zhao, Z. Type A Trichothecene Metabolic Profile Differentiation, Mechanisms, Biosynthetic Pathways, and Evolution in *Fusarium* Species—A Mini Review. *Toxins* **2023**, *15*, 446. [CrossRef]
252. McCormick, S.P.; Stanley, A.M.; Stover, N.A.; Alexander, N.J. Trichothecenes: From Simple to Complex Mycotoxins. *Toxins* **2011**, *3*, 802–814. [CrossRef] [PubMed]
253. Choi, Y.J.; Shin, H.W.; Chun, Y.S.; Leutou, A.S.; Son, B.W.; Park, J.W. Diacetoxyscirpenol as a New Anticancer Agent to Target Hypoxiainducible Factor 1. *Oncotarget* **2016**, *7*, 62107–62122. [CrossRef]
254. Wu, Q.; Wu, W.; Kuca, K. From Hypoxia and Hypoxia-Inducible Factors (HIF) to Oxidative Stress: A New Understanding of the Toxic Mechanism of Mycotoxins. *Food Chem. Toxicol.* **2020**, *135*, 110968. [CrossRef] [PubMed]
255. Arai, M.; Kawachi, T.; Sato, H.; Setiawan, A.; Kobayashi, M. Marine Spongian Sesquiterpene Phenols, Dictyoceratin-C and Smenospondiol, Display Hypoxia-Selective Growth Inhibition against Cancer Cells. *Bioorg. Med. Chem. Lett.* **2014**, *24*, 3155–3157. [CrossRef]
256. Nakamura, H.; Deng, S.; Kobayashi, J.; Ohizumi, Y.; Hirata, Y. Dictyoceratin-A and -B, Novel Antimicrobial Terpenoids from the Okinawan Marine Sponge *Hipposponqia* Sp. *Tetrahedron* **1986**, *42*, 4197–4201. [CrossRef]
257. Kushlan, D.M.; Faulkner, D.J.; Parkanyi, L.; Clardy, J. Metabolites of the Palauan Sponge *Dactylospongia* Sp. *Tetrahedron* **1989**, *45*, 3307–3312. [CrossRef]
258. Shen, Y.C.; Hsieh, P.W. New Sesquiterpene Hydroquinones from a Taiwanese Marine Sponge *Polyfibrospongia australis*. *J. Nat. Prod.* **1997**, *60*, 93–97. [CrossRef] [PubMed]
259. Cao, S.; Gao, Z.; Thomas, S.J.; Hecht, S.M.; Lazo, J.S.; Kingston, D.G.I. Marine Sesquiterpenoids That Inhibit the Lyase Activity of DNA Polymerase Beta. *J. Nat. Prod.* **2004**, *67*, 1716–1718. [CrossRef] [PubMed]
260. Sumii, Y.; Kotoku, N.; Fukuda, A.; Kawachi, T.; Arai, M.; Kobayashi, M. Structure-Activity Relationship and in Vivo Anti-Tumor Evaluations Ofdictyoceratin-A and-C,Hypoxia-Selective Growth Inhibitors from Marine Sponge. *Mar. Drugs* **2015**, *13*, 7419–7432. [CrossRef] [PubMed]
261. Sumii, Y.; Kotoku, N.; Fukuda, A.; Kawachi, T.; Sumii, Y.; Arai, M.; Kobayashi, M. Enantioselective Synthesis of Dictyoceratin-A (Smenospondiol) and -C, Hypoxia-Selective Growth Inhibitors from Marine Sponge. *Bioorg. Med. Chem.* **2015**, *23*, 966–975. [CrossRef] [PubMed]
262. Kawachi, T.; Tanaka, S.; Fukuda, A.; Sumii, Y.; Setiawan, A.; Kotoku, N.; Kobayashi, M.; Arai, M. Target Identification of the Marine Natural Products Dictyoceratin-A and -C as Selective Growth Inhibitors in Cancer Cells Adapted to Hypoxic Environments. *Mar. Drugs* **2019**, *17*, 163. [CrossRef] [PubMed]
263. Ravi, B.N.; Perzanowski, H.P.; Ross, R.A.; Erdman, T.R.; Scheuer, P.J.; Finer, J.; Clardy, J. Recent Research in Marine Natural Products: The Puupehenones. *Pure Appl. Chem.* **1979**, *51*, 1893–1900. [CrossRef]
264. Amade, P.; Chevelot, L.; Perzanowski, H.P.; Scheuer, P.J. A Dimer of Puupehenone. *Helv. Chim. Acta* **1983**, *66*, 1672–1675. [CrossRef]
265. Nasu, S.S.; Yeung, B.K.S.; Hamann, M.T.; Scheuer, P.J.; Kelly-Borges, M.; Goins, K. Puupehenone-Related Metabolites from Two Hawaiian Sponges, *Hyrtios* Spp. *J. Org. Chem.* **1995**, *60*, 7290–7292. [CrossRef]
266. Piña, I.C.; Sanders, M.L.; Crews, P. Puupehenone Congeners from an Indo-Pacific *Hyrtios* Sponge. *J. Nat. Prod.* **2003**, *66*, 2–6. [CrossRef]
267. Robinson, S.J.; Hoobler, E.K.; Riener, M.; Loveridge, S.T.; Tenney, K.; Valeriote, F.A.; Holman, T.R.; Crews, P. Using Enzyme Assays to Evaluate the Structure and Bioactivity of Sponge-Derived Meroterpenes. *J. Nat. Prod.* **2009**, *72*, 1857–1863. [CrossRef]
268. Kohmoto, S.; McConnell, O.J.; Wright, A.; Koehn, F.; Thompson, W.; Lui, M.; Snader, K.M. Puupehenone, a Cytotoxic Metabolite from a Deep Water Marine Sponge, *Stronglyophora hartmani*. *J. Nat. Prod.* **1987**, *50*, 336. [CrossRef]
269. Coval, S.J.; Conover, M.A.; Mierzwa, R.; King, A.; Puar, M.S.; Phife, D.W.; Pai, J.-K.; Burrier, R.E.; Ahn, H.-S.; Boykow, G.C.; et al. Wiedendiol-A and -B, Cholesteryl Ester Transfer Protein Inhibitors from the Marine Sponge *Xestospongia wiedenmayeri*. *Bioorg. Med. Chem. Lett.* **1995**, *5*, 605–610. [CrossRef]
270. Ueda, K.; Ueta, T.; Siwu, E.R.O.; Kita, M.; Uemura, D. Haterumadienone: A New Puupehenone Congener from an Okinawan Marine Sponge, *Dysidea* Sp. *Chem. Lett.* **2005**, *34*, 1530–1531. [CrossRef]
271. Utkina, N.K.; Denisenko, V.A.; Krasokhin, V.B. Diplopuupehenone, a New Unsymmetrical Puupehenone-Related Dimer from the Marine Sponge *Dysidea* Sp. *Tetrahedron Lett.* **2011**, *52*, 3765–3768. [CrossRef]

272. Hagiwara, K.; Garcia Hernandez, J.E.; Harper, M.K.; Carroll, A.; Motti, C.A.; Awaya, J.; Nguyen, H.-Y.; Wright, A.D. Puupehenol, a Potent Antioxidant Antimicrobial Meroterpenoid from a Hawaiian Deep-Water *Dactylospongia* Sp. Sponge. *J. Nat. Prod.* **2015**, *78*, 325–329. [CrossRef] [PubMed]
273. Amagata, T.; Whitman, S.; Johnson, T.A.; Stessman, C.C.; Loo, C.P.; Lobkovsky, E.; Clardy, J.; Crews, P.; Holman, T.R. Exploring Sponge-Derived Terpenoids for Their Potency and Selectivity against 12-Human, 15-Human, and 15-Soybean Lipoxygenases. *J. Nat. Prod.* **2003**, *66*, 230–235. [CrossRef] [PubMed]
274. Castro, M.E.; González-Iriarte, M.; Barrero, A.F.; Salvador-Tormo, N.; Muñoz-Chápuli, R.; Medina, M.A.; Quesada, A.R. Study of Puupehenone and Related Compounds as Inhibitors of Angiogenesis. *Int. J. Cancer* **2004**, *110*, 31–38. [CrossRef] [PubMed]
275. Douat-Casassus, C.; Marchand-Geneste, N.; Diez, E.; Aznar, C.; Picard, P.; Geoffre, S.; Huet, A.; Bourguet-Kondracki, M.-L.; Gervois, N.; Jotereau, F.; et al. Covalent Modification of a Melanoma-Derived Antigenic Peptide with a Natural Quinone Methide. Preliminary Chemical, Molecular Modelling and Immunological Evaluation Studies. *Mol. BioSyst.* **2006**, *2*, 240–249. [CrossRef]
276. Mohammed, K.A.; Hossain, C.F.; Zhang, L.; Bruick, R.K.; Zhou, Y.D.; Nagle, D.G. Laurenditerpenol, a New Diterpene from the Tropical Marine Alga *Laurencia intricata* That Potently Inhibits HIF-1 Mediated Hypoxic Signaling in Breast Tumor Cells. *J. Nat. Prod.* **2004**, *67*, 2002–2007. [CrossRef]
277. Braekman, J.C.; Daloze, D.; Hulot, G.; Tursch, B.; Declercq, J.P.; Germain, G.; van Meerssche, M. Chemical Studies of Marine Invertebrates. XXXVII(1). Three Novel Meroditerpenoids from the Sponge Strongylophora Durissima(2). *Bull. Sociétés Chim. Belg.* **1978**, *87*, 917–926. [CrossRef]
278. McHardy, L.M.; Warabi, K.; Andersen, R.J.; Roskelley, C.D.; Roberge, M. Strongylophorine-26, a Rho-Dependent Inhibitor of Tumor Cell Invasion That Reduces Actin Stress Fibers and Induces Nonpolarized Lamellipodial Extensions. *Mol. Cancer Ther.* **2005**, *4*, 772–778. [CrossRef] [PubMed]
279. Noda, A.; Sakai, E.; Kato, H.; Losung, F.; Mangindaan, R.E.P.; de Voogd, N.J.; Yokosawa, H.; Tsukamoto, S. Strongylophorines, Meroditerpenoids from the Marine Sponge *Petrosia corticata*, Function as Proteasome Inhibitors. *Bioorg. Med. Chem. Lett.* **2015**, *25*, 2650–2653. [CrossRef] [PubMed]
280. Mohammed, K.A.; Jadulco, R.C.; Bugni, T.S.; Harper, M.K.; Sturdy, M.; Ireland, C.M. Strongylophorines: Natural Product Inhibitors of Hypoxia-Inducible Factor-1 Transcriptional Pathway. *J. Med. Chem.* **2008**, *51*, 1402–1405. [CrossRef] [PubMed]
281. Dai, J.; Liu, Y.; Zhou, Y.-D.; Nagle, D.G. Hypoxia-Selective Antitumor Agents: Norsesterterpene Peroxides from the Marine Sponge *Diacarnus levii* Preferentially Suppress the Growth of Tumor Cells under Hypoxic Conditions. *J. Nat. Prod.* **2007**, *70*, 130–133. [CrossRef]
282. Erdogan-Orhan, I.; Sener, B.; de Rosa, S.; Perez-Baz, J.; Lozach, O.; Leost, M.; Rakhilin, S.; Meijer, L. Polyprenyl-Hydroquinones and -Furans from Three Marine Sponges Inhibit the Cell Cycle Regulating Phosphatase CDC25A. *Nat. Prod. Res.* **2004**, *18*, 1–9. [CrossRef]
283. Tasdemir, D.; Bugni, T.S.; Mangalindan, G.C.; Concepción, G.P.; Harper, M.K.; Ireland, C.M. Cytotoxic Bromoindole Derivatives and Terpenes from the Philippine Marine Sponge *Smenospongia* Sp. *Z. Naturforsch. C* **2002**, *57*, 914–922. [CrossRef]
284. Cimino, G.; De Stefano, S.; Minale, L. Polyprenyl Derivatives from the Sponge *Ircinia spinosula*: 2-Polyprenylbenzoquinones, 2-Polyprenylbenzoquinols, Prenylated Furans and a C-31 Difuranoterpene. *Tetrahedron* **1972**, *28*, 1315–1324. [CrossRef]
285. McPhail, K.; Davies-Coleman, M.T.; Coetzee, P. A New Furanosesterterpene from the South African Nudibranch *Hypselodoris capensis* and a Dictyoceratida Sponge. *J. Nat. Prod.* **1998**, *61*, 961–964. [CrossRef] [PubMed]
286. Erdoğan, I.; Şener, B. Two Metabolites from Tbe Marine Sponge *Spongia officinalis* L. *Acta Pharm. Turc.* **2001**, *43*, 17–19.
287. Prawat, H.; Mahidol, C.; Kaweetripob, W.; Wittayalai, S.; Ruchirawat, S. Iodo–Sesquiterpene Hydroquinone and Brominated Indole Alkaloids from the Thai Sponge *Smenospongia* Sp. *Tetrahedron* **2012**, *68*, 6881–6886. [CrossRef]
288. Arai, M.; Kawachi, T.; Setiawan, A.; Kobayashi, M. Hypoxia-Selective Growth Inhibition of Cancer Cells by Furospinosulin-1, a Furanosesterterpene Isolated from an Indonesian Marine Sponge. *ChemMedChem* **2010**, *5*, 1919–1926. [CrossRef] [PubMed]
289. Arai, M.; Kawachi, T.; Kotoku, N.; Nakata, C.; Kamada, H.; Tsunoda, S.; Tsutsumi, Y.; Endo, H.; Inoue, M.; Sato, H.; et al. Furospinosulin-1, Marine Spongean Furanosesterterpene, Suppresses the Growth of Hypoxia-Adapted Cancer Cells by Binding to Transcriptional Regulators P54(Nrb) and LEDGF/P75. *ChemBioChem* **2016**, *17*, 181–189. [CrossRef] [PubMed]
290. Kashman, Y.; Zviely, M. Furospongolide, a New C21 Furanoterpene from a Marine Organism. *Experientia* **1980**, *36*, 1279. [CrossRef]
291. Liu, Y.; Liu, R.; Mao, S.-C.; Morgan, J.B.; Jekabsons, M.B.; Zhou, Y.-D.; Nagle, D.G. Molecular-Targeted Antitumor Agents. 19. Furospongolide from a Marine *Lendenfeldia* Sp. Sponge Inhibits Hypoxia-Inducible Factor-1 Activation in Breast Tumor Cells. *J. Nat. Prod.* **2008**, *71*, 1854–1860. [CrossRef]
292. Manzo, E.; Ciavatta, M.L.; Villani, G.; Varcamonti, M.; Sayem, S.M.A.; van Soest, R.; Gavagnin, M. Bioactive Terpenes from Spongia Officinalis. *J. Nat. Prod.* **2011**, *74*, 1241–1247. [CrossRef]
293. Li, J.; Du, L.; Kelly, M.; Zhou, Y.-D.; Nagle, D.G. Structures and Potential Antitumor Activity of Sesterterpenes from the Marine Sponge *Hyrtios communis*. *J. Nat. Prod.* **2013**, *76*, 1492–1497. [CrossRef]
294. Albizati, K.F.; Holman, T.; Faulkner, D.J.; Glaser, K.B.; Jacobs, R.S. Luffariellolide, an Anti-Inflammatory Sesterterpene from the Marine Sponge *Luffariella* Sp. *Experientia* **1987**, *43*, 949–950. [CrossRef]
295. Tasdemir, D.; Concepción, G.P.; Mangalindan, G.C.; Harper, M.K.; Hajdu, E.; Ireland, C.M. New Terpenoids from a *Cacospongia* Sp. from the Philippines. *Tetrahedron* **2000**, *56*, 9025–9030. [CrossRef]

296. Elkhayat, E.; Edrada, R.; Ebel, R.; Wray, V.; van Soest, R.; Wiryowidagdo, S.; Mohamed, M.H.; Müller, W.E.G.; Proksch, P. New Luffariellolide Derivatives from the Indonesian Sponge *Acanthodendrilla* Sp. *J. Nat. Prod.* **2004**, *67*, 1809–1817. [CrossRef] [PubMed]
297. Cao, S.; Foster, C.; Lazo, J.S.; Kingston, D.G.I. Sesterterpenoids and an Alkaloid from a *Thorectandra* Sp. as Inhibitors of the Phosphatase Cdc25B. *Bioorg. Med. Chem.* **2005**, *13*, 5094–5098. [CrossRef]
298. Blanchard, J.L.; Epstein, D.M.; Boisclair, M.D.; Rudolph, J.; Pal, K. Dysidiolide and Related γ-Hydroxy Butenolide Compounds as Inhibitors of the Protein Tyrosine Phosphatase, CDC25. *Bioorg. Med. Chem. Lett.* **1999**, *9*, 2537–2538. [CrossRef] [PubMed]
299. Wang, S.; Wang, Z.; Lin, S.; Zheng, W.; Wang, R.; Jin, S.; Chen, J.; Jin, L.; Li, Y. Revealing a Natural Marine Product as a Novel Agonist for Retinoic Acid Receptors with a Unique Binding Mode and Inhibitory Effects on Cancer Cells. *Biochem. J.* **2012**, *446*, 79–87. [CrossRef] [PubMed]
300. Minamida, Y.; Matsuura, H.; Ishii, T.; Miyagi, M.; Shinjo, Y.; Sato, K.; Kamada, T.; Mihara, Y.; Togashi, I.; Sugimoto, K.; et al. New Acetogenin Katsuurallene from Laurencia Saitoi Collected from Katsuura, Japan. *Nat. Prod. Bioprospect.* **2022**, *12*, 10. [CrossRef] [PubMed]
301. Lorenzo-Morales, J.; Díaz-Marrero, A.R.; Cen-Pacheco, F.; Sifaoui, I.; Reyes-Batlle, M.; Souto, M.L.; Daranas, A.H.; Piñero, J.E.; Fernández, J.J. Evaluation of Oxasqualenoids from the Red Alga *Laurencia viridis* against *Acanthamoeba*. *Mar. Drugs* **2019**, *17*, 420. [CrossRef]
302. Koutsaviti, A.; Daskalaki, M.G.; Agusti, S.; Kampranis, S.C.; Tsatsanis, C.; Duarte, C.M.; Roussis, V.; Ioannou, E. Thuwalallenes A–E and Thuwalenynes A–C: New C_{15} Acetogenins with Anti-Inflammatory Activity from a Saudi Arabian Red Sea *Laurencia* Sp. *Mar. Drugs* **2019**, *17*, 644. [CrossRef] [PubMed]
303. Li, X.-D.; Miao, F.-P.; Li, K.; Ji, N.-Y. Sesquiterpenes and Acetogenins from the Marine Red Alga *Laurencia okamurai*. *Fitoterapia* **2012**, *83*, 518–522. [CrossRef]
304. Ji, N.-Y.; Li, X.-M.; Xie, H.; Ding, J.; Li, K.; Ding, L.-P.; Wang, B.-G. Highly Oxygenated Triterpenoids from the Marine Red Alga *Laurencia mariannensis* (Rhodomelaceae). *Helv. Chim. Acta* **2008**, *91*, 1940–1946. [CrossRef]
305. Blunt, J.W.; Hartshorn, M.P.; McLennan, T.J.; Munro, M.H.G.; Robinson, W.T.; Yorke, S.C. Thyrsiferol: A Squalene-Derived Metabolite of Laurencia Thyrsifera. *Tetrahedron Lett.* **1978**, *19*, 69–72. [CrossRef]
306. Mahdi, F.; Falkenberg, M.; Ioannou, E.; Roussis, V.; Zhou, Y.D.; Nagle, D.G. Thyrsiferol Inhibits Mitochondrial Respiration and HIF-1 Activation. *Phytochem. Lett.* **2011**, *4*, 75–78. [CrossRef]
307. Rudi, A.; Goldberg, I.; Stein, Z.; Benayahu, Y.; Schleyer, M.; Kashman, Y. Sodwanones A-C, Three New Triterpenoids from a Marine Sponge. *Tetrahedron Lett.* **1993**, *34*, 3943–3944. [CrossRef]
308. Rudi, A.; Kashman, Y.; Benayahu, Y.; Schleyer, M. Sodwanones A-F, New Triterpenoids from the Marine Sponge *Axinella weltneri*. *J. Nat. Prod.* **1994**, *57*, 1416–1423. [CrossRef]
309. Rudi, A.; Goldberg, I.; Stein, Z.; Kashman, Y.; Benayahu, Y.; Schleyer, M.; Garcia Gravalos, M.D. Sodwanones G, H, and I, New Cytotoxic Triterpenes from a Marine Sponge. *J. Nat. Prod.* **1995**, *58*, 1702–1712. [CrossRef]
310. Rudi, A.; Aknin, M.; Gaydou, E.M.; Kashman, Y. Sodwanones K, L, and M; New Triterpenes from the Marine Sponge *Axinella weltneri*. *J. Nat. Prod.* **1997**, *60*, 700–703. [CrossRef]
311. Rudi, A.; Yosief, T.; Schleyer, M.; Kashman, Y. Several New Isoprenoids from Two Marine Sponges of the Family Axinellidae. *Tetrahedron* **1999**, *55*, 5555–5566. [CrossRef]
312. Carletti, I.; Long, C.; Funel, C.; Amade, P. Yardenone A and B: New Cytotoxic Triterpenes from the Indian Ocean Sponge *Axinella* Cf. *Bidderi*. *J. Nat. Prod.* **2003**, *66*, 25–29. [CrossRef]
313. Funel, C.; Berrué, F.; Roussakis, C.; Fernandez Rodriguez, R.; Amade, P. New Cytotoxic Steroids from the Indian Ocean Sponge *Axinella* Cf. *Bidderi*. *J. Nat. Prod.* **2004**, *67*, 491–494. [CrossRef]
314. Dai, J.; Fishback, J.A.; Zhou, Y.-D.; Nagle, D.G. Sodwanone and Yardenone Triterpenes from a South African Species of the Marine Sponge *Axinella* Inhibit Hypoxia-Inducible Factor-1 (HIF-1) Activation in Both Breast and Prostate Tumor Cells. *J. Nat. Prod.* **2006**, *69*, 1715–1720. [CrossRef]
315. Rudi, A.; Stein, Z.; Goldberg, I.; Yosief, T.; Kashman, Y.; Schleyer, M. Yardenone and Abudinol Two New Triterpenes from the Marine Sponge *Ptilocaulis spiculifer*. *Tetrahedron Lett.* **1998**, *39*, 1445–1448. [CrossRef]
316. Tabudravu, J.N.; Jaspars, M. Stelliferin Riboside, a Triterpene Monosaccharide Isolated from the Fijian Sponge *Geodia globostellifera*. *J. Nat. Prod.* **2001**, *64*, 813–815. [CrossRef]
317. Liu, W.K.; Ho, J.C.K.; Che, C.T. Apoptotic Activity of Isomalabaricane Triterpenes on Human Promyelocytic Leukemia HL60 Cells. *Cancer Lett.* **2005**, *230*, 102–110. [CrossRef]
318. Wang, R.; Zhang, Q.; Peng, X.; Zhou, C.; Zhong, Y.; Chen, X.; Qiu, Y.; Jin, M.; Gong, M.; Kong, D. Stellettin B Induces G1 Arrest, Apoptosis and Autophagy in Human Non-Small Cell Lung Cancer A549 Cells via Blocking PI3K/Akt/MTOR Pathway. *Sci. Rep.* **2016**, *6*, 27071. [CrossRef]
319. Chen, Y.; Zhou, Q.; Zhang, L.; Zhong, Y.; Fan, G.; Zhang, Z.; Wang, R.; Jin, M.; Qiu, Y.; Kong, D. Stellettin B Induces Apoptosis in Human Chronic Myeloid Leukemia Cells via Targeting PI3K and Stat5. *Oncotarget* **2017**, *8*, 28906–28921. [CrossRef]
320. Tasdemir, D.; Mangalindan, G.C.; Concepción, G.P.; Verbitski, S.M.; Rabindran, S.; Miranda, M.; Greenstein, M.; Hooper, J.N.A.; Harper, M.K.; Ireland, C.M. Bioactive Isomalabaricane Triterpenes from the Marine Sponge *Rhabdastrella globostellata*. *J. Nat. Prod.* **2002**, *65*, 210–214. [CrossRef] [PubMed]

321. Chang, C.H.; Lin, B.J.; Chen, C.H.; Nguyen, N.L.; Hsieh, T.H.; Su, J.H.; Chen, M.C. Stellettin B Induces Cell Death in Bladder Cancer via Activating the Autophagy/DAPK2/Apoptosis Signaling Cascade. *Mar. Drugs* **2023**, *21*, 73. [CrossRef]
322. Tsai, T.C.; Wu, W.T.; Lin, J.J.; Su, J.H.; Wu, Y.J. Stellettin B Isolated from *Stelletta* Sp. Reduces Migration and Invasion of Hepatocellular Carcinoma Cells through Reducing Activation of the MAPKs and FAK/PI3K/AKT/MTOR Signaling Pathways. *Int. J. Cell Biol.* **2022**, *2022*, 4416611. [CrossRef] [PubMed]
323. Li, Y.; Tang, H.; Tian, X.; Lin, H.; Wang, M.; Yao, M. Three New Cytotoxic Isomalabaricane Triterpenes from the Marine Sponge *Stelletta tenuis*. *Fitoterapia* **2015**, *106*, 226–230. [CrossRef] [PubMed]
324. Tang, S.-A.; Zhou, Q.; Guo, W.-Z.; Qiu, Y.; Wang, R.; Jin, M.; Zhang, W.; Li, K.; Yamori, T.; Dan, S.; et al. In Vitro Antitumor Activity of Stellettin B, a Triterpene from Marine Sponge *Jaspis stellifera*, on Human Glioblastoma Cancer SF295 Cells. *Mar. Drugs* **2014**, *12*, 4200–4213. [CrossRef]
325. Cheng, S.Y.; Chen, N.F.; Lin, P.Y.; Su, J.H.; Chen, B.H.; Kuo, H.M.; Sung, C.S.; Sung, P.J.; Wen, Z.H.; Chen, W.F. Anti-Invasion and Antiangiogenic Effects of Stellettin B through Inhibition of the Akt/Girdin Signaling Pathway and VEGF in Glioblastoma Cells. *Cancers* **2019**, *11*, 220. [CrossRef] [PubMed]
326. Kuo, T.J.; Jean, Y.H.; Shih, P.C.; Cheng, S.Y.; Kuo, H.M.; Lee, Y.T.; Lai, Y.C.; Tseng, C.C.; Chen, W.F.; Wen, Z.H. Stellettin B-Induced Oral Cancer Cell Death via Endoplasmic Reticulum Stress–Mitochondrial Apoptotic and Autophagic Signaling Pathway. *Int. J. Mol. Sci.* **2022**, *23*, 8813. [CrossRef]
327. Bukowski, R.; Vaughn, C.; Bottomley, R.; Chen, T. Phase II Study of Anguidine in Gastrointestinal Malignancies: A Southwest Oncology Group Study. *Cancer Treat. Rep.* **1982**, *66*, 381–383. [PubMed]
328. Yap, H.Y.; Murphy, W.K.; DiStefano, A.; Blumenschein, G.R.; Bodey, G.P. Phase II Study of Anguidine in Advanced Breast Cancer. *Cancer Treat. Rep.* **1979**, *63*, 789–791. [PubMed]
329. Dosik, G.M.; Barlogie, B.; Johnston, D.A.; Murphy, W.K.; Drewinko, B. Lethal and Cytokinetic Effects of Anguidine on a Human Colon Cancer Cell Line. *Cancer Res.* **1978**, *38*, 3304–3309. [PubMed]
330. Chang, A.Y.; Kim, K.; Boucher, H.; Bonomi, P.; Stewart, J.A.; Karp, D.D.; Blum, R.H. A Randomized Phase II Trial of Echinomycin, Trimetrexate, and Cisplatin plus Etoposide in Patients with Metastatic Nonsmall Cell Lung Carcinoma: An Eastern Cooperative Oncology Group Study (E1587). *Cancer* **1998**, *82*, 292–300. [CrossRef]
331. Schilsky, R.L.; Faraggi, D.; Korzun, A.; Vogelzang, N.; Ellerton, J.; Wood, W.; Henderson, I.C. Phase II Study of Echinomycin in Patients with Advanced Breast Cancer: A Report of Cancer and Leukemia Group B Protocol 8641. *Investig. New Drugs* **1991**, *9*, 269–272. [CrossRef]
332. Marshall, M.E.; Wolf, M.K.; Crawford, E.D.; Taylor, S.; Blumenstein, B.; Flanigan, R.; Meyers, F.J.; Hynes, H.E.; Barlogie, B.; Eisenberger, M. Phase II Trial of Echinomycin for the Treatment of Advanced Renal Cell Carcinoma. A Southwest Oncology Group Study. *Investig. New Drugs* **1993**, *11*, 207–209. [CrossRef]
333. Bailey, C.M.; Liu, Y.; Peng, G.; Zhang, H.; He, M.; Sun, D.; Zheng, P.; Liu, Y.; Wang, Y. Liposomal Formulation of HIF-1α Inhibitor Echinomycin Eliminates Established Metastases of Triple-Negative Breast Cancer. *Nanomedicine* **2020**, *29*, 102278. [CrossRef]
334. Comas, L.; Polo, E.; Domingo, M.P.; Hernández, Y.; Arias, M.; Esteban, P.; Martínez-Lostao, L.; Pardo, J.; Martínez de la Fuente, J.; Gálvez, E.M. Intracellular Delivery of Biologically-Active Fungal Metabolite Gliotoxin Using Magnetic Nanoparticles. *Materials* **2019**, *12*, 1092. [CrossRef]
335. Manh Hung, L.V.; Song, Y.W.; Cho, S.K. Effects of the Combination of Gliotoxin and Adriamycin on the Adriamycin-Resistant Non-Small-Cell Lung Cancer A549 Cell Line. *Mar. Drugs* **2018**, *16*, 105. [CrossRef]
336. Turbyville, T.J.; Wijeratne, E.M.K.; Liu, M.X.; Burns, A.M.; Seliga, C.J.; Luevano, L.A.; David, C.L.; Faeth, S.H.; Whitesell, L.; Gunatilaka, A.A.L. Search for Hsp90 Inhibitors with Potential Anticancer Activity: Isolation and SAR Studies of Radicicol and Monocillin I from Two Plant-Associated Fungi of the Sonoran Desert. *J. Nat. Prod.* **2006**, *69*, 178–184. [CrossRef] [PubMed]
337. Dethe, D.H.; Sau, S.K. Total Synthesis of (+)-Strongylophorines 2 and 9. *Org. Lett.* **2019**, *21*, 3799–3803. [CrossRef]

marine drugs

Review

Shark IgNAR: The Next Broad Application Antibody in Clinical Diagnoses and Tumor Therapies?

Xiaofeng Jiang [1,2,3,*], Ling Sun [1,2], Chengwu Hu [1,2], Feijian Zheng [3], Zhengbing Lyu [1,2] and Jianzhong Shao [4,*]

1 College of Life Sciences, Zhejiang Sci-Tech University, Hangzhou 310018, China; 202120801057@mails.zstu.edu.cn (L.S.); 202220901018@mails.zstu.edu.cn (C.H.); zhengbingl@zstu.edu.cn (Z.L.)
2 Zhejiang Provincial Key Laboratory of Silkworm Bioreactor and Biomedicine, Zhejiang Sci-Tech University, Hangzhou 310018, China
3 Jiangsu Baiying Biotech Co., Ltd., Taizhou 225300, China; zhengfeijian@biointron.com
4 College of Life Sciences, Zhejiang University, Hangzhou 310058, China
* Correspondence: xfjiang@zstu.edu.cn (X.J.); shaojz@zju.edu.cn (J.S.); Tel.: +86-(571)-86843199 (X.J.); +86-(571)-88206582 (J.S.)

Abstract: Antibodies represent a relatively mature detection means and serve as therapeutic drug carriers in the clinical diagnosis and treatment of cancer—among which monoclonal antibodies (mAbs) currently occupy a dominant position. However, the emergence and development of small-molecule monodomain antibodies are inevitable due to the many limitations of mAbs, such as their large size, complex structure, and sensitivity to extreme temperature, and tumor microenvironments. Thus, since first discovered in Chondroid fish in 1995, IgNAR has become an alternative therapeutic strategy through which to replace monoclonal antibodies, thus entailing that this novel type of immunoglobulin has received wide attention with respect to clinical diagnoses and tumor therapies. The variable new antigen receptor (VNAR) of IgNAR provides an advantage for the development of new antitumor drugs due to its small size, high stability, high affinity, as well as other structural and functional characteristics. In that respect, a better understanding of the unique characteristics and therapeutic potential of IgNAR/VNAR in clinical and anti-tumor treatment is needed. This article reviews the advantages of its unique biochemical conditions and molecular structure for clinical diagnoses and novel anti-tumor drugs. At the same time, the main advantages of the existing conjugated drugs, which are based on single-domain antibodies, are introduced here, thereby providing new ideas and methods for the development of clinical diagnoses and anti-tumor therapies in the future.

Keywords: single-domain antibody; immunodiagnostic; shark; VNAR; antibody–drug conjugate; anti-tumor therapy

1. Preface

Cancer and chronic inflammatory diseases are currently the main indications for antibody therapy; this is due, in part, to the systemic accessibility of the target antigens. To date, the clinically approved therapeutic drug market is still dominated by mAbs of the traditional IgG type, and they continue to show great commercial impact and sustainable market growth [1]. The intrinsic advantages of mAbs include high levels of specificity in terms of a target, reduced off-site toxicity, the efficacy benefits of induced cell death, and a long serum half-life [2,3]. Despite this success, biological limitations and economic barriers remain obstacles to overcome in the many forms of mAb drugs used in clinical diagnoses and tumor therapies [2,4].

Antibody fragments with a smaller molecular weight, which have been shown to have a more uniform distribution than mAbs in tissues, can improve diffusivity and vascular permeability [5]. In diagnostic and therapeutic applications, smaller and more flexible therapeutic antibody formats with exciting therapeutic potential have been considered and developed for optical imaging both in vitro and in vivo [6], viruses [7,8], tumors [9], and other human disease therapies [10].

In 1989, two variable domains of an antibody heavy chain with antigen-binding abilities were screened out from mice by Ward et al. [11]; they were only able to determine the heavy chains and named them single-domain antibodies (sdAbs). An antibody family called the heavy-chain antibodies (HCAbs), which naturally lack light chains, was initially found in the humoral immune system of mammalian camelids in 1993 [12]. Two years later, an immunoglobulin (Ig)-based new antigen receptor (IgNAR) of the same type was also found in cartilaginous fish in 1995 [13]. As a new therapeutic strategy to replace monoclonal antibodies, the major types of naturally occurring single-domain antibodies are, thus far, derived from the antigen-binding variable domain of camelids and sharks, which are referred to as the variable domain of the heavy chain of heavy-chain antibodies (VHHs) and variable new antigen receptors (VNARs), respectively. These both function as two members of the most ancient antigen recognition receptors [14–16].

Structurally, the conventional antibodies (IgG) are mostly heterodimers of 150–160 kDa, with two heavy chains (VHs) and two light chains (VLs) [17]. By contrast, the form of the IgNAR molecule is a heavy-chain dimer, and each heavy chain of IgNAR comprises five constant domains that follow a single variable domain, VNAR. The VNARs of IgNAR are truly smaller, with a molecular mass of ~12 kDa, than the camel-derived monodomain antibody because each carries only two CDRs (CDR1 and CDR3) and a deleted CDR2 region (Figure 1). In addition, VNARs have two additional high-variable loops (hypervariable 2 and hypervariable 4), and their small and simple domain generates four diversity loops [14,18]. Although CDR1 and CDR3 are considered the two major determinants for antigen binding by VNAR domains, other hypervariable regions—such as HV2 and HV4—show an increased frequency of somatic mutations, indicating their potential involvement in antigen recognition [19]. Due to their unique structures and binding modes, shark VNARs may have unique therapeutic potential.

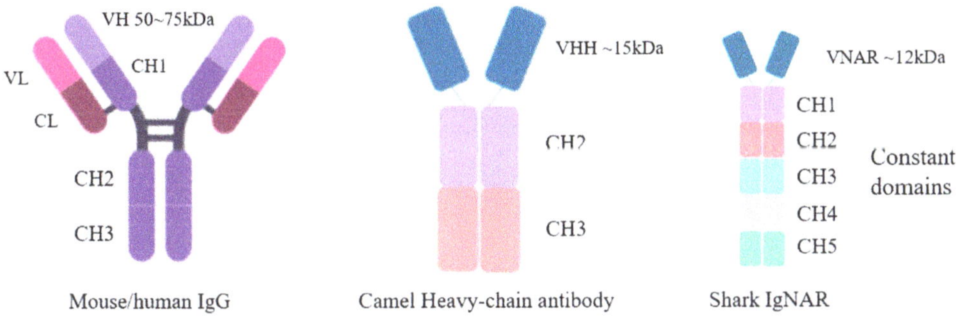

Figure 1. Size and structure of IgG and Ig–like biologics. Schematic representation of molecular models depicting the relative structure and size of different antibodies showing different options for treatment.

2. Structural Characteristics and Advantages of IgNAR

2.1. Limitations of mAbs

Certain limitations in monoclonal antibody treatments have existed in the clinical diagnosis and treatment stages. First, mammalian IgG, as a drug, is unstable and orally unachievable; at the same time, it is often blocked when penetrating solid tumors [20] and crossing the blood–brain barrier (BBB) [21]. Second, due to the size of mAbs, which are approximately 150 kDa, the action site within the human body is limited to the cell surface molecules with minimal tissue penetration, as well as a variety of antigens, including epitopes located in clefts on protein surfaces (e.g., enzyme active sites) that are non-accessible [22,23], thus resulting in poor binding affinity (approximately ten times weaker than VNAR) [19] and low tissue infiltration ability [24]. Finally, the inconvenience, discomfort, and cost of treatment that mAb drug application brings considerably affect the patients. With traditional mAb drug treatments, inconsistent clinical effects exist in different diseases and patients. Moreover, it is ineffective for medium- and advanced-stage cancer patients. In addition, the high cost of treatment is required for producing complex, large globular glycoproteins [2]. In addition, due to the sensitivity of mAbs to temperature and humidity, maintaining their optimal performance is difficult, particularly when the drugs must be used in developing resource-poor countries with insufficient electricity supply [4,25].

In addition to its own limitations, a potential predominance of shark-derived VNAR therapeutic efficacy and response over that of mAbs has been observed in emerging viruses or new acute infectious diseases [7,26]. The COVID-19 pandemic, caused by severe acute respiratory syndrome coronavirus 2 (SARS-CoV-2), has led to a devastating global health crisis. SARS-CoV-2 has rapidly evolved into a highly infectious variant around the world. Researchers have suggested that the novel variants may reduce the sensitivity of SARS-CoV-2 to antibody therapies and vaccines, which would then complicate the development of antibodies [27]. Finding facilities equipped to administer an IV infusion that can manage anaphylaxis while not exposing uninfected patients to SARS-CoV-2 may be difficult [28].

Therefore, due to the limitations of traditional antibodies in clinical applications, developing diagnostic reagents and therapeutic drugs based on new types of antibody molecules is necessary.

2.2. *Advantages of Shark-Derived VNAR*

Newly developed biologics should overcome the inherent limitations of traditional antibodies. Furthermore, they have the ability to quickly cross the tissue barrier while retaining the specificity and affinity of antibodies, making them a meaningful supply for current monoclonal antibody therapies. Meanwhile, the activity of antibody drugs in vivo should be further optimized to increase their efficacy and expand their clinical applications. One of the candidate biological inhibitors with potential is based on the discovery of VNAR, which was found in the antigen-binding variable region of IgNAR in chondroid fish (Table 1). It has multiple natural and downstream attributes, such as small size, high solubility, thermal stability, folding ability, good tissue permeability in vivo, reduced propensity to aggregate, and high target-binding ability. VNARs have become attractive candidates for drug development due to these attributes.

Table 1. Comparison of the advantages and disadvantages of the V region of mAbs, VHHs, and VNARs.

		V Region of mAbs	VHH	VNAR
Structural complexity	Complex post-translational modifications (glycoproteins)	+++	—	—
Molecular weight	Expression in prokaryotic cells	—	+++	+++
	molecular weight (~kDa)	50~75	~15	~12
	Tissue penetration (BBB, ocular model, placental barrier)	—	++	+++
Structural stability	Physiological and biochemical environment (high temperature, pH, urea)	—	+++	+++
Shortcomings	Difficulty of humanization	—	+	+++

In the comparison of strengths and weaknesses, +++ represents the highest degree, + represents a slightly weaker ability, — represents no or less ability.

2.2.1. Structural Characteristics of Shark Monodomain Antibodies

The immunoglobulin neoantigen receptor antibody (IgNAR) from sharks is a heavy-chain protein dimer without associated light chains [29]. The specificity of the molecules is defined by the variable region of IgNAR, and VNAR types are defined in terms of cysteine number, CDR3 length, and amino acid variability. The single-domain natural lack of CDR2 in VNARs heightens the requirement for CDR1 and CDR3 to provide specific and high-affinity binding to prospective antigens [30]. It was observed that the VNAR domain with four antigen-binding coils over a single chain possessed the ability to bind antigens with relatively higher affinity than conventional antibodies containing six loops across two chains [31,32].

In a natural VNAR phage library constructed from six naive nurse sharks [15], the presence of two canonical cysteines located at amino acids 21 and 82 was used as a key criterion for type I-IV VNAR; moreover, the sequences that did not contain one or both cysteines were considered other types (Figure 2). The high variability in CDR3 length and cysteine amount is critical for VNAR diversity because binding diversity is mainly dependent on the CDR3 structures [15]. Different from conventional antibodies, VNAR has a CDR2 region that is replaced by short-chain HV2 [29]. Therefore, to compensate for this condition, sequence diversity is reflected in the CDR3 region. VNARs encode unusually long and structurally complex CDR3s, which display a high degree of variability, to compensate for the reduced size of variable regions in IgNARs [33]. CDR3, which is more variable in terms of sequence, length, and conformation, plays a key role in antigen recognition. It has a maximum of 100+ amino acid residues [34], an unusual topological structure (which can bind relatively hidden epitopes of target antigens, such as pockets or grooves), and the ability to penetrate rapidly [35]. Each VNAR covers less area than standard bivalent antibodies but still maintains precise target specificity. Ubah et al. proved that two amino acid residues from the HV2 region are involved in the association of VNAR with SARS-CoV-2 receptor-binding domains (RBDs) in addition to the binding of the CDR region with the RBD. Their study provided additional evidence for the functional significance of the HV2 domain [27].

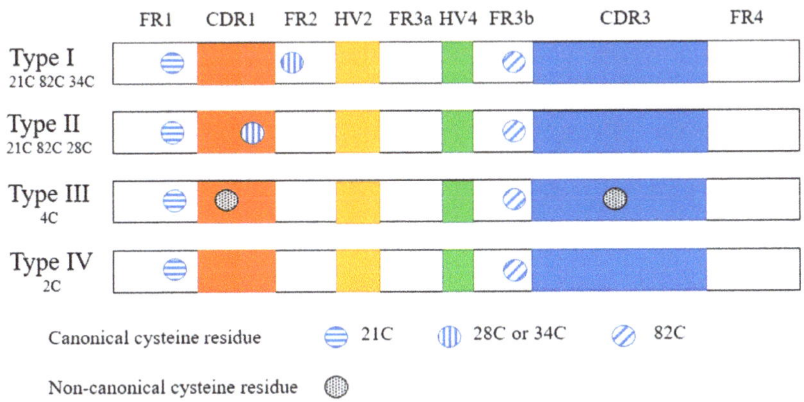

Figure 2. Illustration of VNAR isotypes showing the similarities and differences between different isotypes of VNAR domain. This schematic is based on the specific sequence and classification methods by Feng et al. [15].

2.2.2. Biochemical Characteristics of IgNAR

VNARs have high chemical and thermal stability. Influenced by the critical evolutionary environment, IgNARs are resistant to chemical denaturants that can be more stable than classical antibodies. This option is attractive for drug delivery, diagnostics, and imaging. It is stable in the blood of sharks that contain 350 mmol/L urea and 1000 mOsm/kg osmotic salt ions. It can also maintain great stability at high temperatures in liquid, lyophilized, and immobilized forms for a long time. Katherine et al. exposed recombinant VNARs to mouse gastric scraping (pH = 5) and intestinal samples (proteinase-rich environment) and showed no evident signs of degradation after 1 h of incubation, thus demonstrating the stability of VNARs in extreme pH environments and their ability to resist proteinase hydrolytic cleavage [2,36]. In addition, Dooley et al. incubated VNARs at high temperatures (85–97 °C), and they still maintained binding activity after 3 h [31]. These characteristics provide great conditions for the development and improvement of mAb drugs and the potential of field immunodetection reagents [29,37,38]. Another advantage of sdAbs is the multiple ways in which they can be administrated, given their small size and stable biochemistry. For example, they can be directly entered into the lungs by aerosolization, which is particularly useful in combating respiratory viruses, such as SARS-CoV-2 [39].

2.2.3. IgNAR Can Be Humanized

VNARs are distinct from typical Ig VH and VL domains as well as camelid VHH domains. They share higher structural homology with immunoglobulin VL and T-cell receptor V domains than with immunoglobulin VH [30]. The total area of 25–30% amino acid homology was found between VNARs and the variable region of human antibodies via sequence homolog analysis; the results showed low overall sequence identity [40] (Figure 3). At the same time, shark VNARs were conserved in certain key antigen-specific binding functional domains, thus suggesting that shark VNARs have antigen-binding properties that are similar to mammalian IgGs and VHHs. In addition, shark VNARs have their own unique sequence and structure, which may be different from other types of antibodies. However, based on the existing VNAR crystal data, the structure of VNARs has a high similarity to that of the variable region of human antibodies. Regarding in vivo therapeutic applications, shark VNARs need to be humanized to limit potential immunogenicity [41], as well as to improve thermodynamic stability, folding, and expression properties without reducing their favorable antigen-binding and structural stability characteristics [30,42]. CDR grafting is the most straight-forward and widely used humanization approach: the CDRs of a non-human antibody of interest are grafted onto an appropriate human germline framework, and the binding and functional properties of the original antibody are thus retained.

In 2013, on the basis of screening specific VNARs [32], Kovalenko et al. focused on the VNAR domain of anti-human serum albumin (HSA), which was isolated from immunized sharks and could be humanized by converting over 60% of non-complementarity-determining region residues to a human germline sequence. In addition, within this process, the resulting molecules largely retain their specificity and affinity for the antigen binding of the parental VNAR [30]. In this study, conducting random mutagenesis on the resulting molecules was followed by the refinement of clones through an off-rate ranking-based selection of target antigens. After analysis, VNAR—which was selected in the aforementioned method—exhibited negligible antigenicity, high stability, and high affinity, which may meet clinical requirements [42]. Zhang et al. showed VNAR CDRs based on an analysis of currently available VNAR antigen structure complexes in the global Protein Data Bank archive of 3D structure data. They described a detailed protocol through which to humanize VNARs via CDR grafting [43]. Fischer et al. concluded that a structural and dynamic understanding of the VNAR binding site upon humanization is a key aspect of antibody humanization [44]. Based on existing research, the humanized transformation of VNAR can be realized via frame transplantation without losing functions. Meanwhile, Martin et al. proposed that, in this area, further work for VNAR humanization is needed to maximize human sequence content while avoiding a loss of binding affinity and/or immunogenicity that would result from aggregation or decreased stability [45].

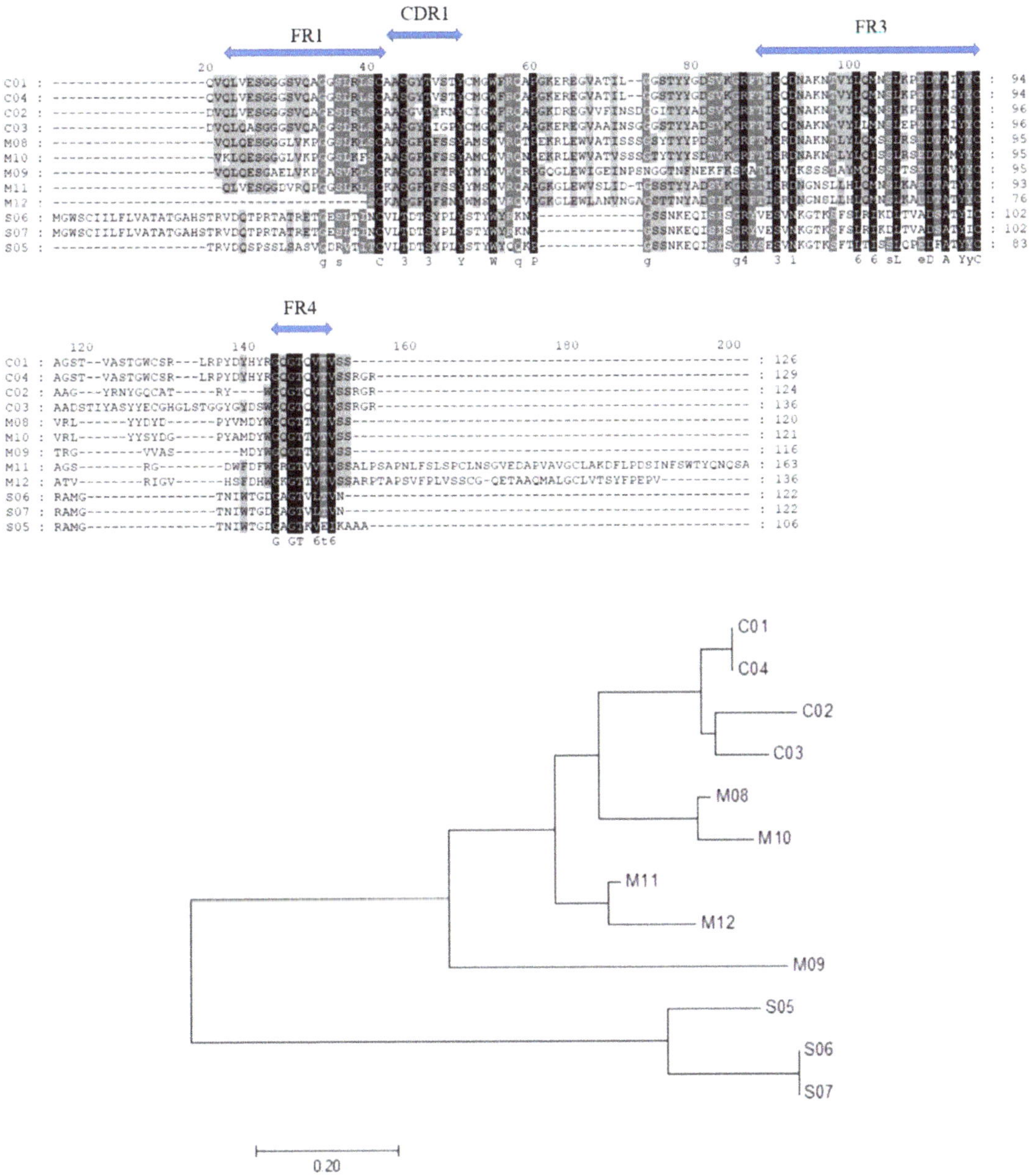

Figure 3. Sequence comparisons of heavy chains of antibodies from different species are shown, including the analysis of phylogenetic tree. C01–C04 stand for Camelidae VHHs, S05–S07 for shark VNARs, and M08–M12 for mice and other mammals' IgG heavy-chain antibodies.

2.3. Preparation and Mass Production of Specific VNARs

2.3.1. Use of Chiloscyllium plagiosum as a Model Organism for VNAR Preparation

Early studies on sdAbs mainly focused on camelids because raising camelids is easier than raising sharks [46,47]. Contrary to mammals, the immune cycle in sharks is usually long [48]. Fewer than 10 shark species are currently being studied for the development of

VNAR-immunized libraries, such as the nurse shark (*Ginglymostoma cirratum*) [7], wobbegong shark (*Orectolobus ornatus*) [49], and horn shark (*Heterodontus francisci*) [50], etc., with nurse sharks being the most common.

However, the generation of VNARs is hindered by the high cost and cumbersome care process of large shark breeding. They are difficult to maintain in captivity because of their endangered state, large body size, slow maturity, aggressive temper, and fast movement. In addition, certain cartilaginous fish fail to produce antigen-specific IgNARs, such as the small spotted catshark [51]. Compared with these options, *Chiloscyllium plagiosum* (white-spotted bamboo shark) is an attractive alternative ideal model to study and obtain antigen-specific VNARs through immunization as it has stable VNAR production, easy breeding conditions, as well as better maneuverability and repeatability of antigen immunization.

Bamboo shark is a small, demersal species that seldom bites, has a strong body shape, and matures quickly [52]. It can be fed with an artificial diet, and it is easy to keep [35] and immunize in a laboratory environment [53]. Found in their genome, transcriptome, and plasma, bamboo sharks are the first shark species whose chromosomes are the complete configuration of all IgNAR family structures [35]. The recent discovery of shear forms in bamboo sharks has broadened the understanding of IgNAR properties [29], and their genome has revealed chromosomal rearrangements and the presence of rapidly evolving immune genes in cartilaginous fishes [54]. The presence of strong and rapid IgNAR recall was also observed when undergoing a response following a re-encounter with antigens. Many biological explorations on bamboo sharks, which serve as a promising small animal model for high-affinity sdAb generation, have been conducted [26,35,55–57].

2.3.2. Phage Library Screening of Specific VNARs

The production of sdAbs is important for the detection and identification of potential candidate proteins for further drug studies [15,39]. In recent years, it has been demonstrated that sdAbs are highly amendable to a variety of modifications without losing their structural integrity; in addition, they are compatible with a variety of high-throughput screening platforms such as yeast [58], phage [27], bacteria [59], and ribosome displays [60,61]—with the phage display being the most established one because of its large storage capacity, simple operation, and the ability to be manipulated at the gene level. Meanwhile, besides the employment of phage libraries derived from immunized specimens, naïve [15,62] and synthetic libraries [63–65] have been explored as additional, less time-consuming options. It needs to be emphasized that IgNARs have experienced iterative affinity maturation in immunized sharks upon immunization [18]; therefore, VNARs from immunized libraries generally have higher affinities and specificities than those from semi-synthetic libraries and naïve libraries.

Currently, the most popular and broadest approach through which to isolate target antigens for shark VNAR is through phage display (Figure 4). Using this technology, the gene encoding the antibody binding domain is fused with the phage coat protein gene to display the antibody on the phage surface for the selection of antigen recognition binding proteins [66]. Existing phages are built from stock in two forms. First, after repeated immune processes, simple blood samples are collected from animals to enhance and extract RNA, and then the VNAR sequence is amplified from the cDNA generated from the total information [67]. Antibodies with strong specificity and high affinity for immune antigens can usually be obtained with this method. Second, natural or semi-synthetic phage display libraries are constructed based on the VNAR domain produced by natural animals, and these usually contain additional diversity in the CDR region [68–71]. Feng et al. [15], based on EASeL technology, extracted RNA from six nurse sharks to construct a phage display natural library with a library capacity of up to 1.2×10^{10}, from which antibodies with high affinity and those with a specific recognition of tumor treatment-related antigens and viruses could be obtained.

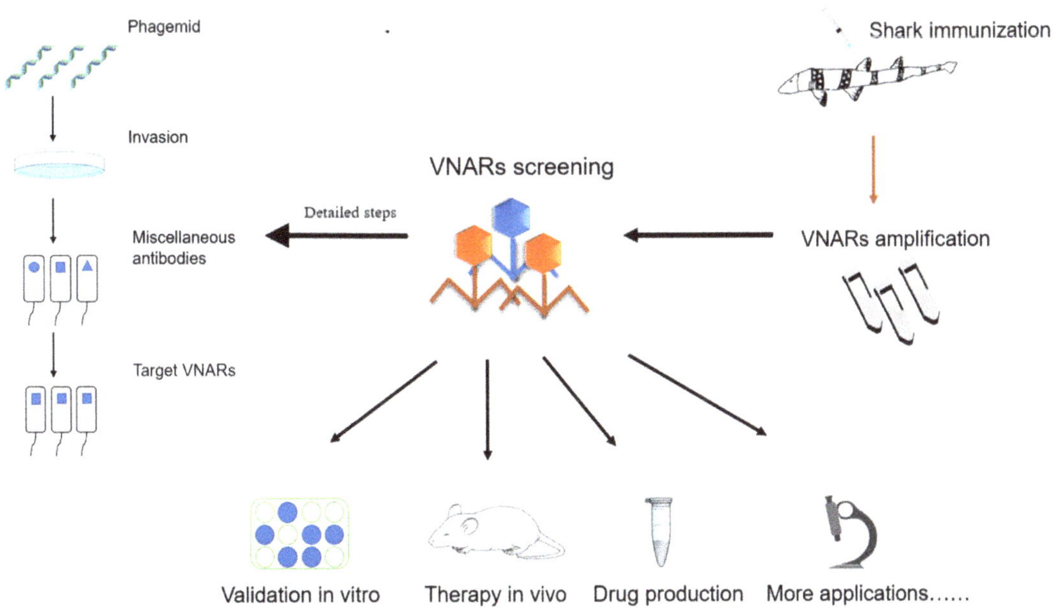

Figure 4. VNAR production using a phage display library. Specific antigens were used to immunize sharks and induce an immune response for approximately three to six months. After which, the screened VNAR sequences were cloned into phage vectors for phage antibody display, and phage libraries were made. The antibodies identified after screening can be used to assess their potency in vitro and in vivo.

2.3.3. Recombinant VNAR Production

Duan et al. [72] transformed phages containing antibody sequences into expressing the HV2151 strain instead. In addition, they obtained large amounts of VNAR from the bacterial liquid lysate via purification in order to compare how to obtain sdAbs with high yield, quality, and purity. At the same time, they attempted to produce sdAbs using the mammalian cell line Expi293F. The advantage of mammalian cell expression is that it allows posttranslational modifications, especially glycosylation. However, monodomain antibodies do not require post-translational modification, and recombinant VNAR is highly soluble [73] and stable because hydrophilic residues are present on its surface. It also lacks glycosylation modification, which is easy to clone and express in bacteria [38], and it does not cost much compared with the production of traditional monoclonal antibodies [74]. Experiments have proven that the small-scale and large-scale production of recombinant monodomain antibodies have excellent biological functions [72]. Thus, the bacterial expression system is suitable for the production of large quantities of recombinant monodomain antibodies [75]. Experiments have proven that the yield of shark VNARs in Escherichia coli ranges from 2 mg/L to 15 mg/L [72] and that such a low cost can bring considerable economic benefits.

3. Potential Applications of VNAR in Preclinical Test

Intact mAbs dominate clinically approved therapeutic drugs. However, due to the inherent characteristics that limit the development of these antibodies, antibody fragments that are smaller and easier to permeate tissues have been developed for in vivo imaging and clinical treatments [2]. In terms of drug targeting, based on their ability to interact with demanding epitopes such as receptor domains, sdAbs have gradually become promising candidates for biomedical applications [76], many of which have been proven successful in early-stage clinical trials [60,77–79]. The drug delivery system, given the unique properties of sdAbs (Table 2), can maximize the delivery of drugs to the necessary sites and minimize off-target toxicity. VNARs have been modified and adapted to satisfy the requirements of drug discovery and development. Through this, a number of important additional attributes have been demonstrated, thereby leading to the belief that it will also become a valuable platform for multiple medical treatments [2].

Table 2. The first marketed single-domain VHH-based antibody drugs and current VNAR-based drugs in development.

Drug	Application	Source	Clinical Trial Phase	Ref.
Caplacizumab	aTTP	VHH	2019 FDA-approved	[76]
AD214	Idiopathic pulmonary fibrosis	VNAR	Phase I	[77]
TXB4	Primary central nervous system Lymphoma	VNAR	Preclinical	[78]

3.1. Advantages in Drug Development and Clinical Treatment

When combined with traditional antibodies, VNARs have high affinity and clearly high tissue penetration. Based on its unique structure, the potential of VNAR technology as a powerful "engine" for novel drug discovery is evident. The small size and unique topology of shark VNARs provide an opportunity through which to penetrate tissues and bind to novel and hidden targets that are difficult to access through the larger spherical binding domains that are currently available. VNARs demonstrate a surprising ability for specific and high-affinity binding to diverse antigens by using just two variable domains per molecule. VNARs have evident advantages in developing highly specific and effective drugs against specific targets given their ability and versatility [80]; they also provide a new idea for the development of bis-specificity antibodies because VNARs can be easily fused [81].

Rapid distribution and elimination are desirable features of disease-specific biologics [82]; as such, the small size of VNARs provides extensive applicability for in vivo diagnostic imaging. Therefore, their excellent molecular characteristics make VNAR a potential substitute for the defects of traditional antibody drugs, thus allowing them to become a highly effective new targeted therapy agent. The screening of semi-synthetic [83] and CDR3-randomized VNAR libraries allows for the rapid and convenient identification of anti-idiotypic VNAR domains against monoclonal antibodies. The resulting VNAR variant does not cross-react with unrelated antibodies and was able to maintain its excellent target recognition in human and mouse sera. Molecular engineering and phage display technologies could be potentially used in molecular imaging, drug delivery, and the treatment of several major diseases [84].

Due to the large number of recombinant VNAR proteins that can be expressed in prokaryotes and the low cost of preparation, although there are still many challenges for the development of VNAR-based drugs, such as the need for humanization of the sequence and the short half-life of the vector, the price is much lower than that of traditional antibody drugs, and this serves as the basis for their widespread use. Increasing numbers of next-generation antibodies and novel scaffolds have been introduced into the research of biotechnology and biopharmaceutical companies to overcome the limitations of traditional antibodies, as well as provide additional opportunities for new disease-targeting and alternative drug delivery methods.

The advantages of VNARs, such as their stable quality, low production cost, easy storage, and long half-life, are beneficial to the efficacy of their clinical applications. Ongoing preclinical developments, such as immunoassay [85], medical imaging [86], in vitro diagnosis [87], and disease treatment [88], will help define the utility of shark VNARs as a novel family of drug candidates for treating cancer and other human diseases [14].

3.2. Exploration and Development of VNAR-Based New Drugs

VNARs may be an effective neutralizing agent against mutated virus strains based on their ability to bind highly variable influenza viruses (which cause great immunogenicity). In 2021, Gauhar et al. [89] reported the identification of neutralizing single-domain VNAR antibodies that were selected against the severe acute respiratory syndrome coronavirus 2 spike protein (which was derived from the Wuhan variant with the phage display approach). And then, Obinna et al. [27] and Valdocino et al. [90] compared the binding of VNARs that were selected from phage libraries and mutant virus strains. It was shown that the mutation of the virus had been proven to barely affect the affinity of VNARs. A crystallographic analysis of VNARs found that they recognized separate epitopes on the RBD and had distinctly different mechanisms of virus neutralization—ones that were unique to VNARs. VNARs were reported as showing picomolar affinity binding and a wide range of neutralizing activity toward the receptor binding domain (RBD) of SARS-CoV-2 variants [91]. In addition, they can be isolated from the SARS-CoV-2 RBD-immunized *Chiloscyllium plagiosum* [26] due to their ability to cope with evolving and evading COVID-19 [7]. The intranasal administration of VNARs can effectively protect mice from the challenges of SARS-CoV-2, as demonstrated by their advantages of small size and high bioavailability [91]. These results showed that VNARs offer unique binding capabilities to the RBD protein, especially in regions that are not readily susceptible to conventional mAbs. Thus, they should be a useful adjunct to existing antibody approaches in terms of treating COVID-19 as detectors and in therapeutics. Broadly speaking, these findings also suggest the potential druggability and assay reagent iteration of VNARs, which would provide these molecules with the potential for extensive use in human diseases.

Currently, three companies in the world are engaged in the research and development of shark antibody drugs: Ossianix, Elasmogen, and AdAlta. Only Ad-214 from AdAlta has been used in clinical practice thus far [92]. Ad-214 is an i-body developed by AdAlta that specifically binds to CXR4. Meanwhile, Ad-314 is fused with human Fc for the treatment of idiopathic pulmonary fibrosis. A phase I intravenous administration safety study has been successfully completed. At the same time, AdAlta is working on developing Ad-214 inhalable preparations so as to improve the bioavailability of the drug, improve patient convenience, and reduce the cost. Non-immunoglobulin VNARs were fused with anti-hTNF-α biologics (Quad-X™ and D1-NDure™-C4) to determine the effect of anti-drug antibodies (ADAs) on preclinical in vivo efficacy [75], and the promising applications of VNARs in the biomedical industry were also indicated.

3.3. Application of VNAR as an Enzyme Inhibitor

When antibodies are used as enzyme inhibitors, they can inhibit enzyme activity by changing the conformation of the active site(s) or directly binding to the active site(s) of the enzyme [93]. Burgess et al. [94] identified a VNAR that specifically recognized Aurora-A kinase by constructing a VNAR semi-synthetic library, and proved, via crystal structure analysis, that the VNAR could destroy the salt bridge, change the conformation, and inactivate the enzyme. The goal of replicating the precise targeting specificity of the antibodies and increasing added value through differential qualities, such as small size, has been the core aim in the development and progress of several alternative drugs in recent years.

3.4. VNARs Can Penetrate Tissues and Deliver Drugs across the Blood–Brain Barrier

A well-defined high tissue penetration was verified in VNAR treatment. Drug delivery across the BBB remains an important barrier for the development of biopharmaceuticals with therapeutic effects on the central nervous system. On the basis of the small size of VNARs and their extended CDR3 loop, Pawel et al. [95] screened the synthetic VNAR phage display library for antibodies that can penetrate the brain parenchyma of mice and can be specifically taken into TfR1-positive neurons to address issues such as retention when using TfR1 receptor antibodies to cross the BBB. In subsequent assays [96], they demonstrated that the TfR1-targeting VNAR shuttle protein could be fused with the agonist antibodies, as well as be effectively transported to the BBB and delivered into the brain parenchyma at physiologically relevant concentrations. In addition, systemic treatments with VNARs can prevent neuronal loss. The experimental results proved that VNARs can rapidly cross the BBB with excellent pharmacokinetics and safety and that they can adapt to carry various biological therapeutic drugs from blood to brain at any time, thus making them the first of the next generation of brain-penetrating agonist antibodies with therapeutic potential in a wide range of brain diseases.

Given the special structure of the corneas, Kocaleva et al. [97] administered the drug to the mouse model of corneal scratches via dropping; they proved that VNARs have the ability to penetrate the cornea and overcome the drawbacks of traditional antibodies, such as the fact that they could only be administered via vitreous injection, accompanied by infection and retinal detachment. Camacho et al. [98] also proved that VNARs penetraurface abrasion or discomfort and that they may become a new drug candidate for the treatment of vascular ophthalmopathy. These findings suggested that VNARs have good adaptability and penetration to host tissues.

The success of these applications showed that VNARs are druggable after perfect design and adjustment and that they satisfy the requirements of drug discovery and development, thus ensuring that VNARs could become a valuable platform for various medical treatments.

4. Applications in Anti-Tumor Preclinical Studies

Antibody drugs are mostly used in the treatment of cancers, autoimmune diseases, as well as infectious diseases, cardiovascular diseases, and organ transplant rejection. Antibody drugs are widely used in clinical treatment as targeted drugs; in addition, they account for a large proportion of the new FDA-approved drugs. Cancers and chronic inflammatory diseases are currently the main indications for antibody therapy, and this is in part due to the systemic accessibility of the target antigens [2]. As an emerging tumor treatment in recent years, immune antibody therapy can improve the ability of the immune system to recognize antigens on the tumor surface by changing the expression of immune regulatory factors in the tumor microenvironment [99,100].

The main limitation to the wide clinical use of ADCs is their non-uniform distribution in solid tumors. Another major factor affecting the efficacy of ADCs is the heterogeneity of their intratumoral distribution [101]. In addition to the complicated and harsh tumor microenvironment [102], massive neovascularization [103], variable antigen expression [104], and low clearance rate [105], the physicochemical characteristics of monoclonal antibodies—such as their large size and high binding affinity—slow down the penetration of these drugs into tumors [106,107]. Improving the intratumoral distribution of ADCs is critical to increasing their in vivo efficacy [108]. Early diagnosis is particularly important for the timely detection and treatment of diseases, especially for serious diseases such as tumors. The utilization of VNARs against various tumor markers has also been successfully developed to date (Figure 5).

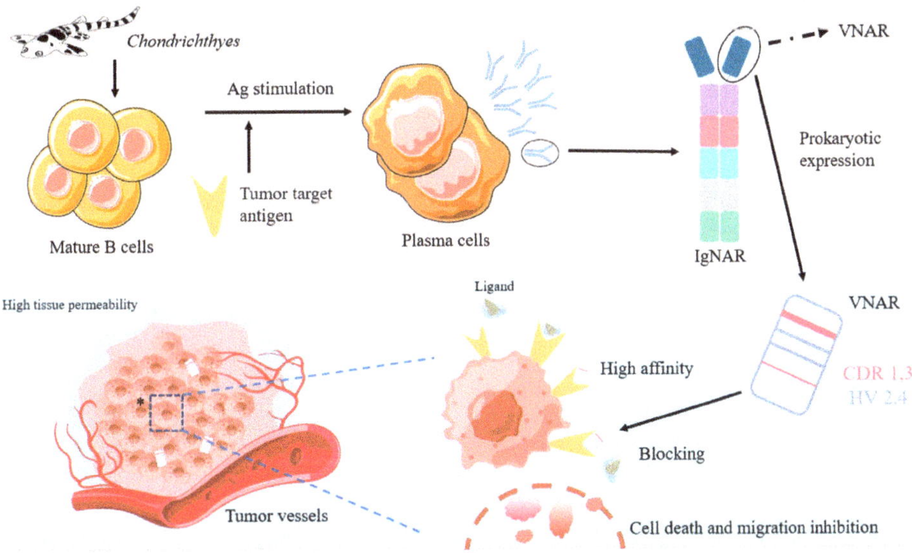

Figure 5. The production of IgNAR and its advantages and applications in the treatment of solid tumors.

4.1. VNARs Have Stronger Affinity to Cancer-Specific Targeting Antigens

Torchia et al. [83] chemically synthesized a small peptide through phage display library screening and then attached it to the amino terminus of a pre-prepared IgG Fc protein. They identified a small peptide with an affinity for a unique tumor type and demonstrated its ability to kill tumor cells specifically and trigger macrophages to phagocytose tumor cells. The effective clearance of human lymphoma in a mouse xenograft model demonstrated that this approach can be used to personalize and precisely target tumors. On this basis, Arturo et al. [65] screened VNAR libraries that were displayed by yeast through fluorescence-activated cell sorting (FACS) so as to enrich antigen-bound VNARs against the BCRS of different lymphoma cell lines. Five VNARs were expressed as Fc fusion proteins and revealed binding constants in the low one-digit nanomolar range.

Meanwhile, a proof-of-concept study based on the generation of VNAR antibody–drug conjugates has been reported. The high specificity of VNAR antibodies provides a therapeutic window for the eradication of lymphoma B cells, and future experiments may result in VNAR-Fc antibody formats with a higher binding valence. Treatment with VNARs has many advantages over monoclonal antibodies [60]. VNARs have a much smaller molecular weight than monoclonal antibodies, and this may allow greater tissue permeability. A molecule in the form of a polypeptide body can carry more than two antigen-binding domains, thus resulting in a higher affinity for the target.

4.2. Strong and Rapid Tissue Permeability

As potential chemotherapeutic agents, sdAds may passively target and penetrate tumor tissue with their excellent permeability, all the while their clearance by the lymphatic system is reduced. Adam et al. [109] proposed a new concept in the nanoparticle targeting of sdAds, i.e., anti-DLL4 VNARs were specifically conjugated with a target in DLL4 and used as a new treatment for pancreatic cancer. The studies demonstrated that VNARs can specifically bind to DLL4 with high affinity and are preferentially internalized by pancreatic cancer cell lines and endothelial cells that express DLL4. In addition, anti-DLL4 VNARs have significant anti-angiogenic effects. Arturo et al. [65] screened a yeast library for soluble anti-idiotypic VNAR targeting lymphoma cells and generated VNAR antibody–

drug conjugates that induced lymphoma cell-specific killing at low concentrations of ~20 pM to 1 μM without significant cytotoxicity—even at higher three-digit nanomolar concentrations.

4.3. The Next-Generation Antibody for Anti-Tumor Applications

In 2017, Ubah et al. [110] immunized nurse sharks and screened anti-rhTNF-α (a recombinant homo tumor necrosis factor) sdAbs via phage display technology. An in vitro assay confirmed that the candidate VNAR obtained was as effective as adalimumab in the treatment of intestinal epithelial barrier dysfunction. In the follow-up animal experiments in 2019, the mouse arthritis model (Tg197) even indicated that VNARs are more superior to IgG in their in vivo binding capacity [111]. In 2022, Zhao et al. [53] identified 15 specific mouse TNF VNARs from a phage display VNAR library after immunizing a bamboo shark. Their findings indicated that VNARs showing affinity to mTNF-α were successfully enriched and identified by iterative biological screening. These results showed that VNARs can fulfill the requirements for next-generation antibody drugs in clinical tumor treatment.

Favorable therapeutic effects have been achieved in hematological malignancies since the introduction of chimeric antigen receptor (CAR) T cell therapy in this field. However, solid tumors remain a challenge due to the lack of appropriate antigen targets and immunosuppressive tumor microenvironments.

VNARs can overcome the disadvantages of traditional IgG drugs and effectively penetrate solid tumors with the help of their small size and high antigen-binding affinity. The PD-L1 immune pathway is crucial for tumor cells to escape from immune surveillance in the human body. Broos [112] stated, in their publication in 2019, that the antigen-binding component of this pathway should be further developed. Hpd-l1-binding sdAbs were prepared and injected intravenously in mice, and results confirmed that this antibody was able to block PD-1/PD-L1, enhance the T cell receptor signaling pathway, and kill tumor cells. Subsequently, bivalent and trivalent sdAbs were constructed using a glycine-serine linker, and their activities were 313 and 135 times those of a monovalent single-domain antibody, respectively. In addition, an attempt was made to link the identified high-affinity sdAbs fragment to the human IgG Fc fragment, and this modified Fc domain was found to effectively enhance the anti-tumor effect [113].

Dan Li et al. [20] constructed a semi-synthetic VNAR phage library and identified anti-PD-L1 sdAbs. These antibodies showed cross-reactivity with human, mouse, and dog PD-L1s, as well as partially blocking the interaction between human PD-1 and PD-L1. Through this process, to a certain extent, the prevention of tumor metastasis and the induction of tumor regression were achieved.

5. Conclusions

The progress of research into sdAbs as valuable drug conjugates is summarized in this review. The structural characteristics and potential applications in clinical tests, as well as the anti-tumor drugs, were highlighted to reveal the value of sdAbs as biomedical reagents. Biological agents predominate the market for therapeutic drugs, and innovation drives the development of the next generation of medical products. The development of therapeutic antibodies has focused on smaller, more stable, and more flexible products to improve the efficacy of the drugs and expand their clinical use. The structure of shark sdAbs brings about specific functions for these molecules, including a small size, excellent thermal stability, penetration into tumor epitopes, and a low production cost. These advantages will hopefully lead to the development of highly specific, stable, and effective drugs in the future [114]. These characteristics will enable sdAbs to become the focus of various clinical uses.

Shark-derived sdAbs and their conjugates can still be improved in terms of their stability, expression level, protease resistance, and the aggregation caused by synthetic linkers. Small-size proteins are usually associated with short serum half-lives. Generally, any molecules smaller than the threshold for glomerular filtration (approximately 60 kDa) will be rapidly eliminated from the body. Fusion to the Fc domain can solve this problem. However, if a small size is advantageous, then the addition of several extra domains (i.e., Fc) would counteract the advantage of a small size. Although a large number of preclinical studies on shark-derived sdAbs have been conducted, their progress into clinical use has been slow. Considering the great evolutionary distance between cartilaginous fishes and humans, potential immunogenicity should be considered prior to clinical application. However, the feasibility of humanizing VNAR domains to prevent xenoreactivity has been demonstrated in previous studies [2]. Although Fc fragments lack the ability to mediate the ADCC effect and to guide immune cells to clean the targeted tumor cells, VNAR structural characteristics and their high affinity for target antigens make it possible for them to be used as effective antigen-binding therapeutic drugs.

This study also indicated that bamboo shark, as a model organism for the preparation of high-affinity VNARs, may contribute to paving the path for VNAR application as a clinical drug candidate. However, in the process of IgNAR preparation, identifying methods to dynamically monitor IgNARs in sharks for observation and recording is still necessary.

The main direction of antibody development at present is to reduce the size and complexity of antibodies while maintaining their affinity and selectivity for their targets. This approach includes natural antibodies (such as single-domain antibodies), antibody-like domains, and scaffolds. sdAbs should still be modified and clinically verified for their aspects, such as with respect to their immunogenicity and functionalization, even though these antibodies can efficiently expand potential drug targets due to their unique structural characteristics [84]. Envafolimab is the first camel-derived humanized PD-L1-IgG Fc single-domain fusion antibody drug to enter phase I clinical studies [9]. However, drugs based on shark-derived VNARs have rarely been clinically studied. The mechanism of action of VNARs with their molecular targets in vivo should be further investigated for VNAR antibody drugs to clarify their function, benefits, and efficacy in tumor immunodiagnosis and treatment. Shark VNARs are promising in the treatment and early diagnosis of tumors, especially solid tumors, due to their superior molecular structure characteristics and their objective advantages over VHH. Further development of VNAR antibody drugs may change the future of biological agents.

Author Contributions: X.J. writing—original draft, writing—review and editing; L.S. conceptualization, design, writing—original draft, writing—review and editing; C.H. data curation, visualization; F.Z. data curation, visualization; Z.L. resources, supervision, writing—review and editing; J.S. validation, writing—review and editing. All authors have read and agreed to the published version of the manuscript.

Funding: This research was funded by Zhejiang Provincial Public Welfare Technology Application Research Project, China, grant number: LGF18H090012.

Institutional Review Board Statement: Not applicable.

Data Availability Statement: Not applicable.

Conflicts of Interest: The authors declare that there are no conflicts of interest regarding the publication of this paper.

References

1. Kaplon, H.; Crescioli, S.; Chenoweth, A.; Visweswaraiah, J.; Reichert, J.M. Antibodies to watch in 2023. *MAbs* **2023**, *15*, 2153410. [CrossRef] [PubMed]
2. Kovaleva, M.; Ferguson, L.; Steven, J.; Porter, A.; Barelle, C. Shark variable new antigen receptor biologics—A novel technology platform for therapeutic drug development. *Expert Opin. Biol. Ther.* **2014**, *14*, 1527–1539. [CrossRef]
3. Adams, G.P.; Weiner, L.M. Monoclonal antibody therapy of cancer. *Nat. Biotechnol.* **2005**, *23*, 1147–1157. [CrossRef] [PubMed]
4. Murray, C.K.; Gasser, R.A.; Magill, A.J.; Miller, R.S. Update on rapid diagnostic testing for malaria. *Clin. Microbiol. Rev.* **2008**, *21*, 97–110. [CrossRef] [PubMed]
5. Dreher, M.R.; Liu, W.; Michelich, C.R.; Dewhirst, M.W.; Yuan, F.; Chilkoti, A. Tumor vascular permeability, accumulation, and penetration of macromolecular drug carriers. *J. Natl. Cancer Inst.* **2006**, *98*, 335–344. [CrossRef]

6. Sokolov, P.; Nifontova, G.; Samokhvalov, P.; Karaulov, A.; Sukhanova, A.; Nabiev, I. Nontoxic Fluorescent Nanoprobes for Multiplexed Detection and 3D Imaging of Tumor Markers in Breast Cancer. *Pharmaceutics* **2023**, *15*, 946. [CrossRef] [PubMed]
7. Chen, W.-H.; Hajduczki, A.; Martinez, E.J.; Bai, H.; Matz, H.; Hill, T.M.; Lewitus, E.; Chang, W.C.; Dawit, L.; Peterson, C.E.; et al. Shark nanobodies with potent SARS-CoV-2 neutralizing activity and broad sarbecovirus reactivity. *Nat. Commun.* **2023**, *14*, 580. [CrossRef]
8. Kok, B.H.; Lim, H.T.; Lim, C.P.; Lai, N.S.; Leow, C.Y.; Leow, C.H. Dengue virus infection—A review of pathogenesis, vaccines, diagnosis and therapy. *Virus Res.* **2023**, *324*, 17. [CrossRef] [PubMed]
9. Papadopoulos, K.P.; Harb, W.; Peer, C.J.; Hua, Q.; Xu, S.Y.; Lu, H.L.; Lu, N.; He, Y.; Xu, T.; Dong, R.P.; et al. First-in-Human Phase I Study of Envafolimab, a Novel Subcutaneous Single-Domain Anti-PD-L1 Antibody, in Patients with Advanced Solid Tumors. *Oncologist* **2021**, *26*, E1514–E1525. [CrossRef]
10. Andre, A.S.; Dias, J.N.R.; Aguiar, S.; Nogueira, S.; Bule, P.; Carvalho, J.I.; Antonio, J.P.M.; Cavaco, M.; Neves, V.; Oliveira, S.; et al. Rabbit derived VL single-domains as promising scaffolds to generate antibody-drug conjugates. *Sci. Rep.* **2023**, *13*, 4837. [CrossRef]
11. Ward, E.S.; Gussow, D.; Griffiths, A.D.; Jones, P.T.; Winter, G. Binding activities of a repertoire of single immunoglobulin variable domains secreted from *Escherichia coli*. *Nature* **1989**, *341*, 544–546. [CrossRef]
12. Hamers-Casterman, C.; Atarhouch, T.; Muyldermans, S.; Robinson, G.; Hamers, C.; Songa, E.B.; Bendahman, N.; Hamers, R. Naturally occurring antibodies devoid of light chains. *Nature* **1993**, *363*, 446–448. [CrossRef]
13. Greenberg, A.S.; Avila, D.; Hughes, M.; Hughes, A.; McKinney, E.C.; Flajnik, M.F. A new antigen receptor gene family that undergoes rearrangement and extensive somatic diversification in sharks. *Nature* **1995**, *374*, 168–173. [CrossRef]
14. English, H.; Hong, J.; Ho, M. Ancient species offers contemporary therapeutics: An update on shark VNAR single domain antibody sequences, phage libraries and potential clinical applications. *Antib. Ther.* **2020**, *3*, 1–9. [CrossRef] [PubMed]
15. Feng, M.; Bian, H.; Wu, X.; Fu, T.; Fu, Y.; Hong, J.; Fleming, B.D.; Flajnik, M.F.; Ho, M. Construction and next-generation sequencing analysis of a large phage-displayed VNAR single-domain antibody library from six naive nurse sharks. *Antib. Ther.* **2019**, *2*, 1–11. [CrossRef] [PubMed]
16. Van Bockstaele, F.; Holz, J.B.; Revets, H. The development of nanobodies for therapeutic applications. *Curr. Opin. Investig. Drugs* **2009**, *10*, 1212–1224.
17. Zinn, S.; Vazquez-Lombardi, R.; Zimmermann, C.; Sapra, P.; Jermutus, L.; Christ, D. Advances in antibody-based therapy in oncology. *Nat. Cancer* **2023**, *4*, 165–180. [CrossRef]
18. Dooley, H.; Stanfield, R.L.; Brady, R.A.; Flajnik, M.F. First molecular and biochemical analysis of in vivo affinity maturation in an ectothermic vertebrate. *Proc. Natl. Acad. Sci. USA* **2006**, *103*, 1846–1851. [CrossRef] [PubMed]
19. Stanfield, R.L.; Dooley, H.; Verdino, P.; Flajnik, M.F.; Wilson, I.A. Maturation of shark single-domain (IgNAR) antibodies: Evidence for induced-fit binding. *J. Mol. Biol.* **2007**, *367*, 358–372. [CrossRef]
20. Li, D.; English, H.; Hong, J.; Liang, T.Y.Z.; Merlino, G.; Day, C.P.; Ho, M. A novel PD-L1-targeted shark V-NAR single-domain-based CAR-T cell strategy for treating breast cancer and liver cancer. *Mol. Ther. Oncolytics* **2022**, *24*, 849–863. [CrossRef]
21. Pothin, E.; Lesuisse, D.; Lafaye, P. Brain Delivery of Single-Domain Antibodies: A Focus on VHH and VNAR. *Pharmaceutics* **2020**, *12*, 937.
22. Henderson, K.A.; Streltsov, V.A.; Coley, A.M.; Dolezal, O.; Hudson, P.J.; Batchelor, A.H.; Gupta, A.; Bai, T.; Murphy, V.J.; Anders, R.F.; et al. Structure of an IgNAR-AMA1 complex: Targeting a conserved hydrophobic cleft broadens malarial strain recognition. *Structure* **2007**, *15*, 1452–1466. [CrossRef] [PubMed]
23. Barelle, C.; Gill, D.S.; Charlton, K. Shark Novel Antigen Receptors-The Next Generation of Biologic Therapeutics? In *Pharmaceutical Biotechnology*; Guzman, C.A., Feuerstein, G.Z., Eds.; Springer: Berlin/Heidelberg, Germany, 2009; pp. 49–62.
24. Zielonka, S.; Empting, M.; Grzeschik, J.; Konning, D.; Barelle, C.J.; Kolmar, H. Structural insights and biomedical potential of IgNAR scaffolds from sharks. *MAbs* **2015**, *7*, 15–25. [CrossRef]
25. Jorgensen, P.; Chanthap, L.; Rebueno, A.; Tsuyuoka, R.; Bell, D. Malaria rapid diagnostic tests in tropical climates: The need for a cool chain. *Am. J. Trop. Med. Hyg.* **2006**, *74*, 750–754. [CrossRef] [PubMed]
26. Chen, Y.L.; Lin, J.J.; Ma, H.; Zhong, N.; Xie, X.X.; Yang, Y.R.; Zheng, P.Y.; Zhang, L.J.; Jin, T.C.; Cao, M.J. Screening and Characterization of Shark-Derived VNARs against SARS-CoV-2 Spike RBD Protein. *Int. J. Mol. Sci.* **2022**, *23*, 10904. [CrossRef] [PubMed]
27. Ubah, O.C.; Lake, E.W.; Gunaratne, G.S.; Gallant, J.P.; Fernie, M.; Robertson, A.J.; Marchant, J.S.; Bold, T.D.; Langlois, R.A.; Matchett, W.E.; et al. Mechanisms of SARS-CoV-2 neutralization by shark variable new antigen receptors elucidated through X-ray crystallography. *Nat. Commun.* **2021**, *12*, 7325. [CrossRef] [PubMed]
28. An EUA for Bamlanivimab-A Monoclonal Antibody for COVID-19. *Med. Lett. Drugs Ther.* **2021**, *325*, 880–881.
29. Juma, S.N.; Gong, X.X.; Hu, S.J.; Lv, Z.B.; Shao, J.Z.; Liu, L.L.; Chen, G.Q. Shark New Antigen Receptor (IgNAR): Structure, Characteristics and Potential Biomedical Applications. *Cells* **2021**, *10*, 1140. [CrossRef]
30. Kovalenko, O.V.; Olland, A.; Piche-Nicholas, N.; Godbole, A.; King, D.; Svenson, K.; Calabro, V.; Muller, M.R.; Barelle, C.J.; Somers, W.; et al. Atypical Antigen Recognition Mode of a Shark Immunoglobulin New Antigen Receptor (IgNAR) Variable Domain Characterized by Humanization and Structural Analysis. *J. Biol. Chem.* **2013**, *288*, 17408–17419. [CrossRef]
31. Dooley, H.; Flajnik, M.F.; Porter, A.J. Selection and characterization of naturally occurring single-domain (IgNAR) antibody fragments from immunized sharks by phage display. *Mol. Immunol.* **2003**, *40*, 25–33. [CrossRef] [PubMed]

32. Muller, M.R.; Saunders, K.; Grace, C.; Jin, M.; Piche-Nicholas, N.; Steven, J.; O'Dwyer, R.; Wu, L.Y.; Khetemenee, L.; Vugmeyster, Y.; et al. Improving the pharmacokinetic properties of biologics by fusion to an anti-HSA shark VNAR domain. *MAbs* **2012**, *4*, 673–685. [CrossRef] [PubMed]
33. Streltsov, V.A.; Carmichael, J.A.; Nuttall, S.D. Structure of a shark IgNAR antibody variable domain and modeling of an early-developmental isotype. *Protein Sci.* **2005**, *14*, 2901–2909. [CrossRef]
34. Jia, L.; Wang, Y.; Shen, Y.J.; Zhong, B.; Luo, Z.; Yang, J.J.; Chen, G.D.; Jiang, X.F.; Chen, J.Q.; Lyu, Z. IgNAR characterization and gene loci identification in whitespotted bamboo shark (*Chiloscyllium plagiosum*) genome. *Fish Shellfish Immunol.* **2023**, *133*, 9. [CrossRef]
35. Wei, L.K.; Wang, M.N.; Xiang, H.T.; Jiang, Y.; Gong, J.H.; Su, D.; Al Azad, M.A.R.; Dong, H.M.; Feng, L.M.; Wu, J.J.; et al. Bamboo Shark as a Small Animal Model for Single Domain Antibody Production. *Front. Bioeng. Biotechnol.* **2021**, *9*, 16. [CrossRef] [PubMed]
36. Griffiths, K.; Dolezal, O.; Parisi, K.; Angerosa, J.; Dogovski, C.; Barraclough, M.; Sanalla, A.; Casey, J.; González, I.; Perugini, M.; et al. Shark Variable New Antigen Receptor (VNAR) Single Domain Antibody Fragments: Stability and Diagnostic Applications. *Antibodies* **2013**, *2*, 66–81. [CrossRef]
37. Ho, M. Inaugural Editorial: Searching for Magic Bullets. *Antib. Ther.* **2018**, *1*, 1–5. [CrossRef]
38. Muyldermans, S. Nanobodies: Natural Single-Domain Antibodies. In *Annual Review of Biochemistry*; Kornberg, R.D., Ed.; Annual Reviews: Palo Alto, CA, USA, 2013; Volume 82, pp. 775–797.
39. Ho, M. Perspectives on the development of neutralizing antibodies against SARS-CoV-2. *Antib. Ther.* **2020**, *3*, 109–114. [CrossRef] [PubMed]
40. Dooley, H.; Flajnik, M.F. Antibody repertoire development in cartilaginous fish. *Dev. Comp. Immunol.* **2006**, *30*, 43–56. [CrossRef] [PubMed]
41. Nuttall, S.D. Overview and discovery of IgNARs and generation of VNARs. *Single Domain Antibodies Methods Protoc.* **2012**, *911*, 27–36.
42. Steven, J.; Muller, M.R.; Carvalho, M.F.; Ubah, O.C.; Kovaleva, M.; Donohoe, G.; Baddeley, T.; Cornock, D.; Saunders, K.; Porter, A.J.; et al. In Vitro Maturation of a humanized shark Vnar Domain to improve its Biophysical Properties to Facilitate clinical Development. *Front. Immunol.* **2017**, *8*, 15. [CrossRef]
43. Zhang, Y.-F.; Sun, Y.; Hong, J.; Ho, M. Humanization of the Shark VNAR Single Domain Antibody Using CDR Grafting. *Curr. Protoc.* **2023**, *3*, e630. [CrossRef] [PubMed]
44. Fernandez-Quintero, M.L.; Fischer, A.L.M.; Kokot, J.; Waibl, F.; Seidler, C.A.; Liedl, K.R. The influence of antibody humanization on shark variable domain (VNAR) binding site ensembles. *Front. Immunol.* **2022**, *13*, 11. [CrossRef] [PubMed]
45. Rossotti, M.A.; Belanger, K.; Henry, K.A.; Tanha, J. Immunogenicity and humanization of single-domain antibodies. *FEBS J.* **2022**, *289*, 4304–4327. [CrossRef] [PubMed]
46. De Greve, H.; Virdi, V.; Bakshi, S.; Depicker, A. Simplified monomeric VHH-Fc antibodies provide new opportunities for passive immunization. *Curr. Opin. Biotechnol.* **2020**, *61*, 96–101. [CrossRef]
47. Liu, H.P.; Schittny, V.; Nash, M.A. Removal of a Conserved Disulfide Bond Does Not Compromise Mechanical Stability of a VHH Antibody Complex. *Nano Lett.* **2019**, *19*, 5524–5529. [CrossRef]
48. Flajnik, M.F. A cold-blooded view of adaptive immunity. *Nat. Rev. Immunol.* **2018**, *18*, 438–453. [CrossRef]
49. Leow, C.H.; Fischer, K.; Leow, C.Y.; Braet, K.; Cheng, Q.; McCarthy, J. Isolation and characterization of malaria PfHRP2 specific V-NAR antibody fragments from immunized shark phage display library. *Malar. J.* **2018**, *17*, 15. [CrossRef]
50. Burciaga-Flores, M.; Marquez-Aguirre, A.L.; Duenas, S.; Gasperin-Bulbarela, J.; Licea-Navarro, A.F.; Camacho-Villegas, T.A. First pan-specific vNAR against human TGF-beta as a potential therapeutic application: In silico modeling assessment. *Sci. Rep.* **2023**, *13*, 3596. [CrossRef]
51. Crouch, K.; Smith, L.E.; Williams, R.; Cao, W.; Lee, M.; Jensen, A.; Dooley, H. Humoral immune response of the small-spotted catshark, *Scyliorhinus canicular*. *Fish Shellfish Immunol.* **2013**, *34*, 1158–1169. [CrossRef]
52. Chen, W.K.; Liu, M.K. Reproductive biology of whitespotted bamboo shark Chiloscyllium plagiosum in northern waters off Taiwan. *Fisheries Science.* **2006**, *72*, 1215–1224. [CrossRef]
53. Zhao, L.F.; Chen, M.L.; Wang, X.N.; Kang, S.K.; Xue, W.W.; Li, Z.P. Identification of Anti-TNF alpha VNAR Single Domain Antibodies from Whitespotted Bambooshark (*Chiloscyllium plagiosum*). *Mar. Drugs* **2022**, *20*, 307. [CrossRef] [PubMed]
54. Zhang, Y.L.; Gao, H.Y.; Li, H.B.; Guo, J.; Ouyang, B.J.; Wang, M.N.; Xu, Q.W.; Wang, J.H.; Lv, M.Q.; Guo, X.Y.; et al. The White-Spotted Bamboo Shark Genome Reveals Chromosome Rearrangements and Fast-Evolving Immune Genes of Cartilaginous Fish. *iScience* **2020**, *23*, 53. [CrossRef]
55. Dong, H.M.; Zhang, Y.L.; Wang, J.H.; Xiang, H.T.; Lv, T.H.; Wei, L.K.; Yang, S.S.; Liu, X.P.; Ren, B.Z.; Zhang, X.Q.; et al. Cas9-Based Local Enrichment and Genomics Sequence Revision of Megabase-Sized Shark IgNAR Loci. *J. Immunol.* **2022**, *208*, 181–189. [CrossRef] [PubMed]
56. De Silva, D.P.N.; Tan, E.; Mizuno, N.; Hosoya, S.; Reza, M.S.; Watabe, S.; Kinoshita, S.; Asakawa, S. Transcriptomic analysis of immunoglobulin novel antigen receptor (IgNAR) heavy chain constant domains of brownbanded bamboo shark (*Chiloscyllium punctatum*). *Fish Shellfish Immunol.* **2019**, *84*, 370–376. [CrossRef] [PubMed]

57. Yu, C.D.; Ding, W.; Zhu, L.; Zhou, Y.H.; Dong, Y.K.; Li, L.; Liu, J.J.; Wang, Y.Z.; Li, Z.H.; Zhu, L.N.; et al. Screening and characterization of inhibitory vNAR targeting nanodisc-assembled influenza M2 proteins. *iScience* **2023**, *26*, 21. [CrossRef] [PubMed]
58. Ryckaert, S.; Pardon, E.; Steyaert, J.; Callewaert, N. Isolation of antigen-binding camelid heavy chain antibody fragments (nanobodies) from an immune library displayed on the surface of *Pichia pastoris*. *J. Biotechnol.* **2010**, *145*, 93–98. [CrossRef] [PubMed]
59. Fleetwood, F.; Devoogdt, N.; Pellis, M.; Wernery, U.; Muyldermans, S.; Stahl, S.; Lofblom, J. Surface display of a single-domain antibody library on Gram-positive bacteria. *Cell. Mol. Life Sci.* **2013**, *70*, 1081–1093. [CrossRef]
60. Konning, D.; Zielonka, S.; Grzeschik, J.; Empting, M.; Valldorfl, B.; Krah, S.; Schroter, C.; Sellmann, C.; Hock, B.; Kolmarl, H. Camelid and shark single domain antibodies: Structural features and therapeutic potential. *Curr. Opin. Struct. Biol.* **2017**, *45*, 10–16. [CrossRef] [PubMed]
61. Yau, K.Y.F.; Groves, M.A.T.; Li, S.; Sheedy, C.; Lee, H.; Tanha, J.; MacKenzie, C.R.; Jermutus, L.; Hall, J.C. Selection of hapten-specific single-domain antibodies from a non-immunized llama ribosome display library. *J. Immunol. Methods* **2003**, *281*, 161–175. [CrossRef]
62. Monegal, A.; Ami, D.; Martinelli, C.; Huang, H.; Aliprandi, M.; Capasso, P.; Francavilla, C.; Ossolengo, G.; de Marco, A. Immunological applications of single-domain llama recombinant antibodies isolated from a naive library. *Protein Eng. Des. Sel.* **2009**, *22*, 273–280. [CrossRef]
63. Goldman, E.R.; Anderson, G.P.; Liu, J.L.; Delehanty, J.B.; Sherwood, L.J.; Osborn, L.E.; Cummins, L.B.; Hayhurst, A. Facile generation of heat-stable antiviral and antitoxin single domain antibodies from a semisynthetic llama library. *Anal. Chem.* **2006**, *78*, 8245–8255. [CrossRef] [PubMed]
64. Yan, J.R.; Li, G.H.; Hu, Y.H.; Ou, W.J.; Wan, Y.K. Construction of a synthetic phage-displayed Nanobody library with CDR3 regions randomized by trinucleotide cassettes for diagnostic applications. *J. Transl. Med.* **2014**, *12*, 1–11. [CrossRef] [PubMed]
65. Palacios, A.M.; Grzeschik, J.; Deweid, L.; Krah, S.; Zielonka, S.; Rosner, T.; Peipp, M.; Valerius, T.; Kolmar, H. Specific Targeting of Lymphoma Cells Using Semisynthetic Anti-Idiotype Shark Antibodies. *Front. Immunol.* **2020**, *11*, 15.
66. McCafferty, J.; Griffiths, A.D.; Winter, G.; Chiswell, D.J. Phage antibodies: Filamentous phage displaying antibody variable domains. *Nature* **1990**, *348*, 552–554. [CrossRef]
67. Muller, M.R.; O'Dwyer, R.; Kovaleva, M.; Rudkin, F.; Dooley, H.; Barelle, C.J. Generation and isolation of target-specific single-domain antibodies from shark immune repertoires. *Methods Mol. Biol.* **2012**, *907*, 177–194. [PubMed]
68. Shao, C.Y.; Secombes, C.J.; Porter, A.J. Rapid isolation of IgNAR variable single-domain antibody fragments from a shark synthetic library. *Mol. Immunol.* **2007**, *44*, 656–665. [CrossRef] [PubMed]
69. Walsh, R.; Nuttall, S.; Revill, P.; Colledge, D.; Cabuang, L.; Soppe, S.; Dolezal, O.; Griffiths, K.; Bartholomeusz, A.; Locarnini, S. Targeting the hepatitis B virus precore antigen with a novel IgNAR single variable domain intrabody. *Virology* **2011**, *411*, 132–141. [CrossRef]
70. Ohtani, M.; Hikima, J.; Jung, T.S.; Kondo, H.; Hirono, I.; Aoki, T. Construction of an Artificially Randomized IgNAR Phage Display Library: Screening of Variable Regions that Bind to Hen Egg White Lysozyme. *Mar. Biotechnol.* **2013**, *15*, 56–62. [CrossRef]
71. Ohtani, M.; Hikima, J.; Jung, T.S.; Kondo, H.; Hirono, I.; Takeyama, H.; Aoki, T. Variable domain antibodies specific for viral hemorrhagic septicemia virus (VHSV) selected from a randomized IgNAR phage display library. *Fish Shellfish. Immunol.* **2013**, *34*, 724–728. [CrossRef]
72. Duan, Z.; Buffington, J.; Hong, J.; Ho, M. Production and Purification of Shark and Camel Single-Domain Antibodies from Bacterial and Mammalian Cell Expression Systems. *Curr. Protoc.* **2022**, *2*, e459. [CrossRef]
73. Leow, C.H.; Fischer, K.; Leow, C.Y.; Cheng, Q.; Chuah, C.; McCarthy, J. Single Domain Antibodies as New Biomarker Detectors. *Diagnostics* **2017**, *7*, 52. [CrossRef] [PubMed]
74. Konning, D.; Kolmar, H. Beyond antibody engineering: Directed evolution of alternative binding scaffolds and enzymes using yeast surface display. *Microb. Cell. Fact.* **2018**, *17*, 17. [CrossRef] [PubMed]
75. Ubah, O.C.; Porter, A.J.; Barelle, C.J. In Vitro ELISA and Cell-Based Assays Confirm the Low Immunogenicity of VNAR Therapeutic Constructs in a Mouse Model of Human RA: An Encouraging Milestone to Further Clinical Drug Development. *J. Immunol. Res.* **2020**, *2020*, 1–14. [CrossRef] [PubMed]
76. Scully, M.; Cataland, S.R.; Peyvandi, F.; Coppo, P.; Knobl, P.; Hovinga, J.A.K.; Metjian, A.; de la Rubia, J.; Pavenski, K.; Callewaert, F.; et al. Caplacizumab Treatment for Acquired Thrombotic Thrombocytopenic Purpura. *N. Engl. J. Med.* **2019**, *380*, 335–346. [CrossRef]
77. Cao, Q.H.; Huang, C.L.; Yi, H.; Gill, A.J.; Chou, A.; Foley, M.; Hosking, C.G.; Lim, K.K.; Triffon, C.F.; Shi, Y.; et al. A single-domain i-body, AD-114, attenuates renal fibrosis through blockade of CXCR4. *JCI Insight* **2022**, *7*, 19. [CrossRef]
78. Clarke, E.; Stocki, P.; Sinclair, E.H.; Gauhar, A.; Fletcher, E.J.R.; Krawczun-Rygmaczewska, A.; Duty, S.; Walsh, F.S.; Doherty, P.; Rutkowski, J.L. A Single Domain Shark Antibody Targeting the Transferrin Receptor 1 Delivers a TrkB Agonist Antibody to the Brain and Provides Full Neuroprotection in a Mouse Model of Parkinson's Disease. *Pharmaceutics* **2022**, *14*, 1335. [CrossRef]
79. Jain, S.; Doshi, A.S.; Iyer, A.K.; Amiji, M.M. Multifunctional nanoparticles for targeting cancer and inflammatory diseases. *J. Drug Target* **2013**, *21*, 888–903. [CrossRef]
80. Peyvandi, F.; Scully, M.; Hovinga, J.A.K. Caplacizumab for Acquired Thrombotic Thrombocytopenic Purpura. *N. Engl. J. Med.* **2016**, *374*, 511–522. [CrossRef]

81. Cunningham, S.P.A.; Piedra, F.; Martinon-Torres, H.; Szymanski, B.; Brackeva, E.; Dombrecht, L.; Detalle, C.; Fleurinck, R.S. Grp, Nebulised ALX-0171 for respiratory syncytial virus lower respiratory tract infection in hospitalised children: A double-blind, randomised, placebo-controlled, phase 2b trial. *Lancet Resp. Med.* **2021**, *9*, 21–32. [CrossRef]
82. Kim, G.W.; Lee, N.R.; Pi, R.H.; Lim, Y.S.; Lee, Y.M.; Lee, J.M.; Jeong, H.S.; Chung, S.H. IL-6 inhibitors for treatment of rheumatoid arthritis: Past, present, and future. *Arch. Pharm. Res.* **2015**, *38*, 575–584. [CrossRef]
83. Stanfield, R.L.; Dooley, H.; Flajnik, M.F.; Wilson, I.A. Crystal structure of a shark single-domain antibody V region in complex with lysozyme. *Science* **2004**, *305*, 1770–1773. [CrossRef]
84. Husain, B.; Ellerman, D. Expanding the Boundaries of Biotherapeutics with Bispecific Antibodies. *Biodrugs* **2018**, *32*, 441–464. [CrossRef]
85. Feldwisch, J.; Tolmachev, V. Engineering of affibody molecules for therapy and diagnostics. *Methods Mol. Biol.* **2012**, *899*, 103–126. [PubMed]
86. Torchia, J.; Weiskopf, K.; Levy, R. Targeting lymphoma with precision using semisynthetic anti-idiotype peptibodies. *Proc. Natl. Acad. Sci. USA* **2016**, *113*, 5376–5381. [CrossRef]
87. Mir, M.A.; Mehraj, U.; Sheikh, B.A.; Hamdani, S.S. Nanobodies: The "Magic Bullets" in therapeutics, drug delivery and diagnostics. *Hum. Antibodies* **2020**, *28*, 29–51. [CrossRef] [PubMed]
88. He, T.; Zhu, J.; Nie, Y.; Hu, R.; Wang, T.; Li, P.; Zhang, Q.; Yang, Y. Nanobody Technology for Mycotoxin Detection in the Field of Food Safety: Current Status and Prospects. *Toxins* **2018**, *10*, 180. [CrossRef]
89. Chakravarty, R.; Goel, S.; Cai, W.B. Nanobody: The "Magic Bullet" for Molecular Imaging? *Theranostics* **2014**, *4*, 386–398. [CrossRef]
90. Kong, Q.; Yao, Y.; Chen, R.; Lu, S. Progress in nanobody and its application in diagnosis. *Chin. J. Biotechnol.* **2014**, *30*, 1351–1361.
91. Siontorou, C.G. Nanobodies as novel agents for disease diagnosis and therapy. *Int. J. Nanomed.* **2013**, *8*, 4215–4227. [CrossRef]
92. Gauhar, A.; Privezentzev, C.V.; Demydchuk, M.; Gerlza, T.; Rieger, J.; Kungl, A.J.; Walsh, F.S.; Rutkowski, J.L.; Stocki, P. Single domain shark VNAR antibodies neutralize SARS-CoV-2 infection in vitro. *FASEB J.* **2021**, *35*, 13. [CrossRef]
93. Valdovino-Navarro, B.J.; Duenas, S.; Flores-Acosta, G.I.; Gasperin-Bulbarela, J.; Bernaldez-Sarabia, J.; Cabanillas-Bernal, O.; Cervantes-Luevano, K.E.; Licea-Navarro, A.F. Neutralizing Ability of a Single Domain VNAR Antibody: In Vitro Neutralization of SARS-CoV-2 Variants of Concern. *Int. J. Mol. Sci.* **2022**, *23*, 12267. [CrossRef] [PubMed]
94. Feng, B.; Chen, Z.L.; Sun, J.; Xu, T.T.; Wang, Q.; Yi, H.S.; Niu, X.F.; Zhu, J.B.; Fan, M.Z.; Hou, R.T.; et al. A Class of Shark-Derived Single-Domain Antibodies can Broadly Neutralize SARS-Related Coronaviruses and the Structural Basis of Neutralization and Omicron Escape. *Small Methods* **2022**, *6*, 12. [CrossRef]
95. Lauwereys, M.; Ghahroudi, M.A.; Desmyter, A.; Kinne, J.; Holzer, W.; De Genst, E.; Wyns, L.; Muyldermans, S. Potent enzyme inhibitors derived from dromedary heavy-chain antibodies. *EMBO J.* **1998**, *17*, 3512–3520. [CrossRef] [PubMed]
96. Burgess, S.G.; Oleksy, A.; Cavazza, T.; Richards, M.W.; Vernos, I.; Matthews, D.; Bayliss, R. Allosteric inhibition of Aurora-A kinase by a synthetic vNAR domain. *Open Biol.* **2016**, *6*, 10. [CrossRef]
97. Stocki, P.; Szary, J.; Rasmussen, C.L.M.; Demydchuk, M.; Northall, L.; Logan, D.B.; Gauhar, A.; Thei, L.; Moos, T.; Walsh, F.S.; et al. Blood-brain barrier transport using a high affinity, brain-selective VNAR antibody targeting transferrin receptor 1. *FASEB J.* **2021**, *35*, 19. [CrossRef]
98. Kovaleva, M.; Johnson, K.; Steven, J.; Barelle, C.J.; Porter, A. Therapeutic Potential of Shark Anti-ICOSL VNAR Domains is Exemplified in a Murine Model of Autoimmune Non-Infectious Uveitis. *Front. Immunol.* **2017**, *8*, 13. [CrossRef]
99. Camacho-Villegas, T.A.; Mata-Gonzalez, M.T.; Garcia-Ubbelohd, W.; Nunez-Garcia, L.; Elosua, C.; Paniagua-Solis, J.F.; Licea-Navarro, A.F. Intraocular Penetration of a vNAR: In Vivo and In Vitro VEGF(165) Neutralization. *Mar. Drugs* **2018**, *16*, 13. [CrossRef]
100. Sanmamed, M.F.; Chen, L.P. A Paradigm Shift in Cancer Immunotherapy: From Enhancement to Normalization. *Cell* **2019**, *175*, 313–326. [CrossRef]
101. Xenaki, K.T.; Dorrestijn, B.; Muns, J.A.; Adamzek, K.; Doulkeridou, S.; Houthoff, H.; Oliveira, S.; Henegouwen, P. Homogeneous tumor targeting with a single dose of HER2-targeted albumin-binding domain-fused nanobody-drug conjugates results in long-lasting tumor remission in mice. *Theranostics* **2021**, *11*, 5525–5538. [CrossRef]
102. Stylianopoulos, T.; Munn, L.L.; Jain, R.K. Reengineering the Physical Microenvironment of Tumors to Improve Drug Delivery and Efficacy: From Mathematical Modeling to Bench to Bedside. *Trends Cancer* **2018**, *4*, 292–319. [CrossRef] [PubMed]
103. Jain, R.K. Normalization of tumor vasculature: An emerging concept in antiangiogenic therapy. *Science* **2005**, *307*, 58–62. [CrossRef] [PubMed]
104. Vasalou, C.; Helmlinger, G.; Gomes, B. A Mechanistic Tumor Penetration Model to Guide Antibody Drug Conjugate Design. *PLoS ONE* **2015**, *10*, 20. [CrossRef]
105. Thurber, G.M.; Schmidt, M.M.; Wittrup, K.D. Antibody tumor penetration: Transport opposed by systemic and antigen-mediated clearance. *Adv. Drug Deliv. Rev.* **2008**, *60*, 1421–1434. [CrossRef] [PubMed]
106. Xenaki, K.T.; Oliveira, S.; Henegouwen, P. Antibody or Antibody Fragments: Implications for Molecular Imaging and Targeted Therapy of Solid Tumors. *Front. Immunol.* **2017**, *8*, 6. [CrossRef]
107. Adams, G.P.; Schier, R.; Marshall, K.; Wolf, E.J.; McCall, A.M.; Marks, J.D.; Weiner, L.M. Increased affinity leads to improved selective tumor delivery of single-chain Fv antibodies. *Cancer Res.* **1998**, *58*, 485–490.

108. Cilliers, C.; Guo, H.; Liao, J.S.; Christodolu, N.; Thurber, G.M. Multiscale Modeling of Antibody-Drug Conjugates: Connecting Tissue and Cellular Distribution to Whole Animal Pharmacokinetics and Potential Implications for Efficacy. *AAPS J.* **2016**, *18*, 1117–1130. [CrossRef] [PubMed]
109. Leach, A.; Smyth, P.; Ferguson, L.; Steven, J.; Greene, M.K.; Branco, C.M.; McCann, A.P.; Porter, A.; Barelle, C.J.; Scott, C.J. Anti-DLL4 VNAR targeted nanoparticles for targeting of both tumour and tumour associated vasculature. *Nanoscale* **2020**, *12*, 14751–14763. [CrossRef]
110. Ubah, O.C.; Steven, J.; Kovaleva, M.; Ferguson, L.; Barelle, C.; Porter, A.J.R.; Barelle, C.J. Novel, Anti-hTNF-alpha Variable New Antigen Receptor Formats with Enhanced Neutralizing Potency and Multifunctionality, Generated for Therapeutic Development. *Front. Immunol.* **2017**, *8*, 13. [CrossRef]
111. Ubah, O.C.; Steven, J.; Porter, A.J.; Barelle, C.J. An Anti-hTNF-alpha Variable New Antigen Receptor Format Demonstrates Superior in vivo Preclinical Efficacy to Humira (R) in a Transgenic Mouse Autoimmune Polyarthritis Disease Model. *Front. Immunol.* **2019**, *10*, 12. [CrossRef]
112. Broos, K.; Lecocq, Q.; Xavier, C.; Bridoux, J.; Nguyen, T.T.; Corthals, J.; Schoonooghe, S.; Lion, E.; Raes, G.; Keyaerts, M.; et al. Evaluating a Single Domain Antibody Targeting Human PD-L1 as a Nuclear Imaging and Therapeutic Agent. *Cancers* **2019**, *11*, 872. [CrossRef]
113. Awad, R.M.; Lecocq, Q.; Zeven, K.; Ertveldt, T.; De Beck, L.; Ceuppens, H.; Broos, K.; De Vlaeminck, Y.; Goyvaerts, C.; Verdonck, M.; et al. Formatting and gene-based delivery of a human PD-L1 single domain antibody for immune checkpoint blockade. *Mol. Ther. Methods Clin. Dev.* **2021**, *22*, 11. [CrossRef] [PubMed]
114. Tanaka, Y.; Nishikawa, M.; Kamisaki, K.; Hachiya, S.; Nakamura, M.; Kuwazuru, T.; Tanimura, S.; Soyano, K.; Takeda, K. Marine-derived microbes and molecules for drug discovery. *Inflamm. Regen.* **2022**, *42*, 12. [CrossRef] [PubMed]

marine drugs

Article

From Sea to Science: Coral Aquaculture for Sustainable Anticancer Drug Development

Hung-Yu Lin [1,2], Tsen-Ni Tsai [3,4], Kai-Cheng Hsu [5,6], Yu-Ming Hsu [4,7], Lin-Chien Chiang [4], Mohamed El-Shazly [8], Ken-Ming Chang [9], Yu-Hsuan Lin [4], Shang-Yi Tu [4], Tony Eight Lin [5,6], Ying-Chi Du [3], Yi-Chang Liu [3,*] and Mei-Chin Lu [4,10,*]

1 School of Medicine, College of Medicine, I-Shou University, Kaohsiung 824, Taiwan
2 Division of Urology, Department of Surgery, E-Da Cancer Hospital, I-Shou University, Kaohsiung 824, Taiwan
3 Division of Hematology-Oncology, Department of Internal Medicine, Kaohsiung Medical University Hospital, Kaohsiung 807, Taiwan
4 Graduate Institute of Marine Biology, National Dong Hwa University, Pingtung 944, Taiwan
5 Graduate Institute of Cancer Biology and Drug Discovery, College of Medical Science and Technology, Taipei Medical University, Taipei 110, Taiwan
6 Ph.D. Program for Cancer Molecular Biology and Drug Discovery, College of Medical Science and Technology, Taipei Medical University, Taipei 110, Taiwan
7 Research Center for Precision Environmental Medicine, Kaohsiung Medical University, Kaohsiung 807, Taiwan
8 Department of Pharmacognosy, Faculty of Pharmacy, Ain-Shams University, Organization of African Unity Street, Abassia, Cairo 11566, Egypt
9 Department of Pharmacy and Master Program, Tajen University, Pingtung 907, Taiwan
10 National Museum of Marine Biology and Aquarium, Pingtung 944, Taiwan
* Correspondence: ycliu@cc.kmu.edu.tw (Y.-C.L.); jinx6609@nmmba.gov.tw (M.-C.L.)

Abstract: Marine natural products offer immense potential for drug development, but the limited supply of marine organisms poses a significant challenge. Establishing aquaculture presents a sustainable solution for this challenge by facilitating the mass production of active ingredients while reducing our reliance on wild populations and harm to local environments. To fully utilize aquaculture as a source of biologically active products, a cell-free system was established to target molecular components with protein-modulating activity, including topoisomerase II, HDAC, and tubulin polymerization, using extracts from aquaculture corals. Subsequent in vitro studies were performed, including MTT assays, flow cytometry, confocal microscopy, and Western blotting, along with in vivo xenograft models, to verify the efficacy of the active extracts and further elucidate their cytotoxic mechanisms. Regulatory proteins were clarified using NGS and gene modification techniques. Molecular docking and SwissADME assays were performed to evaluate the drug-likeness and pharmacokinetic and medicinal chemistry-related properties of the small molecules. The extract from *Lobophytum crassum* (LCE) demonstrated potent broad-spectrum activity, exhibiting significant inhibition of tubulin polymerization, and showed low IC_{50} values against prostate cancer cells. Flow cytometry and Western blotting assays revealed that LCE induced apoptosis, as evidenced by the increased expression of apoptotic protein-cleaved caspase-3 and the populations of early and late apoptotic cells. In the xenograft tumor experiments, LCE significantly suppressed tumor growth and reduced the tumor volume (PC3: 43.9%; Du145: 49.2%) and weight (PC3: 48.8%; Du145: 7.8%). Additionally, LCE inhibited prostate cancer cell migration, and invasion upregulated the epithelial marker E-cadherin and suppressed EMT-related proteins. Furthermore, LCE effectively attenuated TGF-β-induced EMT in PC3 and Du145 cells. Bioactivity-guided fractionation and SwissADME validation confirmed that LCE's main component, 13-acetoxysarcocrassolide (13-AC), holds greater potential for the development of anticancer drugs.

Keywords: apoptosis; epithelial–mesenchymal transition (EMT); prostate cancer; tubulin polymerization; 13-acetoxysarcocrassolide

1. Introduction

Historically, human medicine has relied heavily on plants and animals, harnessing their secondary metabolites for therapeutic purposes. Secondary metabolites, although not essential for the organism's survival, carry out significant biological activities and have been utilized as dietary supplements and therapeutic agents. Ancient texts like Shennong's Classic of Materia Medica and the Compendium of Materia Medica by Li Shizhen document numerous marine organisms and their medicinal properties [1]. Recently, marine natural products have been shown to show potent biological activity, with antitumor properties surpassing those of terrestrial sources, largely due to their unique stereochemical structures and special elemental compositions [1].

Soft corals are a prolific source of terpenoids, especially cembrane diterpenoids, which exhibit a broad spectrum of pharmacological activities, including anti-inflammatory, anticancer, antibacterial, and immunomodulatory effects [2,3]. Taiwan, boasting one of the world's highest densities and diversities of marine corals, has significant expertise in developing and establishing aquaculture systems [4]. This technical prowess positions Taiwan to be able to advance sustainable marine environment conservation and develop marine-derived medicines targeting many diseases, especially cancer.

Topoisomerases are crucial enzymes in the DNA metabolism, making them prime targets for anticancer drugs. The pursuit of topoisomerase inhibitors has become a significant focus in cancer drug development. Over the past decade, researchers have identified, synthesized, and evaluated a variety of novel bioactive molecules targeting topoisomerases. These inhibitors have been categorized into several structural classes, including N-heterocycles, quinones, flavonoids, diterpenes, coumarins, lignans, polyphenols, fatty acids, and metal complexes [5–13].

Despite the prevalence of topoisomerase poisons, such as etoposide, in cancer therapy, their associated cardiotoxicity, resistance issues, and potential for causing secondary malignancies necessitate safer alternatives. Catalytic inhibitors, which block the enzyme's function without causing DNA damage, represent a promising research direction [14–18]. Our research identified a marine sesquiterpenoid, 13-acetoxysarcocrassolide (13-AC), which competitively inhibits topoisomerase and the N-terminal ATP binding site of heat shock proteins. This compound holds potential as a less toxic anticancer agent, particularly for blood, oral, and prostate cancers [14]

Microtubules, composed of α-tubulin and β-tubulin subunits, are integral to various cellular functions, including cell shape, division, and intracellular transport. The disruption of tubulin polymerization is a key strategy in cancer treatment as it interferes with cell division [19]. Antitubulin drugs, derived from plants, microbes, and marine organisms, either stabilize or destabilize tubulin. Notable stabilizers, such as Taxol and vinca alkaloids, are widely used in clinical settings [20]. Given the critical role of tubulin in cellular processes and tumorigenesis, targeting tubulin polymerization remains a promising approach in anticancer drug development.

Histone deacetylases (HDACs) regulate gene expression by altering the chromatin structure. HDAC inhibitors (HDACis) are a promising class of anticancer agents, especially when designed as multi-target hybrids that inhibit multiple cancer pathways. These hybrid molecules have garnered significant interest due to their potential to reduce side effects and enhance therapeutic efficacy. Recent developments have seen several HDACi hybrids, such as CUDC-101 and CUDC-907, enter clinical trials, underscoring their therapeutic potential [21]. The research into HDAC inhibitors continues to be a vibrant field, with a focus on developing agents that can synergistically improve the effectiveness of other anticancer drugs.

Epithelial–mesenchymal transition (EMT) is a process where epithelial cells acquire mesenchymal traits, enhancing their motility. This transition is crucial during embryonic development, wound healing, and cancer metastasis. EMT enables cancer cells to invade surrounding tissues and disseminate to distant organs [22,23]. More than 90% of cancer-related deaths are caused by metastatic cancer diseases. Given that over 90% of cancer-related deaths are due to metastasis, understanding and targeting EMT mechanisms are critical for developing therapies to inhibit cancer spread [24,25].

This study investigates the anticancer potential of extracts from aquaculture soft corals, focusing on their effects on topoisomerase II, HDAC, and tubulin polymerization. Using in vitro and in vivo assays, we evaluated the extracts' efficacy against prostate cancer cells and their ability to inhibit cancer cell metastasis and EMT. Specifically, we assessed whether these extracts could inhibit EMT-related protein expression in the presence or absence of TGF-β, an EMT inducer. The goal is to explore the potential of these marine extracts as anticancer and anti-metastatic agents.

2. Results

2.1. Effects of Different Crude Extracts on the Cell Growth of Leukemia and Prostate Cancer Cells

In this study, more than 180 soft corals in the aquaculture system were extracted using ethyl acetate to screen out their cytotoxicity against leukemic and prostate cancer cells. The results showed that six extracts (Figure 1) inhibited the survival of more than half of the cancer cells at the highest dose (40 μg/mL) for 72 treatments (Table 1). C2 showed the most potent activity, with IC_{50} values of less than 0.16 and 0.33 ± 0.05 μg/mL for leukemia Molt4 and K562 cells, respectively. C5 was the most active extract against prostate Du145 and LNCaP cells, with IC_{50} values of 4.96 ± 0.04 and 2.76 ± 0.34 μg/mL, respectively. The use of any of the six crude extracts at a high dose (40 μg/mL) inhibited almost 90% of growth in four cancer cells, except C3 and C4 for Du145 and LNCaP cells, which resulted in IC_{50} values of over 30 μg/mL.

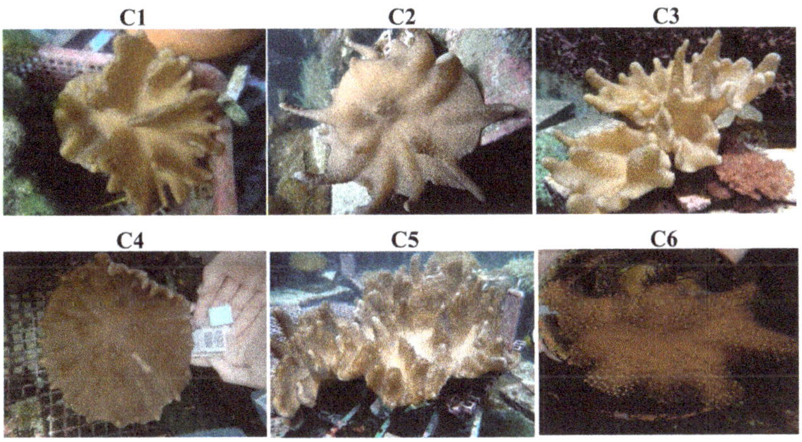

Figure 1. Morphology of aquaculture soft corals.

Table 1. Cytotoxic activity of six coral extracts against different leukemia and prostate cancer cell lines after 72 h using MTT assay. The IC_{50} values were calculated using CalcuSyn software Version 1.1.1.

	IC_{50} (μg/ mL), 72 h			
	Leukemia Cell		Prostate Cancer	
Crude Extracts	**Molt 4**	**K562**	**Du145**	**LNCaP**
C1	4.11 ± 0.99	4.58 ± 0.15	12.39 ± 2.11	17.37 ± 3.86
C2	<0.16	0.33 ± 0.05	14.66 ± 0.79	15.49 ± 4.56
C3	1.87 ± 0.36	6.11 ± 2.28	11.44 ± 4.26	36.18 ± 0.69
C4	0.66 ± 0.084	2.65 ± 0.44	36.9 ± 2.8	37.88 ± 0.21
C5	1.5 ± 0.7	2.29 ± 0.17	4.96± 0.04	2.76 ± 0.34
C6	1.57 ± 0.57	2.27 ± 0.12	5.88 ± 0.48	9.17 ± 0.07

2.2. Effects of the Different Crude Extracts on the Function of Topoisomerase II

The Food and Drug Administration (FDA)-approved chemotherapeutic agents doxorubicin and paclitaxel are topoisomerase inhibitors [26]. A cell-free system assay can be used to detect whether the activity of human topoisomerase II is affected by these coral extracts. The results showed that C1 and C3 increased the level of supercoiled DNA at a dose of 0.16 μg/mL. This indicated that extracts C1 and C3 could diminish the function of topoisomerase II at low doses, and at a dose of 2.5 μg/mL, all the extracts significantly inhibited the formation of relaxed DNA induced by topoisomerase II, while all extracts inhibited topoisomerase II at a high dose of 40 μg/mL (Figure 2). All these extracts dose-dependently decreased the catalytic activity of topoisomerase II, with IC_{50} values of 0.16, 0.55, 0.17, 2.93, 3.10, and 2.35 μg/mL, respectively. Therefore, topoisomerase II could be a potent target of the six coral extracts.

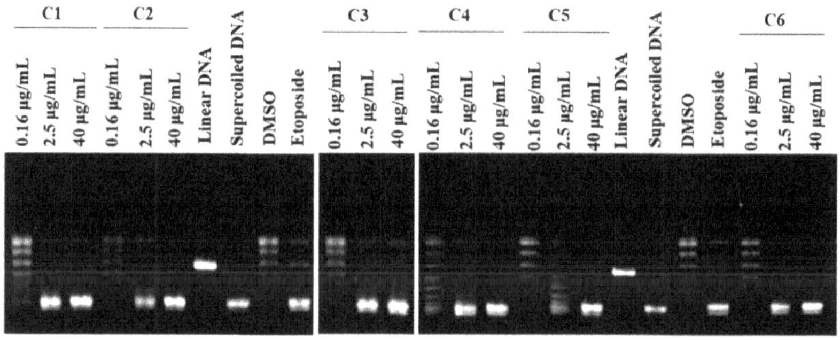

Figure 2. Effects of the six coral extracts (C1–C6) on topoisomerase II activity. Supercoiled DNA was pre-incubated with DNA topoisomerase IIα, and the indicated compounds were added (0.16, 2.5, and 40 μg/mL). After incubation and agarose gel electrophoresis, the bands of linear DNA were analyzed. The result indicated that C1–C6 inhibited TOPO II activity in a dose-dependent manner. Linear and supercoiled DNA were marked. Etoposide was used as the positive control.

2.3. Effects of Different Crude Extracts on HDAC Activity

The inhibition of HDAC is a promising target of cancer therapeutics. We evaluated the effect of six coral extracts on HDAC activity. Treatment with six coral extracts at 10 and 40 μg/mL exhibited moderate inhibition of HDAC, with 0.49 ± 0.07 and 0.35 ± 0.09; 0.83 ± 0.09 and 0.47 ± 0.04; 0.88 ± 0.03 and 0.48 ± 0.02; 0.63 ± 0.09 and 0.48 ± 0.04; 0.82 ± 0.08 and 0.62 ± 0.06; and 0.65 ± 0.06 and 0.55 ± 0.05, respectively. The HDAC inhibitor, trichostatin (TSA), significantly inhibited HDAC activity at 300 μM to 0.24 ± 0.01-fold in comparison with the control (Figure 3). The results indicated that the antiproliferative activity of the six coral extracts does not involve HDAC inhibition. The C6 extract showed a comparable activity to trichostatin at 40 μg/mL.

2.4. Effects of Different Crude Extracts on the Activity of tubulin Polymerization

Taxol, vinca, and colchicine-binding site analogs are therapeutically active anticancer drugs targeting tubulin polymerization [20]. We determined the effects of the six coral extracts on tubulin polymerization. Tubulin polymerization assays are used to study the effects of drugs and proteins on tubulin assembly and measure the ability of tubulin to polymerize into microtubules by observing changes in the optical density at a specific wavelength (OD 350 nm) [27]. As shown in Figure 4, paclitaxel, a classic tubulin-stabilizing agent, induced time-dependent 4.24-, 5.31-, 5.08-, and 4.67-fold tubulin accumulation compared with the control after 5, 10, 15, and 20 min, respectively. In addition, 1.93-, 2.05-, 2.97-, and 2.03-fold tubulin accumulation was also observed in the presence of C4 extract (4 μg/mL) compared with the control after 5, 10, 15, and 20 min, respectively. Nevertheless, the treatment with C1–C3 and C5–C6 extracts (4 μg/mL) decreased tubulin accumulation

0.17-, 0.39-, 0.37-, 0.22-, and 0.19-fold after 5 min. All treatments reached steady-state equilibrium status after 10 min. Less than 1% of tubulin accumulation was observed with the treatment of C5 extract after 10 min. These results indicated that tubulin could be a potent target of the six coral extracts.

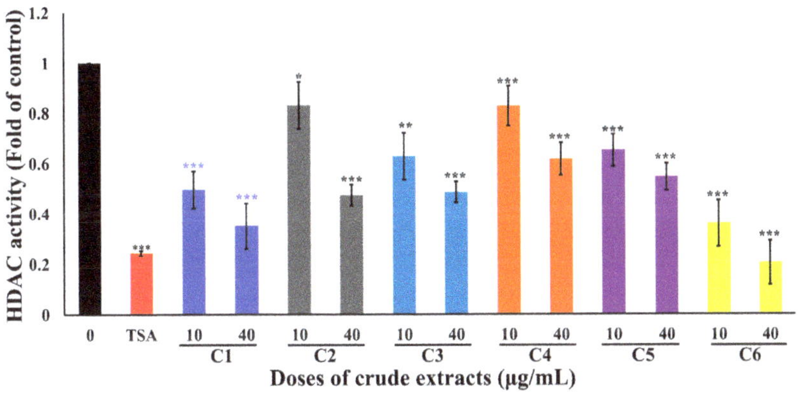

Figure 3. The effect of six coral extracts on histone deacetylase (HDAC) activity in a cell-free system. Trichostatin A (TSA) is a potent reversible inhibitor of HDAC that was used as the positive control. Relative deacetylation of histone was decreased by the treatment with marine organism extracts (10 and 40 μg/mL). (* $p < 0.05$; ** $p < 0.01$; *** $p < 0.005$).

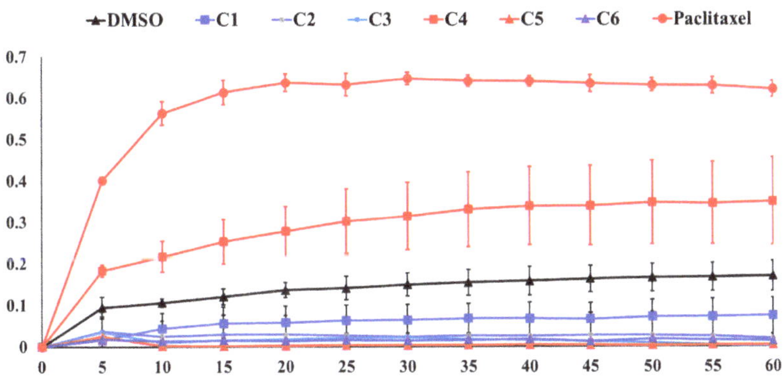

Figure 4. The effects of the coral extracts (4 μg/mL) on the kinetic tubulin polymerization in a cell-free system. Paclitaxel is a tubulin-binding agent and was used as the positive control. The time course of tubulin polymerization and depolymerization at 37 °C was measured in the presence of vehicle (DMSO) or marine organism extracts as indicated. The effect was measured using an ELISA reader at 350 nm. The result indicated that C4 upregulated the level of tubulin polymerization. C1, C2, C3, C5, and C6 upregulated the level of tubulin depolymerization.

2.5. Effect of C5 Extract (LCE) on Cell Growth, Colony Formation, and Apoptosis in Prostate Cancer Cells

Prostate cancer is the fifth leading cause of death in the world, and it is also the second most diagnosed cancer in men, with a high mortality rate. It is usually discovered after being metastasized to other organs, rendering the available treatments ineffective [28]. C5 extract (*Lobophytum crassum* extract, LCE), which showed the most promising antitubulin and antiproliferation activity, was further evaluated against invasive prostate cancer cells using in vitro and in vivo models. The cytotoxic activity of LCE extract was first detected by means of an MTT assay to evaluate its effect on the proliferation of human prostate cancer cells (LNcap, PC3, Du145), and the IC_{50} values were calculated. The results showed that the survival rate of prostate cancer cells decreased when we increased the dose and duration of treatment. The IC_{50} values were 5.70 ± 1.37, 4.14 ± 0.48, and 5.27 ± 2.19 μg/mL after 24 h and 2.76 ± 0.341, 1.92 ± 0.09, and 4.96 ± 0.04 μg/mL at 72 h, respectively (Table 2). Since the MTT results showed that LCE inhibited the growth rate of human prostate cancer cells, the next step was to explore whether different doses of LCE would affect the ability of prostate cancer cells to form colonies under long-term treatment. The results showed that the colony formation of PC3 and Du145, as well as LNCap cells, was significantly decreased at 1.25 μg/mL and 2.5 μg/mL, respectively (Figure 5A). In addition, the apoptosis of LNcap, PC3, and Du145 was dose-dependently induced to 94.5, 92.4, and 57.4% at 10 μg/mL of LCE using flow cytometric analysis (Figure 5B). The results of the Western blotting assay showed that the activation of caspase-3 was increased and the expression of the X-linked inhibitor of apoptosis protein (XIAP) was attenuated at 5 and 10 μg/mL of LCE (Figure 5C). Based on the above results, it can be concluded that LCE could induce apoptosis of prostate cancer cells.

Table 2. Cell growth inhibition of LCE against various prostate cancer cell lines after 24 and 72 h using MTT assay. Values of IC_{50} were calculated using calcuSyn software version 1.1.1.

	Prostate Cencer			Fibroblast
	LNcap	**PC-3**	**Du145**	**CCD966SK**
24 h	5.70 ± 1.37	4.14 ± 0.48	5.27 ± 2.19	>20
72 h	2.76 ± 0.34	1.92 ± 0.09	4.96 ± 0.04	8.21 ± 1.14

2.6. Effect of LCE on Cancer Cellular Invasion Induced with TGFβ

A transwell assay is commonly used to mimic the migration and invasion of cells in organisms. It also demonstrates and analyzes the cells' ability to move in a certain direction in response to various chemoinducers, such as chemokines, growth factors, lipids, or nucleotides [29]. PC3 and Du145 were used to detect the effect of LCE on cell migration and invasion by means of a transwell assay. The migration results showed that the cells' migration to the lower layer of PC3 and Du145 decreased with the increase in the dose of LCE after 48 h of treatment. The quantification graph showed that the migration activity of both PC3 and Du145 cells was significantly reduced with 2.5 μg/mL of LCE (Figure 6A). The quantification graph of the invasion showed that LCE treatment significantly inhibited the invasion of PC3 and Du145. A Western blotting assay was used to investigate the effect of LCE on the expression of EMT-related proteins in PC3 and Du145 cells. The results showed that the adhesion protein E-cadherin, which maintains epithelial cell properties, was increased in PC3 and Du145 following LCE treatment, especially in Du145, and the transcription factor Slug was reduced (Figure 6B). Despite the presence of the protein N-cadherin and the transcription factor Snail in the mesenchymal cells—the hallmark of EMT—E-cadherin was lost, which is an important marker of epithelial cells [30]. LCE showed a potential inhibitory effect against the metastasis and invasion of prostate cancer cells.

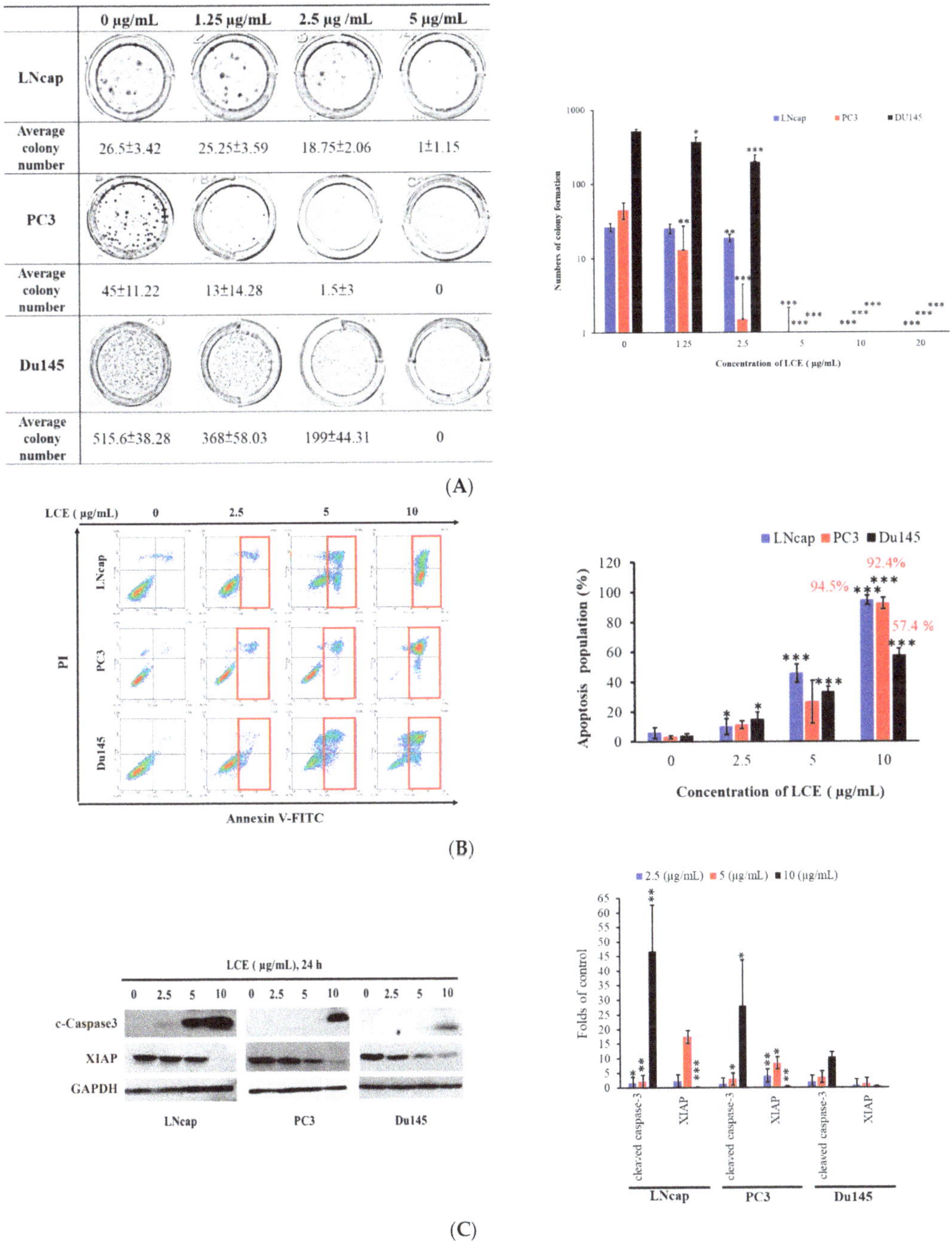

Figure 5. The inhibitory effect of LCE on growth, colony formation, and apoptosis induction in prostate cancer cells. (**A**) Three different cancer cells were treated with different concentrations of LCE in the colony formation assay. (**B**) Apoptosis induction was assessed with annexin-V/PI staining using flow cytometric analysis. (**C**) The expression of apoptosis-regulated proteins was determined

with Western blotting analysis. PCa cells were treated with different doses of LCE for 24 h. Glyceraldehyde-3-phosphate dehydrogenase (GAPDH) was used as the loading control. Quantitative results are presented as means ± SD of three independent experiments (* $p < 0.05$; ** $p < 0.01$; *** $p < 0.005$).

In tumorigenesis and metastasis, the transforming growth factor-β (TGF-β) promotes tumor invasion and metastasis by means of EMT induction [31]. The metastatic invasion activity of the cells is induced by TGF-β. LCE extract was added to detect whether it could influence the transformation of EMT in prostate cancer cells. According to the migration results, LCE treatment (2.5 μg/mL) alone reduced the migration ability in PC3 and Du145 cells, while the number of cell migrations increased by 1.3~1.4 times following TGF-β treatment. The inhibition of cell metastasis was maintained after LCE (2.5 μg/mL) and TGF-β treatment in comparison with the TGF-β group alone. The combined treatment with TGF-β and LCE attenuated metastasis by 46.58% and 79.92% compared with TGF-β treatment, indicating that LCE inhibited metastasis induced by TGF-β treatment. In addition, TGF-β induced an increase in the expression of N-cadherin in prostate cancer cells and decreased the expression of E-cadherin, but it upregulated the performance associated with other EMT biomarkers [32]. LCE treatment reversed the expression of E- and N-cadherin induced by TGF-βin PC3 and Du145 cells, as demonstrated by fluorescent and Western blotting assays, indicating that LCE treatment inhibited the migration and invasion of cancer cells while increasing the expression of E-cadherin and decreasing the expression of N-cadherin (Figure 6D,E).

The proteomic and LC-MS/MS analysis identified six proteins that were changed in LCE-treated PC3 and Du145 cells (Table 3). To verify these proteomic results, a Western blotting assay was used to further determine the expression of six proteins in PC3 and Du145 cells. As shown in Figure 6F, the expression of the six proteins, keratin 1 and 7, dynactin subunit 2 isoform 1 (dynactin 2), proteasome activator compels subunit 1 isoform 1(PSME1), galactoside α-(1,2)-fucosyltransferase 1, and translationally controlled 1 (HRF), was changed in PC3 and Du145 cells after LCE treatment, demonstrating that keratin 1 and 7, dynactin 2, and galactoside α-(1,2)-fucosyltransferase 1 were the principle regulators of the motility and polarity of LCE.

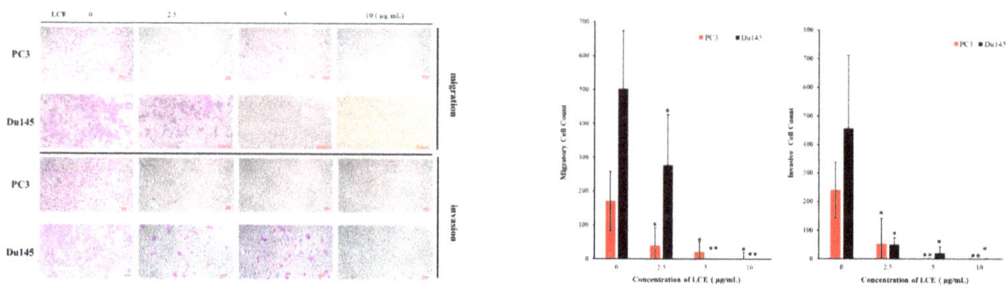

(A)

Figure 6. *Cont.*

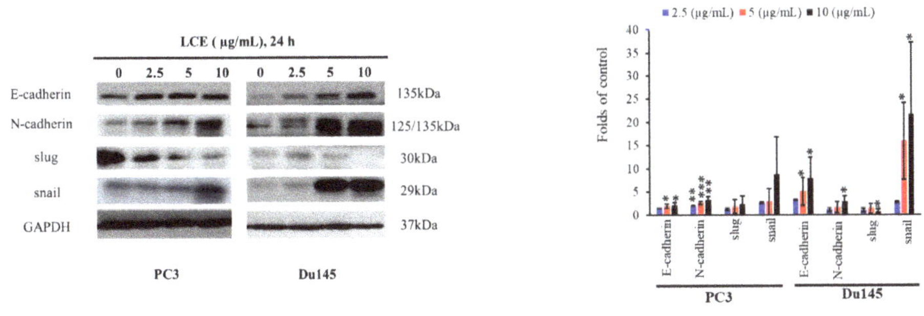

(B)

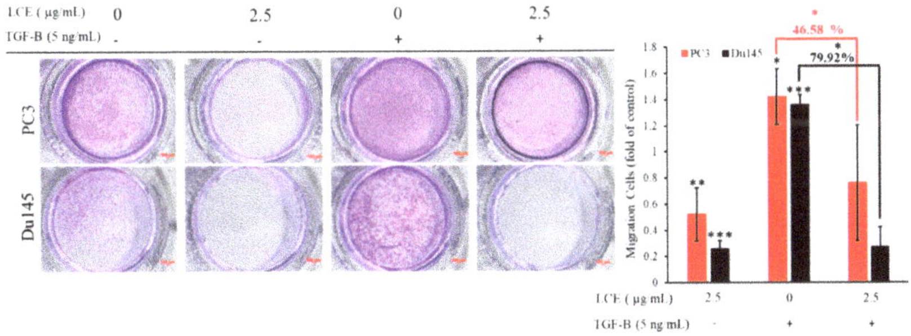

(C)

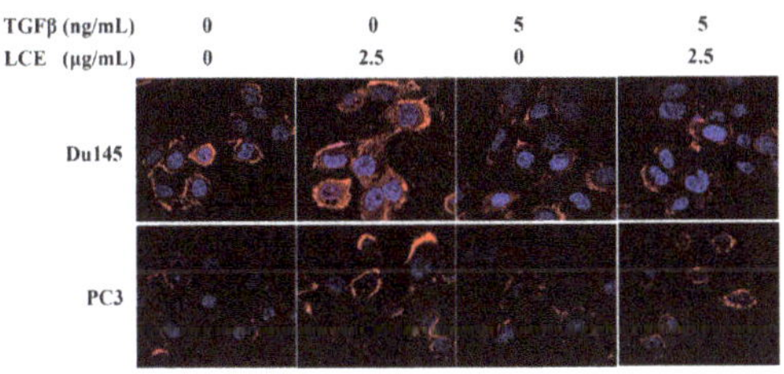

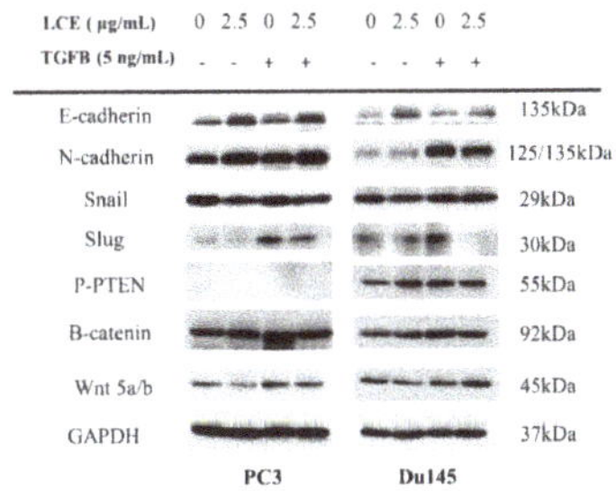

(D)

(E)

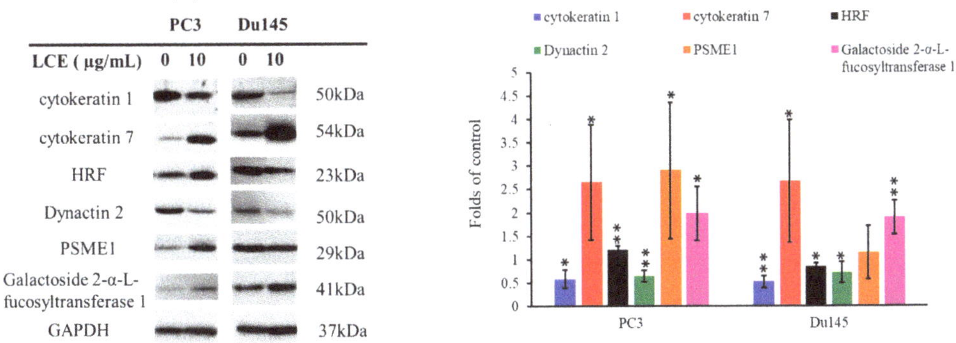

(F)

Figure 6. The effect of LCE on the migration and invasion of prostate cancer PC3 and Du145 cells. (**A**) The effect of LCE on the migration and invasion of PC3 and Du145 cells, demonstrated by transwell assay. Quantitative representation of the migration and invasion cells after LCE treatment for 48 and 72 h. (**B**) LCE treatment reduced EMT-related proteins. The expression of the EMT biomarker was determined with a Western blotting assay. PC3 and Du145 cells were treated with different doses of LCE for 24 h. (**C**) The migration of PC3 and Du145 cells was analyzed by means of a transwell assay. Quantitative representation of migration cells after LCE and TGF-β treatment for 48 h. (**D**) The effect of LCE treatment on the expression of E-cadherin, demonstrated using a fluorescent confocal assay. Scale bar: 10 μm. (**E**) The effect of LCE treatment on the expression of EMT-related biomarkers, detected by Western blotting assay. PC3 and Du145 cells were treated with TGF-β (5 ng/mL) and LCE (2.5 μg/mL) for 24 h. (**F**) The effect of LCE treatment on the expression of targeted proteins, detected with a Western blotting assay. PC3 and Du145 cells were treated with LCE (10 μg/mL) for 6 h. GAPDH was used as the loading control. Scale bar, 100 μm. Quantitative results are presented as means ± SD of three independent experiments (* $p < 0.05$; ** $p < 0.01$; *** $p < 0.005$).

Table 3. Identification of target proteins in PC3 and Du145 treated with LCE by means of proteomic and LC-MS/MS assays.

	Du145		PC3	
Protein	**DMSO**	**LCE**	**DMSO**	**LCE**
Keratin, type II cytoskeletal 7	0.06	0.30	0.53	1.92
Dynactin subunit 2 isoform 1	1.76	1.37	0.53	0.34
Keratin 1	0.61	0.18	1.78	1.44
Proteasome activator complex subunit 1 isoform 1	1.82	1.14	0.60	0.44
Galactoside α-(1,2)-fucosyltransferase 1	0.10	0.66	1.21	2.03
Translationally-controlled 1	0.62	0.49	1.85	1.04

2.7. *Effect of LCE on Gene Profiling*

Next-generation sequencing (NGS) has advanced in the scientific arena in the last few years owing to its high throughput, low cost, scalability, and applicability in different biological disciplines. NGS analyses with FASTQ, HISAT2, FeatureCounts, whole-genome, transcriptome, and exome sequencing were collected and compared with the human reference genome [33]. The volcano plot allowed us to check the differences in the performance of genomes among two groups, as well as the statistical significance of these differences. The X coordinate is a multiple of the difference (fold change) (Figure 7A). Of 16,699 variables, the top 10 target proteins are listed in Table 4. In addition, HMOX1 (heme oxygenase 1, HO-1), HSPA1A (HSP70), and HSPA1B (HSP70) simultaneously increased about 5.56- and 7.46-; 5.10- and 5.58-; and 4.34- and 5.50-fold (Log2FoldChange); however, CXCL1 (C-X-C motif chemokine ligand 1) decreased about 5.35- and 4.30-fold compared with the negative control (Log2FoldChange) in PC3 and Du145 cells, respectively, following LCE treatment (Table 4). Based on the above NGS results, HO-1 and CXCL1 were considered potent regulators of the proliferation inhibition of prostate cancer cells induced by LCE treatment. Gene modification was used to verify the intricate mechanisms by which HO-1 or CXCL1 was involved in the cytotoxic effect of LCE. CXCL1 overexpression experiments revealed that the overexpression of CXCL1 led to an augmented increase in viability by 16% compared with the sole LCE treatment in Du145 cells (Figure 7B). Additionally, SiRNA with HO-1 experiments illuminated that the knockdown of HO-1 led to a significant increase in viability by 7.3% compared with the sole LCE treatment in Du145 cells (Figure 7C). These findings suggested that these two proteins possessed the potential to promote the cytotoxic effect of LCE.

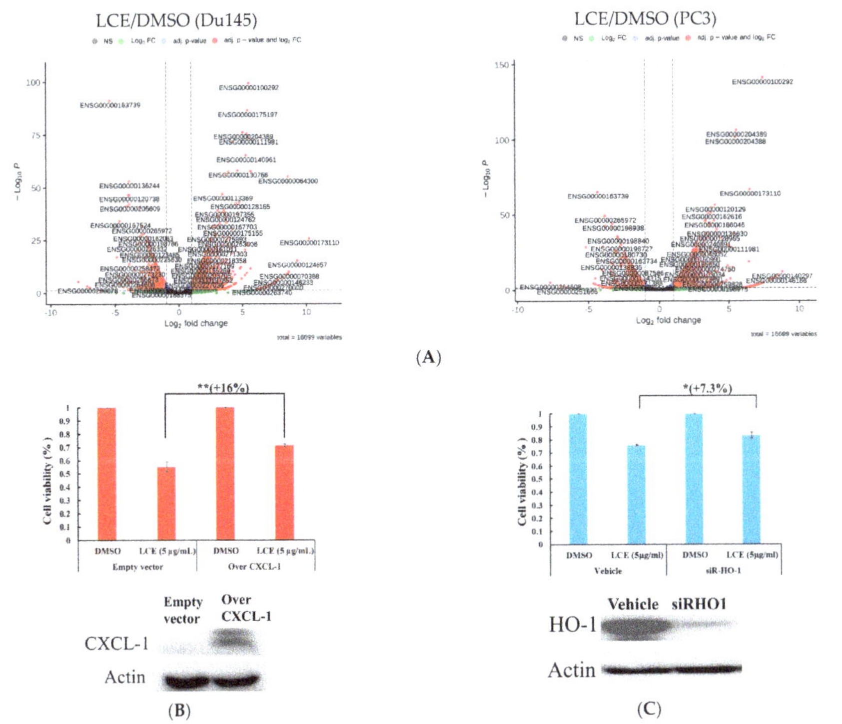

Figure 7. Effect of HO-1 and CXCL1 on the cytotoxic effect of LCE. (**A**) Comparison of genome differences in the two groups of PC3 or Du145 cells treated with LCE using NGS analysis. (**B**,**C**) present the gene modification of CXCL1 (overexpression), and HO-1 (siRNA) was carried out to assess the viability inhibited by LCE treatment. Quantitative results are presented as means ± SD of three independent experiments (* $p < 0.05$; ** $p < 0.01$).

Table 4. Top 10 pharmacological targets of PC3 and Du145 with DMSO and LCE (10 μg/mL) treatment, respectively, using NGS analysis.

PC3 (LCE/DMSO)			Du145 (LCE/DMSO)		
Symbol	**Log^2 Fold Change**	**padj**	**Symbol**	**Log^2 Fold Change**	**padj**
HMOX1	5.56	0	HMOX1	7.46	0
CXCL1	−5.35	0	HSPA1A	5.58	0
DDIT3	5.46	0	HSPA1B	5.50	0
HSPA1A	5.10	0	HSPA6	6.53	0
ATF3	5.41	0	CXCL1	−4.30	0
ULBP1	5.52	0	DUSP1	4.04	0
HSPA1B	4.34	0	BAG3	3.79	0
OSGIN1	5.34	0	DNAJB4	3.76	0
SESN0	4.69	0	DNAJB1	3.54	0
CHAC1	5.7	0	TXNIP	−3.79	0

Heme oxygenase 1 (HMOX1); C-X-C motif chemokine ligand 1 (CXCL1); DNA damage inducible transcript 3 (DDIT3); heat shock protein family A (Hsp70) member 1A (HSPA1); activating transcription factor 3 (ATF3); UL16 binding protein 1 (ULBP1); heat shock protein family A (Hsp70) member 1B (HSPA1B); oxidative stress-induced growth inhibitor 1 (OSGIN1); Sestrin 2 (SESN0); ChaC glutathione-specific gamma-glutamylcyclotransferase 1 (CHAC1); heat shock protein family A (Hsp70) member 6 (HSPA6); dual-specificity phosphatase 1 (DUSP1); BAG cochaperone 3 (BAG3); DnaJ heat shock protein family (Hsp40) member B4 (DNAJB4); DnaJ heat shock protein family (Hsp40) member B1 (DNAJB1); thioredoxin interacting protein (TXNIP).

2.8. 13 Acetoxysarcocrassolide Is the Active Component of LCE and a Potential Candidate for Tubulin Inhibition

Compared with the 1H NMR spectra of 13-acetoxysarcocrossolide (13-AC), the NMR spectra of LCE showed the characteristic signals of 13-AC, including a tertiary methyl group [δ_H 2.0, (3H-13OAc, s)], olefinic protons at C-17 [δ_H 5.60 (1H, d, J = 2 Hz) and 6.24 (1H, 99 d, J = 2 Hz)], and methine proton at C-14 [δ_H 4.58, (1H, t, J = 2.4 Hz)] in α-methyl-γ-lactone ring [34]. Additionally, the HPLC chromatogram of LCE showed a major peak at 39.847 min, coinciding with the retention time of 13-AC (Figure 8A,B). These findings suggested that 13-AC was the major component in the LCE, as demonstrated by the bioactivity-guided fraction.

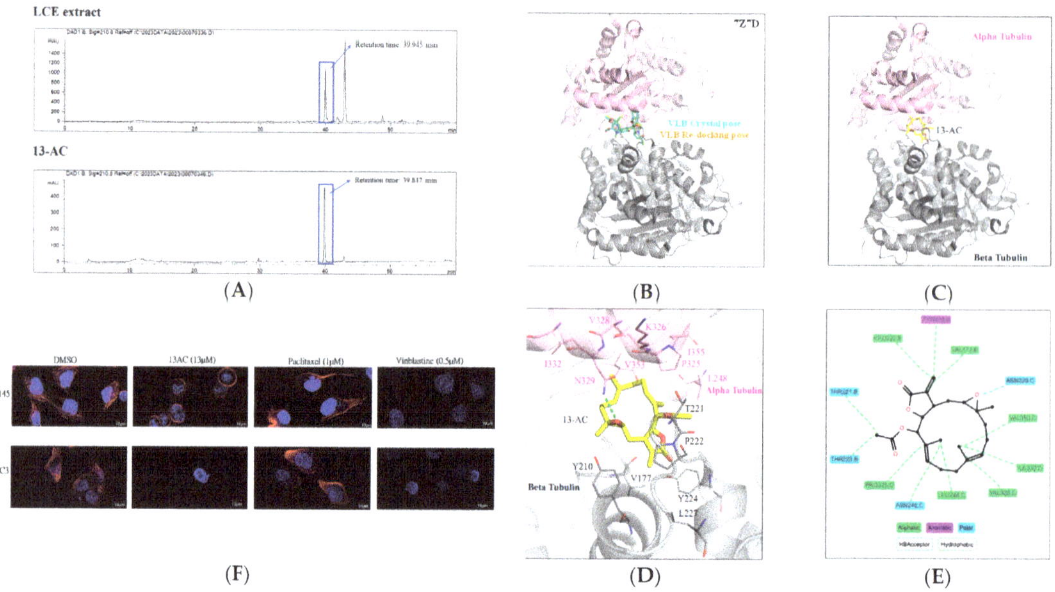

Figure 8. The effect of 13-AC on tubulin depolymerization as demonstrated by means of immunofluorescent and molecular docking assays. (**A**) The HPLC chromatogram of LCE (upper) and 13-AC (lower). (**B–E**) Identification of 13-AC on the interaction of αβtubulins with 2D/3D molecular ducking assay. (**F**) The effect of paclitaxel, vinblastine, and 13-AC on tubulin network according to immunofluorescent staining with confocal examination.

LCE treatment interfered with the tubulin polymerization and disrupted the cytoskeletal network (Figures 4 and 6F and Table 3). To determine protein–ligand interactions that may indicate the potency of, a docking analysis was performed. Vinblastine served as the co-crystal ligand and was redocked to validate the docking procedure used in the study. The docking pose of vinblastine was similar to the crystal pose, suggesting that a reliable docking procedure was used (Figure 8B). The docking result showed that 13-AC can occupy the binding site, which is sandwiched by the alpha and beta tubulins (Figure 8C). Several interactions with the alpha-tubulin were observed (Figure 8D). A hydrogen bond was formed between 13-AC and the side chain of N329 (Figure 8E). As a ring structure, 13-AC facilitated the hydrophobic interactions with residues L248, N249, P325, V328, I332, and V353 located on the alpha-tubulin. The beta tubulin residues V177, Y210, T221, P222, and T223 supplied the additional hydrophobic interactions (Figure 8E). Together, these interactions sandwiched 13-AC within the tubulin-binding site. The identified interactions would be favorable for 13-AC occupation and could potentially result in the inhibition of tubulin polymerization. Moreover, we further examined the integrity of the cytoskeletal microtubules in PC3 and Du145 treated with 13-AC (10 μg/mL; 13 μM) for 6 h with an immunofluorescent assay. Paclitaxel and vinblastine were the positive polymerization and depolymerization agents of tubulin, respectively. The Du145 and PC3 cells of the control group showed the normal structure of microtubulins. Du145 and PC3 treated with paclitaxel possessed a cluster-like phenomenon of microtubulin; conversely, the cells with 13-AC or vinblastine treatment showed a clear outer edge around the cell nucleus, or the microtubulins disappeared (Figure 8F). The results of the molecular docking assay indicated that 13-AC binds to the same site as vinblastine at 7Z7D of αβ-tubulins, suggesting its potential anti-microtubulin effects by disrupting the equilibrium of the tubulin–microtubulin system and ultimately leading to microtubule depolymerization. SwissADME is a web tool designed for the evaluation of the drug-likeness and pharmacokinetic and medicinal chemistry-related properties of small molecules. It is particularly useful in the early stages of drug discovery to assess whether a compound has the necessary characteristics to become a viable drug candidate. SwissADME provides various predictions and analyses, including physicochemical properties, drug-likeness, pharmacokinetics, and medicinal chemistry parameters [35]. As shown in Table 5, 13-AC demonstrated greater potential in drug development, as it could form favorable chemical bonds with the characteristic of small molecules compared with vinblastine. Gastrointestinal absorption (GIA) and water solubility analysis indicated that 13-AC will be highly absorbed in the gastrointestinal tract and more water-soluble than vinblastine. Combined with its high bioavailability score of 13-AC (0.55), the potential of developing 13-AC for oral administration was suggested, indicating that a larger portion of the administered dose reaches the systemic circulation intact [36]. Additionally, 13-AC is not a substrate for the five major isoforms of cytochrome P (CYP) enzymes. This suggests that it may have reduced toxicity and fewer adverse drug reactions compared to vinblastine, which could be metabolized by these enzymes [37,38]. Moreover, the synthetic accessibility (SA) of 13-AC (5.66) is lower than vinblastine (9.65), and it does not trigger any PAINS 0#Alert, suggesting a solution to synthetic challenges regarding insufficient coral sources and making it suitable for lead optimization. Based on these points, it is suggested that 3-AC holds more potential for development as an oral anticancer drug compared with vinblastine due to its favorable pharmacokinetic and chemical properties.

Table 5. Pharmacokinetic and drug-likeness predictions of vinblastine and 13-AC with SwissADME.

	MW	Water Solubility	GIA	BBB	Log K_p	Bioavailability Score	PAINS#alerts	Synthetic Accessibility
Vinblastine	810.97	Poorly	Low	No	−8.49	0.17	0	9.65
13-AC	374.47	Soluble	High	Yes	−6.39	0.55	0	5.66

2.9. Effect of LCE on Tumor Growth in Xenograft Human PC3 and Du145 Model

The above results showed that LCE had a cytotoxic effect on prostate cancer cells (Figure 5A–C), so the impact of LCE on the growth of PC3 and Du145 tumors in xenograft animals was further investigated. PC3 and Du145 cells were injected subcutaneously into the upper right thigh of immunodeficient nude mice until the tumor volume was about 100 mm^3, and the DMSO or LCE extract was injected intraperitoneally (the dose was PC3: 5 μg/g, Du145: 12 μg/g), and the drug was administered three times a week for 38 days. Comparing the differences between the control group and the LCE extract treatment group, it was found that there was no significant difference between the two groups (Figure 9A). The tumor volume of PC3 and Du145 was about 537.4 ± 141.7 and 434.3 ± 110.5 mm^3 in the control groups; however, the volumes were 301.4 ± 73.7 and 220.2 ± 87.3 mm^3 in the LCE group (Figure 9B). The pathological examination of tumor sections in the control groups showed that the cancer cells appeared as round-to-spindly epithelial cells and had a high nucleic/cytoplasm ratio with high mitosis (arrow) in both the control groups of

PC3 and Du145 xenograft tumors (Figure 9C). The results of the microscopic examination showed that there were no obvious pathological changes in the heart, kidney, liver, lungs, spleen, and other tissues and organs (Figure 9D).

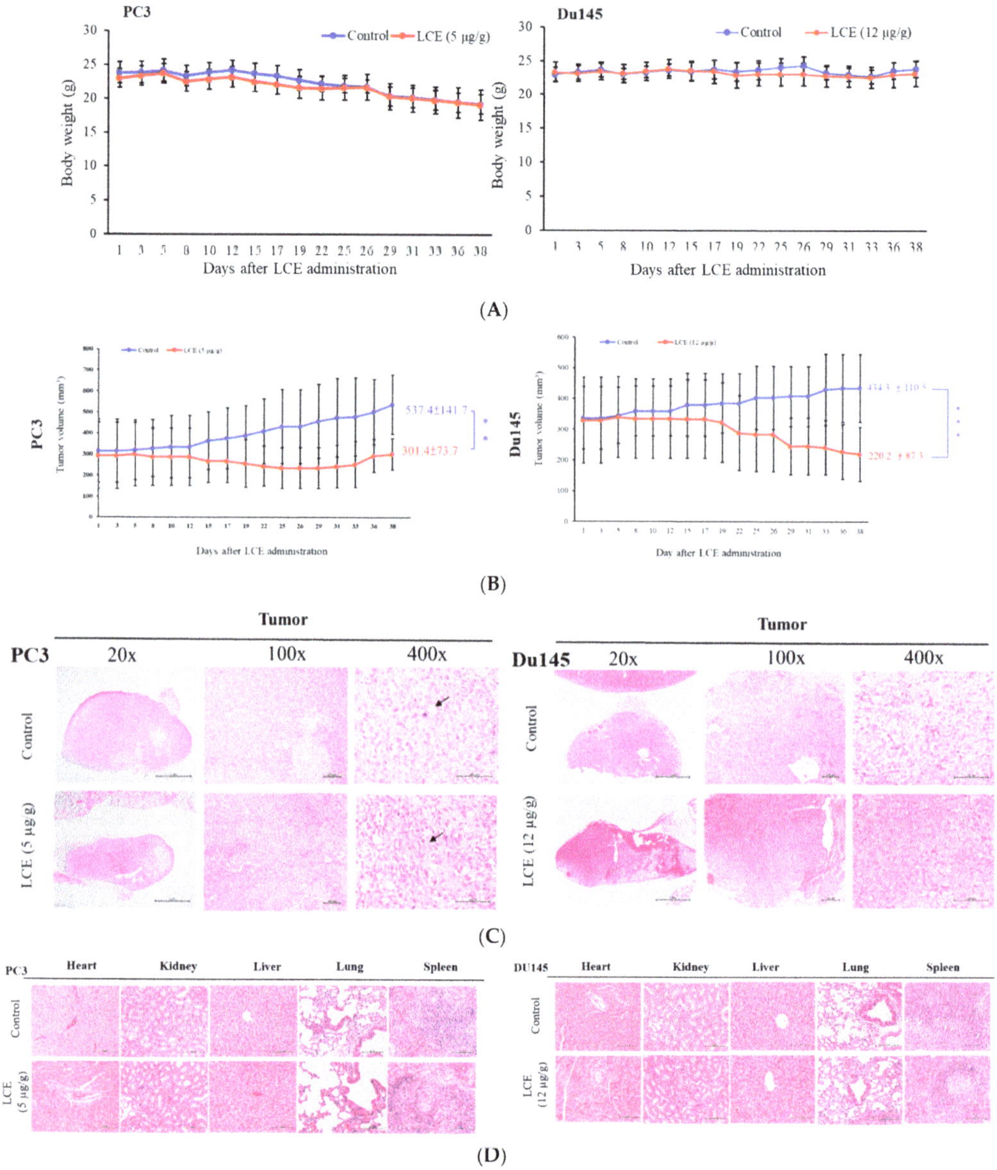

Figure 9. The impact of LCE on tumor growth of PC3 and DU145 in a xenograft model. Tumor-bearing nude mice were fed with solvent control (DMSO), LCE (5 μg/g), and (12 μg/g) for 38 days. (**A**) The body weight and (**B**) tumor volumes were measured every two to three days. Data are shown as mean ± SD. (**C**) Histopathologic features of mice xenograft tumors. Tumor cells expressed round-to-spindly epithelial cells and a high nucleic/cytoplasm ratio with high mitosis (arrow) in both groups. (**D**) No significant lesions of the heart, kidneys, liver, lungs, and spleen were found in either group using H&E staining analysis (400×). (** $p < 0.01$; *** $p < 0.005$).

3. Discussion

Marine natural products hold the potential for drug development, but the supply of marine organisms is a major obstacle to the development of marine natural drugs. Although the problem of drug origin can be solved through chemical synthesis technology, the structure of marine natural substances is complex and diverse, and the use of chemically synthesized compounds does not expand chemical diversity. Aquaculture could provide a good growth environment for soft corals, produce active ingredients, and reduce our dependence on marine environments. We have successfully cultivated a large number of corals using artificial breeding systems to establish a drug-derived coral species database, and in 2023, over 180 species of drug-source corals had been collected, which can be mainly divided into six genera, including *Sinularia*, *Lobophytum*, *Sarcophyton*, *Briareidae*, *Capnella*, and *Xenia*. We screened over 180 extracts of artificial aquaculture soft corals and found that 6 extracts exhibited potent cytotoxicity against leukemia cells at a dose of 10 μg/mL (Table 1). In this study, we demonstrated that these corals possessed anticancer active substances by targeting HDAC, topoisomerase II, and tubulin polymerization within the cell-free system (Figures 2–4). Therefore, exploring effective therapeutic agents from marine natural products has significant potential.

Metastasis is the leading cause of cancer-related mortality [39], and when cancer cells metastasize to other organs, they need to destroy and cross the basal membrane to metastasize to the adjacent tissues and organs. They also need to invade the extracellular matrix and penetrate the blood vessels to flow with the blood. Our study was performed on more malignant androgen-independent cells, PC3 and Du145. The wound healing and transwell tests confirmed that LCE extract had a very significant inhibitory effect on cell migration and invasion (Figure 6A,B). EMT, on the other hand, is a cellular program in which epithelial cells develop the motor and invasion characteristics that are typical of mesenchymal cells, which is an important initiation of cancer progression, invasion, and metastasis [40]. Therefore, EMT is more important in the process of prostate cancer development. During the EMT process, a series of intracellular proteins are altered, including a decrease in the expression of E-cadherin and an increase in the expression of N-cadherin. Unlike E-cadherin, N-cadherin binds loosely to each other, resulting in cell movement t [40]. On the other hand, during EMT, the cytoskeleton and protein complexes change, which affects cell polarity. In this process, the composition of the intermediate filaments is altered by decreasing cytokeratin and increasing vimentin, which in turn leads to cell motility [41,42]. However, the main initiation signal of EMT is certainly represented by the downregulation of E-cadherin, the expression that decreases during EMT, while the loss of function of this protein promotes this transition. Transcriptional repression of E-cadherin has been considered a critical step during EMT [43]. Combined with the significant anti-metastasis and -invasion effects, LCE may have good potential for anti-prostate cancer cell metastasis.

Transforming growth factor β (TGF-β) is a secreted cytokine that is well known for its role as an EMT inducer [44]. In addition, TGF-β promotes tumor cell motility, survival, invasion, and metastasis and the evasion of immune p53 signaling in advanced cancer cells [44]. Therefore, TGF-β was used as an inducer of EMT to promote the expression of excess EMT in this study. The results of the transwell assay showed that the migration transfer ability of PC3 and Du145 was induced under the action of TGF-β, and the migration transfer of both cell lines was significantly inhibited by LCE after treatment with this extract (2.5 μg/mL) and TGF-β at the same time. The inhibition effect of LCE was not reduced by the addition of TGF-β, indicating that LCE still inhibited the metastasis induced by TGF-β in prostate cancer cells with the enhancement of E-cadherin (Figure 6C,D). A possible factor in previous studies suggested a differential effect of TGF-β on Du145 and PC3 cell activation might be related to phosphatase and tensin homologs (PTEN) in the PI3-kinase/AKT pathway, which inhibits PI3-kinase-dependent AKT phosphorylation. In contrast, PTEN has been shown to mutate in many cancers, which can lead to increased levels of pAKT ^{ser473} expression and increased cell survival [45]. In addition, PTEN was active in Du145 cells but inactive in PC3 cells [46,47], and the protein results also showed that PC3 did not express PTEN protein, while Du145 showed the obvious expression of PTEN protein and increased its expression under LCE (Figure 6E), so it was speculated that TGF-β-induced AKT phosphorylation could not be inhibited by PTEN in PC3 cells. TGF-β showed a more obvious effect on the induction of PC3 cells [48].

Based on the results of the 2D protein analysis, six target proteins which LCE possibly affects were screened (Table 3). Keratin 7 and galactoside alpha-(1,2)-fucosyltransferase 1 were increased in PC3 and Du145 treated with LCE (10 μg/mL), and the protein expression of the two cell lines was also consistently increased following treatment with LCE (Figure 6F). Among them, keratin 7 is a type II keratin in cells, a type II intermediate filament (IF) that forms the cytoskeleton in the cytoplasm, which is present in all mammalians epithelial cells and is specifically expressed in epithelial cells in the lumen of internal organs, as well as in glandular ducts and blood vessels. Keratin is an important protein that protects the structural integrity of the epithelial under stress and is thought to be a regulator of many cellular properties and functions, including apical–basal polarization, motility, cell size, protein synthesis, and membrane trafficking and signaling. In cancer cells, keratin is widely used as a diagnostic tumor marker, because epithelial malignancies largely maintain specific keratin patterns associated with the cells of origin, such as lung, adrenocortical, prostate, and liver cancer, which are negative for keratin 7 and keratin 20 [49]. In addition, previous studies indicated that active keratin is involved in cancer cell invasion and metastasis and treatment [50], so the altered keratin expression caused by LCE may in turn affect the physiology of prostate cancer cells, especially in terms of cancer cell invasion and metastasis. Another increased protein is galactoside alpha-(1,2)-fucosyltransferase 1, which is a protease that catalyzes chemical reactions in physiology and participates in cell metabolism-related reactions, and it has been pointed out that the increase in galactoside alpha-(1,2)-fucosyltransferase 1 can inhibit the metastasis of pancreatic cancer cells by regulating glycoproteins [51]. Dynactin subunit 2 is a multi-subunit protein complex that is essential for the movement of cytoplasmic dynein. It binds to microtubules and cytoplasmic dynein in cells and is involved in a variety of cellular functions, including the transport from the ER to the Golgi apparatus, centripetal movement of lysosomes and endosomes, spindle formation, chromosome movement, nuclear localization, and axonogenesis [52]. Thus, it is interesting to mention that LCE exhibited a potent efficiency in terms of EMT and inhibition invasion of prostate cancer cells, with disruption of the cytoskeleton.

With NGS analysis, the result of the volcano plots showed that the important regulators, HO1 and CLCX1, had a consistent effect in PC3 and Du145 cells with LCE treatment (Figure 7A). CXCL1, also known as GROα (growth-regulated oncogene alpha), is a chemokine that plays a role in inflammation and immune responses. In the context of cancer, CXCL1 has been implicated in various aspects of tumor progression and metastasis, making it a potential target for anticancer therapies [53]. CXCL1 can promote tumor growth by stimulating the proliferation of cancer cells. Additionally, it plays a role in angiogenesis, the process by which new blood vessels are formed to supply nutrients and oxygen to tumors. Inhibiting CXCL1 signaling can therefore impede tumor growth and reduce the tumor's ability to access essential nutrients [54]. However, this chemokine is involved in the recruitment of immune cells to the tumor microenvironment, where it can promote tumor cell migration and invasion. By targeting CXCL1 or its receptors, it may be possible to inhibit these processes, thereby preventing cancer cells from spreading to other parts of the body [55]. Given its involvement in multiple aspects of tumor progression and metastasis, CXCL1 has emerged as a potential therapeutic target in cancer treatment. Strategies aimed at inhibiting CXCL1 signaling include the use of monoclonal antibodies, small-molecule inhibitors, and gene therapy approaches. These therapies are being investigated in preclinical studies and clinical trials to assess their safety and efficacy in cancer patients [56]. In this study, the overexpression of CXCL1 reduced viability with 16% in LCE-treated Du145 cells (Figure 7B). In summary, CXCL1 plays a multifaceted role in cancer progression and metastasis, making it an attractive target for anticancer therapies. By inhibiting CXCL1 signaling, it may be possible to impede tumor growth, metastasis, and immune suppression, ultimately improving patient outcomes in various types of cancer. The regulation of heme oxygenase-1 (HO-1), also called heat shock protein 32, plays a significant role in cancer therapy due to its role in cellular responses to oxidative stress and inflammation, especially for detoxification and protection [57]. In addition, the enhancement of HO-1 expression suppressed the growth in androgen-dependent LNCap and androgen-independent PC3 and Du145 cells [58]. The knockdown of HO-1 reversed viability with 7.3% in LCE-treated Du145 cells (Figure 7C). Several studies indicated that HO-1 could be a notable therapeutic target in PCa [59,60]. Both HO-1 and CXCL1 play complex and interconnected roles in cancer progression and represent promising targets for anticancer therapies. Understanding the interplay between these factors and their contributions to the tumor microenvironment is crucial for the development of effective treatment strategies that can disrupt tumor growth, metastasis, and immune evasion in cancer.

Tubulin polymerization, the process by which tubulin proteins assemble into microtubules, plays a crucial role not only in cell division but also in cell migration and invasion, particularly in the context of cancer metastasis. The disruption of tubulin polymerization can impair cell polarization and inhibit efficient migration and invasion [61]. In addition, tubulin polymerization can influence various signaling pathways that regulate cell migration and invasion. For instance, microtubule dynamics can affect the activity and localization of signaling molecules such as Rho GTPases, which play key roles in cytoskeletal rearrangements and cell motility. The disruption of tubulin polymerization can alter the activation of these signaling pathways, impacting cancer cell migration and invasion. Targeting tubulin polymerization and microtubule dynamics has therapeutic implications for cancer metastasis [62]. Microtubule-targeting agents (MTAs), such as taxanes and vinca alkaloids, disrupt tubulin polymerization and inhibit cancer cell proliferation [63,64]. The result of our bioactivity-guided fractionation substantiated that 13-AC was the active component in LCE by means of NMR and HPLC identification (Figure 8A) [34], and we targeted alpha and beta tubulins to disrupt the tubulin dynamics using molecular ducking analysis and confocal examination (Figure 8B–E). Specifically, a hydrogen bond is formed between 13-AC and the side chain of the amino acid N329. Hydrogen bonds are important in molecular recognition and the stabilization of protein–ligand complexes. The ring structure of 13-AC allows it to engage in hydrophobic interactions with specific residues on the alpha-tubulin subunit. These residues (L248, N249, P325, V328, I332, and V353) likely have hydrophobic side chains that can interact favorably with the hydrophobic regions of the ligand. In addition to interacting with alpha-tubulin, 13-AC also engages in hydrophobic interactions with residues on the beta-tubulin subunit (V177, Y210, T221, P222, and T223). These interactions contribute to the overall stability of the protein–ligand complex. Overall, this interaction between 13-AC and tubulin subunits suggests a potential mechanism for the binding of 13-AC to tubulin, which could have implications for drug design or understanding the biological effects of 13-AC. Finally, SwissADME is a web tool developed by the Swiss Institute of Bioinformatics for the prediction of the pharmacokinetic properties and drug-likeness of small molecules [35]. When examining 13-AC (13-acetoxysarcocrassolide) using SwissADME, the tool provides insights into its pharmacokinetic properties and drug-likeness. By comprehensively analyzing these factors, researchers can assess the overall potential of 13-AC as an oral anticancer drug compared to vinblastine. This evaluation provides insights into its suitability for further development and optimization in drug discovery programs.

4. Materials and Methods

4.1. Cell Lines, Chemicals, and Biological Materials

The cell lines, leukemia cells (K562 and Molt4), prostate cancer cells (Du145 and PC3), and normal fibroblasts (CCD-966SK) were purchased from the American Type Culture Collection (ATCC, Manassas, VA, USA). Cells were incubated in a 5% Co2 humidified atmosphere at 37 °C. RPMI 1640 was the growing medium for Molt 4. Minimum essential medium was the growing medium for CCD-966SK, K 562, and Du145. Ham's F-12 medium was the growing medium for PC3. Glutamine (2 mM), antibiotics (100 μg/mL of streptomycin and 100 units/mL of penicillin), and 10% fetal calf serum (FCS) were used to supplement the growing medium. RPMI 1640, minimum essential medium, Ham's F-12 medium, glutamine, antibiotics (streptomycin and penicillin), and FCS were obtained from GibcoBRL (Gaithersburg, MD, USA). 3-(4,5-Dimethylthiazol-2-yl)-2,5-Diphenyltetrazolium Bromide (MTT), dimethyl sulfoxide (DMSO), bovine serum albumin (BSA), and all other chemicals were purchased from Sigma-Aldrich (St. Louis, MO, USA). Antibodies against Slug, snail, p-PTEN, XIAP, and HO-1 were purchased from Santa Cruz Biotechnology (Santa Cruz, CA, USA). Anti E-Cadherin and N-Cadherin antibodies were obtained from ABclonal Technology (Taipei, Taiwan). Antibodies against cleaved caspases-3, cytokeraton 1 and 7, HRF, dynactin 2, PSME, and galactoside 2-α-L fucosynltransferase 1 were obtained from Cell Signaling Technologies (Beverly, MA, USA). HRP-conjugated anti-mouse and anti-rabbit antibodies were harvested from Molecular Probes (Eugene, OR). 4′,6-diamidino-2-phenylindole (DAPI) and fluorescence-conjugate anti-rabbit antibody were bought from Invitrogen technologies (Carlsbad, CA, USA). The topoisomerase II drug screening kit, HDAC activity assay kit (Fluorometric), and tubulin polymerization assay kit were purchased fromTopoGen, Inc (Port Orange, FL, USA), Abcam (Cambridge, UK) and Cytoskeleton (Denver, CO, USA), respectively. Cell Tubulin Staining Kit was obtained from AAT Bioquest (Pleasanton, CA, USA).

4.2. *Preparation of Coral Extracts*

The soft coral was first freeze-dried and then finely ground into powder. The powder was subsequently extracted with ethyl acetate using a weight-to-volume ratio of 1:10 at room temperature for 2 h. This extraction process was repeated three times. The resulting extracts were combined and concentrated under reduced pressure to yield the ethyl acetate extract.

4.3. *In Vitro Proliferation Assay*

Cancer cells were seeded into individual wells of a 96-well plate at a density of 7×10^4 cells/well for Du145 and PC3 and 2×10^5 cells/well for CCD-966SK, Du145, and PC3 in various media conditions. Following treatment with extracts, the cells were incubated for 24, 48, or 72 h. After the respective incubation periods, 50 μL of MTT solution was added to each well for staining. The plates were further incubated at 37 °C for 2–4 h. Absorbance readings at 570 nm and 620 nm were obtained using an ELISA reader (Anthoslabtec instrument, Salzburg, Austria). The IC_{50} value, representing the concentration causing 50% inhibition of cell viability, was subsequently calculated based on these absorbance measurements.

4.4. *Western Blotting Assay*

Equal amounts of protein were separated by means of electrophoresis on 10%, 12%, or 15% SDS-PAGE gels and then electrotransferred to PVDF membranes. The membranes were blocked for 30 min with 5% blocking serum in TBS-T buffer. Specific primary antibodies were then applied, followed by specific secondary antibodies to detect protein expression using an enhanced chemiluminescence kit (Pierce, Rockford, IL, USA).

4.5. *Network Pharmacology with RNASeq Analysis*

The total RNA was purified with TruSeq Stranded mRNA Library Prep kit (Illumina, San Diego, CA, USA). A series of sequencings of FastP [65], SortMeRNA [66], HISAT2 [67] and featureCounts [68] were conducted, and further, an array of DGE, GSEA, WGCNA, and function enrichment was used to determine differences in gene expression in the biological process, molecular function, and cellular component (GENOMICS, Taipei, Taiwan).

4.6. Activities of HDAC, Topoisomerase II, and Tubulin Polymerization in Cell-Free System

4.6.1. Assay of HDAC Activity in Cell-Free System

According to the manufacturer's protocol (BPS Biosciences, San Diego, CA, USA), the extracts (including the carboxylic and hydroxamic acids) were screened for their pan-HDAC-inhibitory activity using an HDAC inhibitor drug screening kit. Different concentrations of the extracts were applied, and the samples were incubated for 30 min at 37 °C to assess the deacetylation of the substrate, which sensitized it. The reaction was halted by means of treatment with 10 μL of lysine developer, and the mixture was further incubated for 30 min at 37 °C to generate a chromophore. Fluorescence measurements were then taken using a spectrofluorometer (Biotek synergy, Winooski, VT, USA) at excitation = 350–380 nm and emission = 440–460 nm.

4.6.2. Assay of Topoisomerase II Activity in Cell-Free System

The assay was performed following the manufacturer's protocol [14,16] and a standard relaxation reaction mix (20 μL) was utilized. This mix contained 50 mM Tris-HCl (pH 8.0), 10 mM MgCl, 200 mM potassium glutamate, 10 mM dithiothreitol, 50 μg/mL bovine serum albumin, 1 mM ATP, 0.3 μg of pHOT1 plasmid DNA, 8 units of human topo II (Topogen, Columbus, OH, USA), and either etoposide (10 mM) or various concentrations of coral extracts. The reaction was carried out at 37 °C for 30 min. The termination of the reaction was achieved by adding 2 μL of 10% SDS, followed by digestion of the bound protein with 2.5 μL of proteinase K (50 μg/mL) and incubation at 37 °C for 15 min. Subsequently, the DNA product was analyzed by means of electrophoresis on a vertical 2% agarose gel at 2 volts/cm in 0.5× TAE buffer, and images were captured using the Eagle Eye II system (Stratagene, La Jolla, CA, USA).

4.6.3. Assay of Tubulin Polymerization in Cell-Free System

According to the manufacturer's protocol, the extracts (including the carboxylic and hydroxamic acids) were screened for tubulin polymerization. Tubulin protein was incubated with GTP and fluorescent-labeled tubulin in a reaction buffer containing 80 mM PIPES (pH 6.8), 1 mM EGTA, 2 mM $MgCl_2$, and 1 mM GTP. The reaction was initiated by adding tubulin to the buffer and monitored over time using a spectrofluorometer (Biotek synergy, Winooski, VT, USA) at excitation/emission wavelengths of 360/420 nm. Changes in fluorescence intensity indicated polymerization activity, which was analyzed to determine the effects of various extracts on microtubule assembly.

4.7. Two-Dimensional Electrophoresis

The cell lysate was precipitated by adding 0.11 g of TCA per 1 mL of acetone (TCA solution) and 20 mM DTT, followed by incubation in a −20 °C freezer for 30 min. The precipitate was then washed twice with TCA solution (supernatant removed by means of centrifugation at 12,000 rpm) and air-dried. Next, the sample was rehydrated with rehydration buffer and incubated at 4 °C overnight. After quantification, 125 μL of the sample was taken for isoelectric focusing (IEF). Following IEF, the strip was rinsed with water and then equilibrated in SDS equilibration buffer (containing 0.5 g DTT) for 15 min. The strip was placed on an SDS-PAGE gel, sealed with 0.5% agarose sealing solution, and subjected to two-dimensional electrophoresis. Finally, the proteins were visualized by means of silver staining.

4.8. Plasmid and siRNA Transfection

Empty vector (EV) pCMV6-AC-GFP and human CXCL1- pCMV6-AC-GFP plasmids (Origene; Rockville, MD, USA) were used for transfection. Cells were grown in a 10 cm dish (2×10^6 cells/dish) for 24 h before transfection, and 5 μg of EV or Human CXCL1-pCMV6-AC-GFP plasmids was transfected using a Lipofectamine 3000 transfection reagent (Invitrogen) following the manufacturer's instructions. After 30 h of transfection, cells were harvested and plated in 96-well culture plates (7000 cells/well) and 10cm dishes

(1×10^6 cells). Cells were treated with LCE for viability analysis and Western blotting after 24h. For siRNA transfection, control siRNA and human HO-1 siRNA were purchased from Origene (Rockville, MD, USA). Cells were seeded at a density of 1.5×10^5 cells/mL in a growth medium for 24 h. Cells were transfected with Lipofectamine RNAiMAX reagent following the manufacturer's protocol. At 48 h after transfection, cells were subcultured and seeded in 96-well culture plates (7000 cells/well) and 10 cm dishes (2×10^6 cells). After 24 h, cells were treated with LCE for viability analysis and Western blotting.

4.9. Immunostaining Confocal Examination

The cells were seeded 7×10^4 cells/mL into 12-well culture plates, and each well had a sterile circular coverslip in the growth medium. After 24 h, cells were treated with DMSO, LCE 2.5 µg/mL, LCE 2.5 µg/mL + TGF-α 5 ng/mL, and TGF-α 5 ng/mL, respectively, for 6 h, followed by immunostaining. For immunostaining and confocal imaging, the cells were rinsed with PBS, followed by fixation with 1% paraformaldehyde for 30 min at room temperature on a shaker. Then, the cells were rinsed three times with PBS and incubated in 0.1% Triton X-100 in PBS for 15 min. The cells were incubated in 300 µL of 1% BSA (bovine serum albumin) (Sigma-Aldrich, Melbourne, Australia) in PBS for 30 min, followed by incubation with the primary antibodies (E-cadherin and N-cadherin; 1:100) overnight at 4 °C. At the end of the incubation step, the cells were washed thrice with PBS, and then the cells were incubated for 1 h with the fluorescence-labeled goat anti-rabbit secondary antibody (Invitrogen) at 1:500 and DAPI 1:1000 in 1% BSA. The cells were washed three times with PBS for 5 min each. Finally, the coverslips were mounted with a fluoro-shield mounting medium (Sigma Aldrich) and sealed with nail polish. The fluorescence images were acquired using an Olympus IX-81 motorized inverted microscope with an FV-1000 laser scanning confocal system using the confocal laser scanning microscope LSM-800 (ZEISS, Göttingen, Germany). Cells were seeded 7×10^4 cells/mL into 4 chambers of Glass-Bottomed Dishes (Cellvis; Sunnyvale, CA, USA). After 24h, the cells were treated with DMSO, LCE, Paclitaxel (1 µM), and Vinoblastin (0.5 µM), respectively, for 6 h, followed by immunostaining. After washing with PBS, the cells were stained with tubulin using a Cell Tubulin Staining Kit (AAT Bioquest, Pleasanton, CA, USA) according to the manufacturer's protocol. The fluorescence images were acquired using an Olympus IX-81 motorized inverted microscope with an FV-1000 laser scanning confocal system using the confocal laser scanning microscope LSM-800 (ZEISS, Germany).

4.10. Molecular Docking and Interaction Analysis

The compound, 13-AC, was molecularly docked using the Schrödinger Maestro molecular software v12.1 suite [69]. The protein structure was obtained from the Protein Data Bank (PDB ID: 7Z7D) repository. Protein preparation and compound preparation were performed using the Maestro Protein Preparation and LigPrep modules in Maestro, respectively. The co-crystal ligand, vinblastine (VLB), was used to define the binding site. Docking analysis was performed using Glide [70]. The extra-precision (XP) setting was used. All other constraint settings were set to default. The docking procedure was validated by redocking the co-crystal ligand, vinblastine, and comparing its spatial positioning to the resulting docking pose. Protein–ligand interactions and the 2D interaction diagram were generated using the ProLIF Python package [71]. The final binding poses were rendered using PyMOL v.2.5.4 software.

4.11. Antitumor Examination of LCE with Xenograft Human Prostate Cancers

The xenograft animal model was established following the existing literature [16]. Five-week-old nude mice (BALB/cAnN.Cgfoxnlnu/CrlNarl) were purchased from the National Laboratory Animal and Research Center. The Animal Care and Treatment Committee of the National Museum of Marin Biology & Aquarium (IACUC Permit Number 201707) approved this study. The Guide for the Care and Use of Laboratory Animals of the National Institutes of Health was followed in all experiments. All efforts were made to minimize animal stress/distress. Human prostate cancer PC3 and Du145 cells were injected subcutaneously into the right leg of the nude mice. LCE was administered by means of intraperitoneal injection in the experimental group, while the control group received solvent only (DMSO). The drug was administered three times a week. The tumor volume was calculated using the following formula: width^2 × length/2. After 38 days of treatment, animals were euthanized with carbon dioxide according to standard protocols. Tumors, heart, liver, spleen, lungs, and kidneys were collected post-euthanasia. The tumor weights were measured, and the organs were fixed with formalin for histochemical staining and microscopic examination.

4.12. Statistical Analysis

All statistics are expressed as the mean ± standard deviation (SD). The comparison of statistically significant data was performed using Student's independent t-test at $p < 0.05$, $p < 0.01$, and $p < 0.001$ for each experiment.

5. Conclusions

As is widely known, soft corals serve as excellent sources of marine-derived natural products. Among them, genera such as Sarcophyton, Sinularia, and Lobophytum are particularly attractive targets for marine natural product research. Six corals were shown to be capable of potent inhibition of the activities of cell growth, HDAC, topoisomerase II, and tubulin polymerization based on screening more than 180 EA extracts of marine soft corals. Particularly, the coral *Lobophytum crassum* exhibited the most effective enhancement of cytotoxicity and suppression of invasion in PCs. Our findings showed that these EA extracts were enriched with active compounds to develop potent inhibitors of HDAC, topoisomerase II, and tubulin polymerization in a cell-free system. Moreover, our research unveils that 13-AC could be a potential candidate with high gastrointestinal absorption (GIA), water solubility, bioavailability score, and synthetic accessibility for cancer therapy. However, the source of marine natural products is a serious problem and a major obstacle to supplying active compounds for the development of clinical drugs. Many still believe that the total synthesis of marine compounds could not provide a sufficient amount for clinical trials. The successful aquaculture of marine corals is an exciting development and represents a potential advancement in the acceleration of lead drug development. Given that these compounds are recognized for their broad spectrum of biological activities, they hold considerable potential for the development of various pharmaceuticals that are beneficial to human health and ecology.

Author Contributions: Conceptualization, T.-N.T. and L.-C.C.; methodology, T.-N.T., Y.-M.H., Y.-H.L., K.-M.C., Y.-C.D., S.-Y.T. and L.-C.C.; software, Y.-M.H., K.-C.H. and T.E.L.; validation, H.-Y.L., Y.-C.L. and M.-C.L.; formal analysis, Y.-M.H. and H.-Y.L.; investigation, T.-N.T. and L.-C.C.; resources, M.-C.L.; data curation, T.-N.T.; writing—original draft preparation, T.-N.T., M.E.-S. and M.-C.L.; writing—review and editing, H.-Y.L.; visualization, H.-Y.L.; supervision, H.-Y.L.; project administration, H.-Y.L., Y.-C.L. and M.-C.L.; funding acquisition, H.-Y.L., Y.-C.L. and M.-C.L. All authors have read and agreed to the published version of the manuscript.

Funding: The authors are grateful to the Ministry of Science and Technology [MOST 110-2320- B-259-001-MY3 (Mei-Chin Lu) and 112-2314-B-037-072 (Yi-Chang Liu)], the Kaohsiung Medical University Hospital (KMUH-DK109006-2 and KMUH-DK(B)110001-3, Y.-C.L.), and the National Health Research Institutes [NHRI-111A1-CACO-03212109 and NHRI-113A1-CACO-03212409 (Yi Chang Liu)], E Da Cancer Hospital [EDCHP 112003 (Hung-Yu Lin), and National Dong Hwa University [111T2560-5 and 113T2951-07 (Mei-Chin Lu)] for financially supporting the work.

Institutional Review Board Statement: The study was approved by the Animal Care and Treatment Committee of Kaohsiung Medical University (IACUC Permit Number 109234).

Data Availability Statement: The data presented in this study are available on request from the corresponding author.

Acknowledgments: The authors would like to thank Jiunn-Wang Liao, the Animal Disease Diagnostic Center (ADDC), College of Veterinary Medicine, National Chung Hsing University, for the examination and evaluation of the histopathologic results report. The authors are also thankful to the aquaculture center, the National Museum of Marine Biology and Aquarium, for the support with coral aquaculture, and the Institutional Animal Center at Kaohsiung Medical University for the support with the xenograft animal and two-dimensional electrophoresis experiment. The work was supported by grants from the National Dong Hwa University, the National Museum of Marine Biology and Aquarium, as well as the Ministry of Science and Technology, Taiwan, awarded to Mei-Chin Lu. All funds are greatly appreciated.

Conflicts of Interest: The authors declare no conflicts of interest.

References

1. Jimenez, P.C.; Wilke, D.V.; Branco, P.C.; Bauermeister, A.; Rezende-Teixeira, P.; Gaudencio, S.P.; Costa-Lotufo, L.V. Enriching cancer pharmacology with drugs of marine origin. *Br. J. Pharmacol.* **2020**, *177*, 3–27. [CrossRef]
2. Chao, C.H.; Wen, Z.H.; Wu, Y.C.; Yeh, H.C.; Sheu, J.H. Cytotoxic and anti-inflammatory cembranoids from the soft coral Lobophytum crassum. *J. Nat. Prod.* **2008**, *71*, 1819–1824. [CrossRef]
3. Hong, J.Y.; Boo, H.J.; Kang, J.I.; Kim, M.K.; Yoo, E.S.; Hyun, J.W.; Koh, Y.S.; Kim, G.Y.; Maeng, Y.H.; Hyun, C.L.; et al. (1S,2S,3E,7E,11E)-3,7,11,15-Cembratetraen-17,2-olide, a cembrenolide diterpene from soft coral Lobophytum sp. inhibits growth and induces apoptosis in human colon cancer cells through reactive oxygen species generation. *Biol. Pharm. Bull.* **2012**, *35*, 1054–1063. [CrossRef] [PubMed]
4. Kulbicki, M.; Parravicini, V.; Bellwood, D.R.; Arias-Gonzalez, E.; Chabanet, P.; Floeter, S.R.; Friedlander, A.; McPherson, J.; Myers, R.E.; Vigliola, L.; et al. Global biogeography of reef fishes: A hierarchical quantitative delineation of regions. *PLoS ONE* **2013**, *8*, e81847. [CrossRef] [PubMed]
5. Liang, X.; Wu, Q.; Luan, S.; Yin, Z.; He, C.; Yin, L.; Zou, Y.; Yuan, Z.; Li, L.; Song, X.; et al. A comprehensive review of topoisomerase inhibitors as anticancer agents in the past decade. *Eur. J. Med. Chem.* **2019**, *171*, 129–168. [CrossRef]
6. Swedan, H.K.; Kassab, A.E.; Gedawy, E.M.; Elmeligie, S.E. Topoisomerase II inhibitors design: Early studies and new perspectives. *Bioorg. Chem.* **2023**, *136*, 106548. [CrossRef] [PubMed]
7. Di Micco, S.; Masullo, M.; Bandak, A.F.; Berger, J.M.; Riccio, R.; Piacente, S.; Bifulco, G. Garcinol and Related Polyisoprenylated Benzophenones as Topoisomerase II Inhibitors: Biochemical and Molecular Modeling Studies. *J. Nat. Prod.* **2019**, *82*, 2768–2779. [CrossRef]
8. Zidar, N.; Secci, D.; Tomasic, T.; Masic, L.P.; Kikelj, D.; Passarella, D.; Argaez, A.N.G.; Hyeraci, M.; Dalla Via, L. Synthesis, Antiproliferative Effect, and Topoisomerase II Inhibitory Activity of 3-Methyl-2-phenyl-1H-indoles. *ACS Med. Chem. Lett.* **2020**, *11*, 691–697. [CrossRef]
9. Jeon, K.H.; Park, S.; Shin, J.H.; Jung, A.R.; Hwang, S.Y.; Seo, S.H.; Jo, H.; Na, Y.; Kwon, Y. Synthesis and evaluation of 7-(3-aminopropyloxy)-substituted flavone analogue as a topoisomerase IIalpha catalytic inhibitor and its sensitizing effect to enzalutamide in castration-resistant prostate cancer cells. *Eur. J. Med. Chem.* **2023**, *246*, 114999. [CrossRef]
10. Alsherbiny, M.A.; Bhuyan, D.J.; Low, M.N.; Chang, D.; Li, C.G. Synergistic Interactions of Cannabidiol with Chemotherapeutic Drugs in MCF7 Cells: Mode of Interaction and Proteomics Analysis of Mechanisms. *Int. J. Mol. Sci.* **2021**, *22*, 10103. [CrossRef]
11. Luan, S.; Gao, Y.; Liang, X.; Zhang, L.; Yin, L.; He, C.; Liu, S.; Yin, Z.; Yue, G.; Zou, Y.; et al. Synthesis and structure-activity relationship of lipo-diterpenoid alkaloids with potential target of topoisomerase IIalpha for breast cancer treatment. *Bioorg. Chem.* **2021**, *109*, 104699. [CrossRef] [PubMed]
12. Emam, S.H.; Hassan, R.A.; Osman, E.O.; Hamed, M.I.A.; Abdou, A.M.; Kandil, M.M.; Elbaz, E.M.; Mikhail, D.S. Coumarin derivatives with potential anticancer and antibacterial activity: Design, synthesis, VEGFR-2 and DNA gyrase inhibition, and in silico studies. *Drug Dev. Res.* **2023**, *84*, 433–457. [CrossRef] [PubMed]
13. Zala, A.R.; Rajani, D.P.; Kumari, P. Synthesis, molecular docking, ADME study, and antimicrobial potency of piperazine based cinnamic acid bearing coumarin moieties as a DNA gyrase inhibitor. *J. Biochem. Mol. Toxicol.* **2023**, *37*, e23231. [CrossRef] [PubMed]
14. Chin, H.K.; Lu, M.C.; Hsu, K.C.; El-Shazly, M.; Tsai, T.N.; Lin, T.Y.; Shih, S.P.; Lin, T.E.; Wen, Z.H.; Yang, Y.S.H.; et al. Exploration of anti-leukemic effect of soft coral-derived 13-acetoxysarcocrassolide: Induction of apoptosis via oxidative stress as a potent inhibitor of heat shock protein 90 and topoisomerase II. *Kaohsiung J. Med. Sci.* **2023**, *39*, 718–731. [CrossRef] [PubMed]
15. Shih, S.P.; Lee, M.G.; El-Shazly, M.; Juan, Y.S.; Wen, Z.H.; Du, Y.C.; Su, J.H.; Sung, P.J.; Chen, Y.C.; Yang, J.C.; et al. Tackling the Cytotoxic Effect of a Marine Polycyclic Quinone-Type Metabolite: Halenaquinone Induces Molt 4 Cells Apoptosis via Oxidative Stress Combined with the Inhibition of HDAC and Topoisomerase Activities. *Mar. Drugs* **2015**, *13*, 3132–3153. [CrossRef] [PubMed]
16. Wang, K.C.; Lu, M.C.; Hsu, K.C.; El-Shazly, M.; Shih, S.P.; Lien, S.T.; Kuo, F.W.; Yang, S.C.; Chen, C.L.; Yang, Y.S.H. The Antileukemic Effect of Xestoquinone, A Marine-Derived Polycyclic Quinone-Type Metabolite, Is Mediated through ROS-Induced Inhibition of HSP-90. *Molecules* **2021**, *26*, 7037. [CrossRef] [PubMed]

17. Lee, M.G.; Liu, Y.C.; Lee, Y.L.; El-Shazly, M.; Lai, K.H.; Shih, S.P.; Ke, S.C.; Hong, M.C.; Du, Y.C.; Yang, J.C.; et al. Heteronemin, a Marine Sesterterpenoid-Type Metabolite, Induces Apoptosis in Prostate LNcap Cells via Oxidative and ER Stress Combined with the Inhibition of Topoisomerase II and Hsp90. *Mar. Drugs* **2018**, *16*, 204. [CrossRef]
18. Lai, K.H.; Liu, Y.C.; Su, J.H.; El-Shazly, M.; Wu, C.F.; Du, Y.C.; Hsu, Y.M.; Yang, J.C.; Weng, M.K.; Chou, C.H.; et al. Antileukemic Scalarane Sesterterpenoids and Meroditerpenoid from Carteriospongia (Phyllospongia) sp. Induce Apoptosis via Dual Inhibitory Effects on Topoisomerase II and Hsp90. *Sci. Rep.* **2016**, *6*, 36170. [CrossRef]
19. Peerzada, M.N.; Dar, M.S.; Verma, S. Development of tubulin polymerization inhibitors as anticancer agents. *Expert. Opin. Ther. Pat.* **2023**, *33*, 797–820. [CrossRef]
20. Naaz, F.; Haider, M.R.; Shafi, S.; Yar, M.S. Anti-tubulin agents of natural origin: Targeting taxol, vinca, and colchicine binding domains. *Eur. J. Med. Chem.* **2019**, *171*, 310–331. [CrossRef]
21. Bass, A.K.A.; El-Zoghbi, M.S.; Nageeb, E.M.; Mohamed, M.F.A.; Badr, M.; Abuo-Rahma, G.E.A. Comprehensive review for anticancer hybridized multitargeting HDAC inhibitors. *Eur. J. Med. Chem.* **2021**, *209*, 112904. [CrossRef] [PubMed]
22. Ribatti, D.; Tamma, R.; Annese, T. Epithelial-Mesenchymal Transition in Cancer: A Historical Overview. *Transl. Oncol.* **2020**, *13*, 100773. [CrossRef] [PubMed]
23. Kalluri, R.; Weinberg, R.A. The basics of epithelial-mesenchymal transition. *J. Clin. Invest.* **2009**, *119*, 1420–1428. [CrossRef] [PubMed]
24. Lambert, A.W.; Pattabiraman, D.R.; Weinberg, R.A. Emerging Biological Principles of Metastasis. *Cell* **2017**, *168*, 670–691. [CrossRef]
25. Mehlen, P.; Puisieux, A. Metastasis: A question of life or death. *Nat. Rev. Cancer* **2006**, *6*, 449–458. [CrossRef] [PubMed]
26. Sharma, N.K.; Bahot, A.; Sekar, G.; Bansode, M.; Khunteta, K.; Sonar, P.V.; Hebale, A.; Salokhe, V.; Sinha, B.K. Understanding Cancer's Defense against Topoisomerase-Active Drugs: A Comprehensive Review. *Cancers* **2024**, *16*, 680. [CrossRef] [PubMed]
27. Das Mukherjee, D.; Kumar, N.M.; Tantak, M.P.; Datta, S.; Ghosh Dastidar, D.; Kumar, D.; Chakrabarti, G. NMK-BH2, a novel microtubule-depolymerising bis (indolyl)-hydrazide-hydrazone, induces apoptotic and autophagic cell death in cervical cancer cells by binding to tubulin at colchicine - site. *Biochim. Biophys. Acta Mol. Cell Res.* **2020**, *1867*, 118762. [CrossRef] [PubMed]
28. Zhang, K.; Bangma, C.H.; Roobol, M.J. Prostate cancer screening in Europe and Asia. *Asian J. Urol.* **2017**, *4*, 86–95. [CrossRef] [PubMed]
29. Liu, L.; Feng, Y.; Xiang, X.; Xu, M.; Tang, G. Biological effect of ETV4 and the underlying mechanism of its regulatory effect on epithelial-mesenchymal transition in intrahepatic cholangiocarcinoma cells. *Oncol. Lett.* **2024**, *28*, 346. [CrossRef]
30. Serrano-Gomez, S.J.; Maziveyi, M.; Alahari, S.K. Regulation of epithelial-mesenchymal transition through epigenetic and post-translational modifications. *Mol. Cancer* **2016**, *15*, 18. [CrossRef]
31. Kim, B.N.; Ahn, D.H.; Kang, N.; Yeo, C.D.; Kim, Y.K.; Lee, K.Y.; Kim, T.J.; Lee, S.H.; Park, M.S.; Yim, H.W.; et al. TGF-beta induced EMT and stemness characteristics are associated with epigenetic regulation in lung cancer. *Sci. Rep.* **2020**, *10*, 10597. [CrossRef]
32. Chen, Q.; Gu, M.; Cai, Z.K.; Zhao, H.; Sun, S.C.; Liu, C.; Zhan, M.; Chen, Y.B.; Wang, Z. TGF-beta1 promotes epithelial-to-mesenchymal transition and stemness of prostate cancer cells by inducing PCBP1 degradation and alternative splicing of CD44. *Cell Mol. Life Sci.* **2021**, *78*, 949–962. [CrossRef]
33. Roy, S.; Mukhopadhyay, A. A randomized optimal k-mer indexing approach for efficient parallel genome sequence compression. *Gene* **2024**, *907*, 148235. [CrossRef]
34. Peng, B.R.; Lu, M.C.; El-Shazly, M.; Wu, S.L.; Lai, K.H.; Su, J.H. Aquaculture Soft Coral Lobophytum crassum as a Producer of Anti-Proliferative Cembranoids. *Mar. Drugs* **2018**, *16*, 15. [CrossRef] [PubMed]
35. Daina, A.; Michielin, O.; Zoete, V. SwissADME: A free web tool to evaluate pharmacokinetics, drug-likeness and medicinal chemistry friendliness of small molecules. *Sci. Rep.* **2017**, *7*, 42717. [CrossRef] [PubMed]
36. Daina, A.; Zoete, V. A BOILED-Egg To Predict Gastrointestinal Absorption and Brain Penetration of Small Molecules. *ChemMedChem* **2016**, *11*, 1117–1121. [CrossRef] [PubMed]
37. Teague, S.J.; Davis, A.M.; Leeson, P.D.; Oprea, T. The Design of Leadlike Combinatorial Libraries. *Angew. Chem. Int. Ed. Engl.* **1999**, *38*, 3743–3748. [CrossRef]
38. van Waterschoot, R.A.; Schinkel, A.H. A critical analysis of the interplay between cytochrome P450 3A and P-glycoprotein: Recent insights from knockout and transgenic mice. *Pharmacol. Rev.* **2011**, *63*, 390–410. [CrossRef]
39. Mrozik, K.M.; Blaschuk, O.W.; Cheong, C.M.; Zannettino, A.C.W.; Vandyke, K. N-cadherin in cancer metastasis, its emerging role in haematological malignancies and potential as a therapeutic target in cancer. *BMC Cancer* **2018**, *18*, 939. [CrossRef]
40. Zhu, G.J.; Song, P.P.; Zhou, H.; Shen, X.H.; Wang, J.G.; Ma, X.F.; Gu, Y.J.; Liu, D.D.; Feng, A.N.; Qian, X.Y.; et al. Role of epithelial-mesenchymal transition markers E-cadherin, N-cadherin, beta-catenin and ZEB2 in laryngeal squamous cell carcinoma. *Oncol. Lett.* **2018**, *15*, 3472–3481.
41. Seyfried, T.N.; Huysentruyt, L.C. On the origin of cancer metastasis. *Crit. Rev. Oncog.* **2013**, *18*, 43–73. [CrossRef] [PubMed]
42. Naderi, R.; Gholizadeh-Ghaleh Aziz, S.; Haghigi-Asl, A.S. Evaluating the effect of Alantolactone on the expression of N-cadherin and Vimentin genes effective in epithelial-mesenchymal transition (EMT) in breast cancer cell line (MDA-MB-231). *Ann. Med. Surg.* **2022**, *73*, 103240. [CrossRef] [PubMed]
43. Sisto, M.; Ribatti, D.; Lisi, S. E-Cadherin Signaling in Salivary Gland Development and Autoimmunity. *J. Clin. Med.* **2022**, *11*, 2241. [CrossRef] [PubMed]

44. Debnath, P.; Huirem, R.S.; Bhowmick, A.; Ghosh, A.; Ghosh, D.; Dutta, P.; Maity, D.; Palchaudhuri, S. Epithelial mesenchymal transition induced nuclear localization of the extracellular matrix protein Fibronectin. *Biochimie* **2024**, *219*, 142–145. [CrossRef] [PubMed]
45. Salmena, L.; Carracedo, A.; Pandolfi, P.P. Tenets of PTEN tumor suppression. *Cell* **2008**, *133*, 403–414. [CrossRef]
46. Dubrovska, A.; Kim, S.; Salamone, R.J.; Walker, J.R.; Maira, S.M.; Garcia-Echeverria, C.; Schultz, P.G.; Reddy, V.A. The role of PTEN/Akt/PI3K signaling in the maintenance and viability of prostate cancer stem-like cell populations. *Proc. Natl. Acad. Sci. USA* **2009**, *106*, 268–273. [CrossRef]
47. Cao, C.; Subhawong, T.; Albert, J.M.; Kim, K.W.; Geng, L.; Sekhar, K.R.; Gi, Y.J.; Lu, B. Inhibition of mammalian target of rapamycin or apoptotic pathway induces autophagy and radiosensitizes PTEN null prostate cancer cells. *Cancer Res.* **2006**, *66*, 10040–10047. [CrossRef] [PubMed]
48. Walker, L.; Millena, A.C.; Strong, N.; Khan, S.A. Expression of TGFbeta3 and its effects on migratory and invasive behavior of prostate cancer cells: Involvement of PI3-kinase/AKT signaling pathway. *Clin. Exp. Metastasis* **2013**, *30*, 13–23. [CrossRef] [PubMed]
49. Chu, P.G.; Weiss, L.M. Keratin expression in human tissues and neoplasms. *Histopathology* **2002**, *40*, 403–439. [CrossRef]
50. Hendrix, M.J.; Seftor, E.A.; Seftor, R.E.; Trevor, K.T. Experimental co-expression of vimentin and keratin intermediate filaments in human breast cancer cells results in phenotypic interconversion and increased invasive behavior. *Am. J. Pathol.* **1997**, *150*, 483–495.
51. Aubert, M.; Panicot, L.; Crotte, C.; Gibier, P.; Lombardo, D.; Sadoulet, M.O.; Mas, E. Restoration of alpha(1,2) fucosyltransferase activity decreases adhesive and metastatic properties of human pancreatic cancer cells. *Cancer Res.* **2000**, *60*, 1449–1456.
52. Echeverri, C.J.; Paschal, B.M.; Vaughan, K.T.; Vallee, R.B. Molecular characterization of the 50-kD subunit of dynactin reveals function for the complex in chromosome alignment and spindle organization during mitosis. *J. Cell Biol.* **1996**, *132*, 617–633. [CrossRef]
53. Korbecki, J.; Bosiacki, M.; Barczak, K.; Lagocka, R.; Chlubek, D.; Baranowska-Bosiacka, I. The Clinical Significance and Role of CXCL1 Chemokine in Gastrointestinal Cancers. *Cells* **2023**, *12*, 1406. [CrossRef]
54. Kaneko, T.; Zhang, Z.; Mantellini, M.G.; Karl, E.; Zeitlin, B.; Verhaegen, M.; Soengas, M.S.; Lingen, M.; Strieter, R.M.; Nunez, G.; et al. Bcl-2 orchestrates a cross-talk between endothelial and tumor cells that promotes tumor growth. *Cancer Res.* **2007**, *67*, 9685–9693. [CrossRef]
55. Ancrile, B.B.; O'Hayer, K.M.; Counter, C.M. Oncogenic ras-induced expression of cytokines: A new target of anti-cancer therapeutics. *Mol. Interv.* **2008**, *8*, 22–27. [CrossRef] [PubMed]
56. Deng, Y.I.; Verron, E.; Rohanizadeh, R. Molecular Mechanisms of Anti-metastatic Activity of Curcumin. *Anticancer Res.* **2016**, *36*, 5639–5647. [CrossRef]
57. Chiang, S.K.; Chen, S.E.; Chang, L.C. A Dual Role of Heme Oxygenase-1 in Cancer Cells. *Int. J. Mol. Sci.* **2018**, *20*, 39. [CrossRef]
58. Gueron, G.; De Siervi, A.; Ferrando, M.; Salierno, M.; De Luca, P.; Elguero, B.; Meiss, R.; Navone, N.; Vazquez, E.S. Critical role of endogenous heme oxygenase 1 as a tuner of the invasive potential of prostate cancer cells. *Mol. Cancer Res.* **2009**, *7*, 1745–1755. [CrossRef] [PubMed]
59. Alaoui-Jamali, M.A.; Bismar, T.A.; Gupta, A.; Szarek, W.A.; Su, J.; Song, W.; Xu, Y.; Xu, B.; Liu, G.; Vlahakis, J.Z.; et al. A novel experimental heme oxygenase-1-targeted therapy for hormone-refractory prostate cancer. *Cancer Res* **2009**, *69*, 8017–8024. [CrossRef] [PubMed]
60. Li, Y.; Su, J.; DingZhang, X.; Zhang, J.; Yoshimoto, M.; Liu, S.; Bijian, K.; Gupta, A.; Squire, J.A.; Alaoui Jamali, M.A.; et al. PTEN deletion and heme oxygenase-1 overexpression cooperate in prostate cancer progression and are associated with adverse clinical outcome. *J. Pathol.* **2011**, *224*, 90–100. [CrossRef]
61. Wu, Q.; Ma, X.; Jin, Z.; Ni, R.; Pan, Y.; Yang, G. Zhuidu Formula suppresses the migratory and invasive properties of triple-negative breast cancer cells via dual signaling pathways of RhoA/ROCK and CDC42/MRCK. *J. Ethnopharmacol.* **2023**, *315*, 116644. [CrossRef] [PubMed]
62. Fife, C.M.; Sagnella, S.M.; Teo, W.S.; Po'uha, S.T.; Byrne, F.L.; Yeap, Y.Y.; Ng, D.C.; Davis, T.P.; McCarroll, J.A.; Kavallaris, M. Stathmin mediates neuroblastoma metastasis in a tubulin-independent manner via RhoA/ROCK signaling and enhanced transendothelial migration. *Oncogene* **2017**, *36*, 501–511. [CrossRef] [PubMed]
63. Abel, A.C.; Muhlethaler, T.; Dessin, C.; Schachtsiek, T.; Sammet, B.; Sharpe, T.; Steinmetz, M.O.; Sewald, N.; Prota, A.E. Bridging the maytansine and vinca sites: Cryptophycins target beta-tubulin's T5-loop. *J. Biol. Chem.* **2024**, *300*, 107363. [CrossRef] [PubMed]
64. Kita, K.; Burdowski, A. Recent clinical trials and optical control as a potential strategy to develop microtubule-targeting drugs in colorectal cancer management. *World J. Gastroenterol.* **2024**, *30*, 1780–1790. [CrossRef] [PubMed]
65. Chen, S.; Zhou, Y.; Chen, Y.; Gu, J. fastp: An ultra-fast all-in-one FASTQ preprocessor. *Bioinformatics* **2018**, *34*, i884–i890. [CrossRef] [PubMed]
66. Kopylova, E.; Noe, L.; Touzet, H. SortMeRNA: Fast and accurate filtering of ribosomal RNAs in metatranscriptomic data. *Bioinformatics* **2012**, *28*, 3211–3217. [CrossRef] [PubMed]
67. Kim, D.; Paggi, J.M.; Park, C.; Bennett, C.; Salzberg, S.L. Graph-based genome alignment and genotyping with HISAT2 and HISAT-genotype. *Nat. Biotechnol.* **2019**, *37*, 907–915. [CrossRef] [PubMed]
68. Liao, Y.; Smyth, G.K.; Shi, W. featureCounts: An efficient general purpose program for assigning sequence reads to genomic features. *Bioinformatics* **2014**, *30*, 923–930. [CrossRef] [PubMed]

69. Jost, W.H. 'Similar to' is not 'identical with', and 'identical with' is not 'the same as'. *Drugs R D* **2015**, *15*, 11–12. [CrossRef]
70. Friesner, R.A.; Murphy, R.B.; Repasky, M.P.; Frye, L.L.; Greenwood, J.R.; Halgren, T.A.; Sanschagrin, P.C.; Mainz, D.T. Extra precision glide: Docking and scoring incorporating a model of hydrophobic enclosure for protein-ligand complexes. *J. Med. Chem.* **2006**, *49*, 6177–6196. [CrossRef]
71. Bouysset, C.; Fiorucci, S. ProLIF: A library to encode molecular interactions as fingerprints. *J. Cheminform.* **2021**, *13*, 72. [CrossRef] [PubMed]

marine drugs

MDPI

Article

Rifamycin-Related Polyketides from a Marine-Derived Bacterium *Salinispora arenicola* and Their Cytotoxic Activity

Cao Van Anh [1,†], Jong Soon Kang [2], Jeong-Wook Yang [2], Joo-Hee Kwon [2], Chang-Su Heo [1,3], Hwa-Sun Lee [1] and Hee Jae Shin [1,3,*]

1 Marine Natural Products Chemistry Laboratory, Korea Institute of Ocean Science and Technology, 385 Haeyang-ro, Yeongdo-gu, Busan 49111, Republic of Korea; caovananh12a1@gmail.com (C.V.A.); science30@kiost.ac.kr (C.-S.H.); hwasunlee@kiost.ac.kr (H.-S.L.)

2 Laboratory Animal Resource Center, Korea Research Institute of Bioscience and Biotechnology, 30 Yeongudanjiro, Cheongju 28116, Republic of Korea; kanjon@kribb.re.kr (J.S.K.); z7v8@kribb.re.kr (J.-W.Y.); juhee@kribb.re.kr (J.-H.K.)

3 Department of Marine Biotechnology, University of Science and Technology (UST), 217 Gajungro, Yuseong-gu, Daejeon 34113, Republic of Korea

* Correspondence: shinhj@kiost.ac.kr; Tel.: +82-51-664-3341; Fax: +82-51-664-3340

† Current address: Vietnam Military Medical University.

Abstract: Eight rifamycin-related polyketides were isolated from the culture broth of a marine-derived bacterium *Salinispora arenicola*, including five known (**2–5** and **8**) and three new derivatives (**1**, **6**, and **7**). The structures of the new compounds were determined by means of spectroscopic methods (HRESIMS and 1D, 2D NMR) and a comparison of their experimental data with those previously reported in the literature. The isolated compounds were evaluated for their cytotoxicity against one normal, six solid, and seven blood cancer cell lines and **1** showed moderate activity against all the tested cell lines with GI_{50} values ranging from 2.36 to 9.96 μM.

Keywords: *Salinispora arenicola*; polyketides; rifamycin; saliniketal; cytotoxicity

1. Introduction

The marine environment covers approximately 70% of planet Earth and hosts a huge biodiversity due to its unique living conditions with high pressure, high salinity, and low oxygen supply [1]. Actinomycetes are the largest reservoir of microbial natural products with interesting bioactivities and have been useful in diverse applications in agriculture and medicine [2]. As an alternative source to the conventionally used terrestrial microorganisms, actinomycetes are ubiquitous in marine environments and are considered an appealing source of novel structures for new drug discovery [3]. The genus *Salinispora* was reported as the first obligate marine actinomycetal genus. Until now, three closely related species from this genus, including *Salinispora tropica*, *S. arenicola*, and *S. pacifica*, have been identified [4]. Members of this genus were commonly found in various substrates in marine environments, including tropical and subtropical sediments, tropical sponges, ascidians, and seaweeds [5]. Although their discovery was relatively late, more than 50 secondary metabolites with a broad range of chemical scaffolds, such as salinosporamides, rifamycins, lomaiviticins, cyclomarins, and salinaphthoquinones, as well as many inspired muta- and semi-synthesis structures, have been reported from this genus [6]. Among the reported compounds, salinosporamide A showed significant activity against various types of cancer and has now entered clinical studies [7]. Based on the unique living conditions and diverse biosynthetic abilities, the genus is considered an emerging source of leading structures for future drug discovery.

Rifamycins are a group of antibiotics produced by several actinomycetes, such as *Amycolatopsis, Streptomyces, Micormonospora, and Salinispora* [8–11]. The rifamycin group, including classic rifamycin drugs and their semi-synthesized derivatives, is widely used in clinical practice for the treatment of tuberculosis [12]. The structures of rifamycins are quite unique and consist of an aromatic moiety bridged by an aliphatic chain. The aromatic part can be a naphthalene or naphthoquinone ring, and the aliphatic chain is called an ansa-chain [13]. The biosynthesis of rifamycins has been well studied, and their structures were confirmed by X-ray crystallography and total synthesis research [14]. To date, the absolute configuration of the ansa-chain was reported to be identical in all rifamycin derivatives [15].

As part of our ongoing research on natural products produced by actinomycetes near Dokdo island, Republic of Korea, the strain 225DD-027 was isolated from a sediment sample and was identified as *Salinispora arenicola* by 16S rRNA gene sequence analysis. The strain produced orange pigments, which were primarily speculated as rifamycin analogs from a literature review. In a small culture (1 L), the production of pigments was relatively low, and it was insufficient for structural elucidation. Therefore, a mass culture was conducted to obtain a sufficient amount and to determine the structures and biological properties of the pigments. As a result, eight rifamycin-related polyketides, including three new compounds (**1**, **6**, and **7**, Figure 1), were isolated, and the details of their isolation, structure determination, and bioactivities are described in this paper.

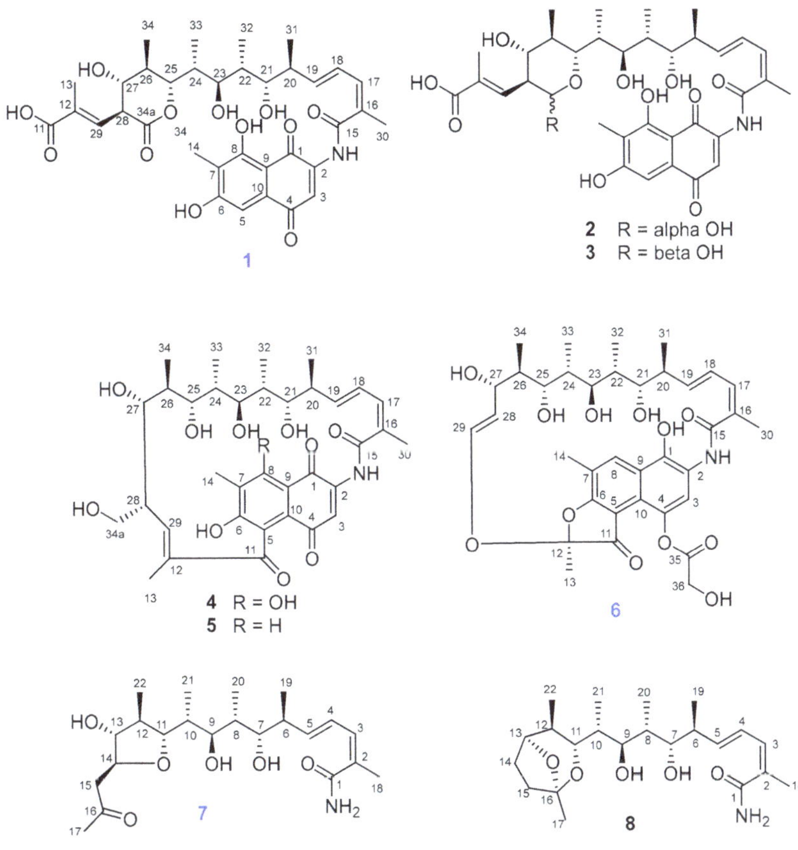

Figure 1. Structures of **1**–**8** isolated from *Salinispora arenicola* 225DD-027.

2. Results and Discussion

Compound **1** was isolated as an orange powder. The molecular formula of **1** was determined as $C_{35}H_{43}NO_{12}$ by HRESIMS data (m/z 670.2852, $[M + H]^+$, calcd for $[C_{35}H_{44}NO_{12}]^+$ 670.2858, −0.9 ppm). The ^1H NMR spectrum of **1** (Table 1) revealed the presence of two singlet aromatic protons at δ_H 7.63 (H-3) and 7.05 (H-5); four olefinic protons at δ_H 6.82 (dd, J = 15.0, 11.2 Hz, H-18), 6.68 (dd, J = 9.6 and 1.2 Hz, H-29), 6.48 (d, J = 11.1 Hz, H-17), and 6.03 (dd, J = 15.1, 8.0 Hz, H-19); four oxygenated methines at δ_H 4.60 (d, J = 11.0 Hz, H-25), 3.76 (d, J = 9.8 Hz, H-21), 3.65 (dd, J = 10.1, 2.6 Hz, H-23), and 3.55 (t, J = 9.6 Hz, H-27); five methines at δ_H 3.45 (t, J = 9.6 Hz, H-28), 2.44 (m, H-20), 2.07 (m, H-24), 1.94 (m, H-22), and 1.93 (m, H-26); and seven methyl groups at δ_H 2.11 (s, H_3-14), 2.09 (s, H_3-30), 1.91 (d, J = 1.3 Hz, H_3-13), 1.10 (d, J = 7.0 Hz, H_3-32), 1.08 (d, J = 6.5 Hz, H_3-34), 1.01 (d, J = 6.8 Hz, H_3-31), and 0.89 (d, J = 6.9 Hz, H_3-33). The ^{13}C and HSQC data of **1** revealed 35 signals of two ketone carbonyls at δ_C 186.5 (C-4) and 183.8 (C-1); three carboxyl groups at δ_C 173.0 (C-34a), 171.4 (C-11), and 169.9 (C-15); two oxygenated sp^2 carbons at δ_C 165.1 (C-8) and 163.8 (C-6); twelve sp^2 carbons at δ_C 108.2-145.7; four oxygenated methines at δ_C 74.5-83.1; five methines at δ_C 35.0-51.6; and seven methyls at δ_C 8.0-20.5. The ^{1}H and ^{13}C NMR data of **1** were almost identical to those of the isolated compound, 34a-α-rifamycin W-M1-hemiacetal (**2**). The only difference was the chemical shift of C-34a ($\delta_{C\text{-}34a}$ 173.0 for **1**, and $\delta_{C\text{-}34a}$ 94.5, $\delta_{H\text{-}34a}$ 5.08 for **2**), indicating the hemiacetal at C-34a of **2** was oxidized to a carbonyl in **1**, which was re-confirmed by HRESIMS data of **1** with one less degree of unsaturation than that of **2**. The presence of a lactone ring between C-25 and C-34a of **1** was also confirmed by the significant downfield chemical shift of C-25 in **1** compared to those of **2** ($\delta_{C\text{-}25}$ 83.1 and $\delta_{H\text{-}25}$ 4.60 for **1**, and $\delta_{C\text{-}25}$ 72.7, $\delta_{H\text{-}25}$ 4.21 for **2**). Further detailed analysis of 2D NMR data (Figure 2) determined the planar structure of **1**, as shown in Figure 1. The NOESY correlation from H-17 to H_3-30 indicated the Z-configuration of $\Delta^{16,17}$, and the large coupling constant of H-18 and H-19 (J = 15.0 Hz) confirmed the E-configuration of $\Delta^{18,19}$. The NOESY correlations of H-27/H_3-29, H-27/H_3-34, and H-25/H_3-34 indicated that H-25, H-27, H_3-29, and H_3-34 were located on the same face of the lactone ring. The large coupling constants of H-27/H-26 and H-27/H-28 (J = 9.6 Hz) confirmed that H-26 and H-28 were located on the opposite face from H-27 (Figure 3). Thus, the relative configuration of the lactone ring was determined to be the same as those of co-isolated compounds (**2** and **3**). The absolute configuration of the ansa-chain was proposed to be the same as that of other rifamycin derivatives by considering their biosynthetic relationship, NMR data, and coupling constants of **1** and **2**. Thus, the structure of **1** was determined, and **1** was given the trivial name of salinisporamycin C.

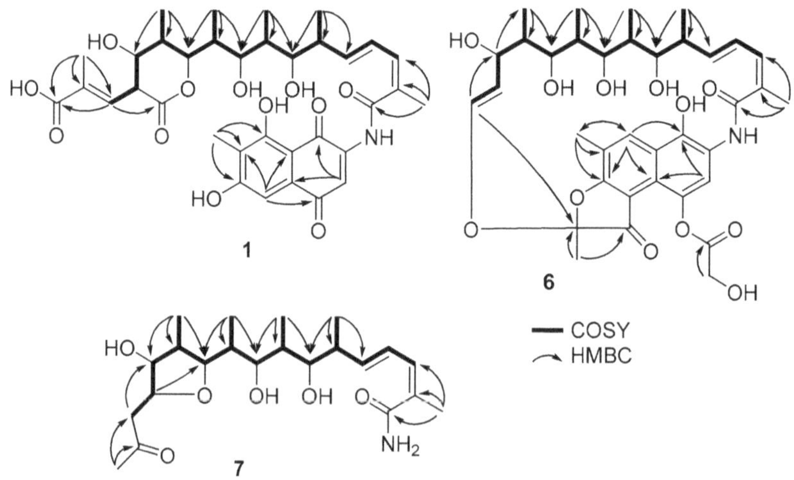

Figure 2. Key ^{1}H-^{1}H COSY and HMBC correlations for **1**, **6**, and **7**.

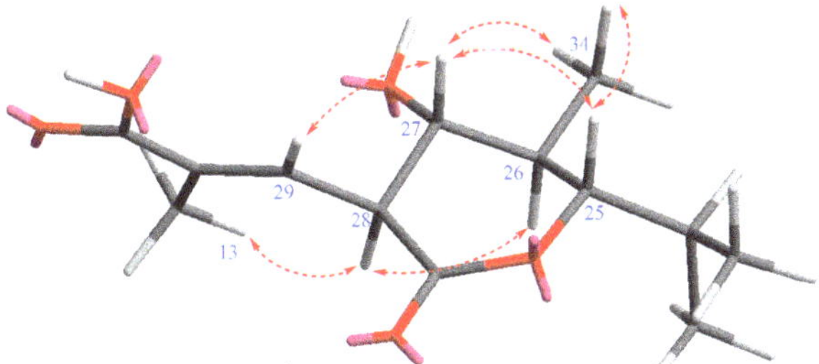

1

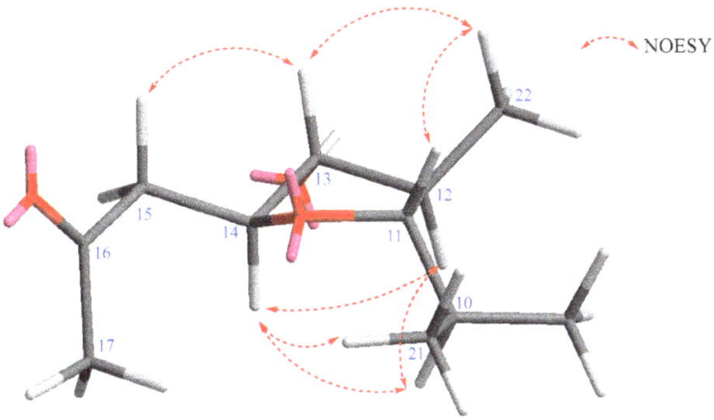

7

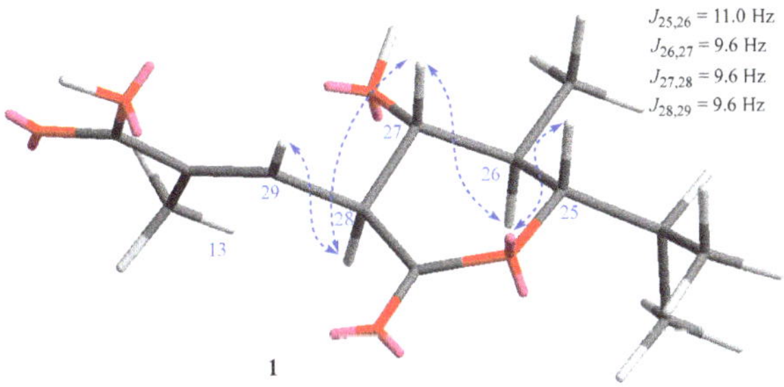

1

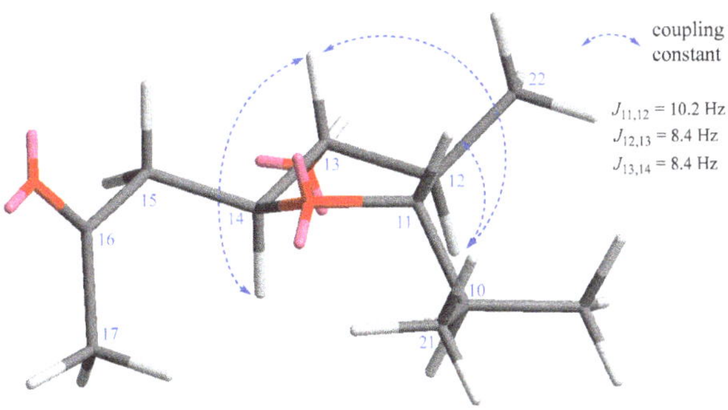

7

Figure 3. Key NOESY correlations and coupling constants for the lactone ring of **1** and tetrahydrofuran ring of **7**.

Table 1. ^{1}H and ^{13}C NMR data for **1** and **6**.

1			6		
No	δ_H, Mult (J in Hz)	δ_C	No	δ_H, Mult (J in Hz)	δ_C
1		183.8	1		144.1
2		142.4	2		125.0
3	7.63, s	117.1	3	7.21, s	119.4
4		186.5	4		139.7
5	7.05, s	108.7	5		121.5
6		163.8	6		175.5
7		118.1	7		125.0
8		165.1	8	8.61, s	137.2
9		108.2	9		122.6
10		132.2	10		112.2
11		171.4	11		197.6
12		134.8	12		108.5
13	1.91, d, (1.3)	13.5	13	1.68, s	21.5
14	2.11, s	8.0	14	2.49, s	15.1
15		169.9	15		172.3
16		129.4	16		132.0
17	6.48, d, (11.1)	138.7	17	6.30, d, (10.7)	134.1
18	6.82, dd, (15.0, 11.2)	127.7	18	6.43, dd, (15.4, 11.2)	124.9
19	6.03, dd, (15.1, 8.0)	145.7	19	5.98, dd, (15.5, 5.7)	141.7
20	2.44. m	42.2	20	2.35, m	39.8
21	3.76, d, (9.8)	75.9	21	3.95, d, (9.4)	73.4
22	1.94, m	35.0	22	1.79, m	34.5
23	3.65, dd, (10.1, 2.6)	77.7	23	3.43, d, (10.3)	78.3
24	2.07. m	38.7	24	1.35, m	39.4
25	4.60, d, (11.0)	83.1	25	3.62, d, (10.6)	71.8
26	1.93, m	39.1	26	1.06, m	41.8
27	3.55, t, (9.6)	74.5	27	4.38, d, (5.6)	68.5
28	3.45, t, (9.6)	51.6	28	5.22, dd, (12.4, 6.0)	125.0
29	6.68, dd, (9.6, 1.2)	137.1	29	6.19, d, (12.5)	142.1
30	2.09, s	20.5	30	2.07, s	20.5
31	1.01, d, (6.8)	16.9	31	0.92, d, (6.9)	18.0
32	1.10, d, (7.0)	11.6	32	1.03, d, (6.9)	11.3
33	0.89, d, (6.9)	9.3	33	0.60, d, (6.8)	8.9
34	1.08, d, (6.5)	13.1	34	−0.64, d, (6.7)	8.8
34a		173.0	35		174.0
			36	4.70, d, (16.9) 4.56, d, (16.9)	62.1

Compound **6** was isolated as an orange powder. The molecular formula of **6** was determined to be $C_{30}H_{45}NO_{12}$ by HRESIMS data (*m*/*z* 706.2809, $[M + Na]^+$, calcd for

$[C_{36}H_{45}NO_{12}Na]^+$ 706.2834, −3.5 ppm). The ^{1}H NMR spectrum showed the presence of two singlet aromatic protons at δ_H 7.21 (H-3) and 8.61 (H-8); five olefinic protons at δ_H 6.30 (d, J = 10.7 Hz, H-17), 6.43 (dd, J = 15.4 and 11.2 Hz, H-18), 5.98 (dd, J = 15.5 and 5.7 Hz, H-19), 5.22 (dd, J = 12.4 and 6.0 Hz, H-28), and 6.19 (d, J = 12.5 Hz, H-29); four oxygenated methines at δ_H 3.95 (d, J = 9.4 Hz, H-21), 3.43 (d, J = 10.3 Hz, H-23), 3.62 (d, J = 10.6 Hz, H-25), and 4.38 (d, J = 5.6 Hz, H-27); four methines at δ_H 2.35 (m, H-20), 1.79 (m, H-22), 1.35 (m, H-24), and 1.06 (m, H-26); oxygenated methylenes at δ_H 4.70 and 4.56 (d, J = 16.9 Hz, H-36a and H-36b); and seven methyl groups at δ_H 1.68 (s, H_3-13), 2.49 (s, H_3-14), 2.07 (s, H_3-30), 0.92 (d, J = 6.9 Hz, H_3-31), 1.03 (d, J = 6.9 Hz, H_3-32), 0.60 (d, J = 6.8 Hz, H_3-33), and -0.64 (d, J = 6.7 Hz, H_3-34). The ^{13}C and HSQC spectra revealed signals of 36 carbons belonging to a ketone at δ_C 197.6 (C-11); two carbonyls at δ_C 172.3 (C-15) and 174.0 (C-35); sixteen sp^2 carbons at δ_C 112.2–175.5; a hemiketal at δ_C 108.5 (C-12); four oxygenated methines at δ_C 68.5–78.3; an oxygenated methylene at δ_C 62.1 (C-36); four methines at δ_C 34.5–41.8; and seven methyls at δ_C 8.8–21.5. The continuous ^{1}H-^{1}H COSY correlations from H-17 to H-29 via H_3-31, H_3-32, H_3-33, and H_3-34, as well as the HMBC correlations from H_3-30 to C-15, C-16, and C-17, established the structure of an ansa-chain. The HMBC correlations from H_3-14 to C-6, C-7, and C-8; from H-3 to C-1 and C-10; from H-8 to C-1, C-6, C-10, and C-14 established a naphthalene ring with three hydroxy groups at the C-1, C-4, and C-6 positions. The HMBC correlations from H-29 to C-12, H_3-13 to C-11, and C-12 confirmed the structure of a furan ring and the connection of the ansa-chain with the aromatic moiety via an ether bond between C-29 and C-12. Further, the HMBC correlations from H-$36_{a,b}$ to C-35 determined the presence of glycolic acid. By comparison with data reported in the literature, the structure of **6** was determined as 8-deoxy-25-desacetyl-27-demethyl-rifamycin L [16] and named salinisporamycin D.

Compound **7** was isolated as a colorless solid. The molecular formula of **7** was determined as $C_{22}H_{37}NO_6$ by HRESIMS data (m/z 434.2496, $[M + Na]^+$, calcd for $[C_{22}H_{37}NO_6Na]^+$ 434.2513, −3.9 ppm), five degrees of unsaturation. The ^{1}H NMR spectrum of **7** (Table 2) revealed the presence of three olefinic protons at δ_H 6.17 (d, J = 11.1 Hz, H-3), 6.58 (dd, J = 15.2 and 11.1 Hz, H-4), and 5.78 (d, J = 15.2 and 8.3 Hz, H-5); five oxygenated methines at δ_H 3.46–4.05; four methines at δ_H 1.81–2.34; a methylene group at δ_H 2.63 and 2.75 (H-15a and H-15b); and six methyls at δ_H 0.95–2.18. The ^{13}C and HSQC NMR spectra demonstrated the presence of 22 carbons, including a ketocarbonyl at δ_C 210.3 (C-16); a carboxyl at δ_C 175.1 (C-1); four olefinic carbons at δ_C 128.3–142.1; five oxygenated methines at δ_C 75.6–83.5; four methines at δ_C 36.3–44.0; a methylene at δ_C 48.5 (C-15); and six methyls at δ_C 10.6–30.6. The ^{1}H and ^{13}C NMR data of **7** were similar to those of the co-isolated known compound, saliniketal A (**8**). The significant downfield chemical shifts of C-11 (δ_C 83.5), C-13 (δ_C 82.7), and C-14 (δ_C 80.8), and the HMBC correlation from H-14 (δ_H 3.95) to C-11 confirmed the partial structure of a tetrahydrofuran ring between C-11 and C-14. The NOESY correlation between H-11, H_3-22, H-13, and H-15a,b indicated their co-facial relationship, and that of H-14/H-12 indicated that H-14 and H-12 were located on the opposite face of the tetrahydrofuran ring. Saliniketals A and B are bicyclic polyketides isolated from a *Salininispora arenicola* strain [15]. Their structures were elucidated by the 2D NMR techniques and were confirmed by total synthesis studies [8]. Saliniketals shared a partially similar structure with the ansa-chain of rifamycin derivatives isolated from the same strain. The biosynthesis studies also confirmed this relationship, and saliniketals and rifamycin derivatives shared the same absolute configuration [9]. By comparing ^{1}H and ^{13}C NMR data and the experimental ECD spectrum of **7** with those of saliniketal A (**8**) and considering their biosynthetic relationship, the absolute configuration of **7** was proposed to be the same as that of saliniketal A (**8**) and named salinifuran A.

Table 2. ^{1}H and ^{13}C NMR data for **7**.

No	δ_H, Mult (J in Hz)	δ_C	No	δ_H, Mult (J in Hz)	δ_C
1		175.1	13	3.46, t (8.4)	82.7
2		131.4	14a	3.95, td (8.7, 3.5)	80.8
3	6.17, br d (11.1)	134.1	14b		
4	6.58, dd (15.2, 11.1)	128.3	15a	2.75 dd (15.6, 3.5)	48.5
5	5.78, dd (15.2, 8.3)	142.1	15b	2.63 dd (15.6, 8.9)	
6	2.34, m	42.3	16		210.3
7	3.73, dd (9.3, 1.3)	75.6	17	2.18, s	30.6
8	1.89, m	36.3	18	1.95, s	20.9
9	3.50, dd (7.9, 4.6)	78.9	19	0.95, d (6.9)	17.1
10	1.81, m	38.5	20	0.98, d (7.0)	10.9
11	4.05, dd (10.2, 1.2)	83.5	21	0.95, d (6.9)	10.6
12	2.00, m	44.1	22	1.05, d (6.5)	14.2

Structures of known compounds were identified as 34a-α-rifamycin W-M1-hemiacetal (**2**), 34a-β-rifamycin W-M1-hemiacetal (**3**) [9], rifamycin W (**4**) [17], protorifamycin I (**5**) [18], and saliniketal A (**8**) [19] by comparison of their spectroscopic data with those reported in the literature.

Rifamycins are a group of antimicrobial drugs, and their mode of action, resistance, and biosynthesis have been well studied [20]. Previous studies showed that the biosynthesis of rifamycins starts with 3-amino-5-hydroxybenzoic acid (AHBA) and chain extension by various rifamycin biosynthetic genes. The ansa-chain was established from two acetates and eight propionates [15]. Numerous structures of naturally occurring rifamycins are mainly due to the extensive post-PKS enzymatic tailoring conducted by enzymes encoded by pathway-specific genes [15]. Similarly, the possible biosynthesis pathway of the new compounds was proposed, as shown in Figure 4. Firstly, proansamycin X was synthesized, and then the compound was converted to rifamycin W. Rifamycin W was oxidized to rifamycin Z, and then this compound was converted to demethly-desacetyl rifamycin SV. Compound **1** could be originated from rifamycin Z by oxidation and decyclization at the C-5 position. Compound **6** could be synthesized from demethly-desacetyl rifamycin SV by deoxidation at C-8 and adding glycolic acid (from an acetate unit) at the C-4 position. The biosynthesis of **7** was proposed to be similar to saliniketals. Rifamycin W was converted to a percussor (**11**) via several steps, and **11** could be reduced and cyclized to give a tetrahydrofuran-containing derivative (**13**), and then the napthoquinone moiety was eliminated to yield salinifuran (**7**).

Some isolated compounds were screened for their cytotoxicity against one normal, six solid, and seven blood cancer cell lines (Table 3). According to the guidelines of NCI, when a compound shows cytotoxicity with an IC_{50} value less than 4 μg/mL or 10 μM, the compound is considered to have cytotoxicity [21]. We defined the potency of compounds as significant (IC_{50} < 1 μM), moderate (IC_{50} = 1–10 μM), weak (IC_{50} = 10–30 μM), and non-cytotoxic (IC_{50} > 30 μM). Compound **1** showed moderate activity against all the tested cell lines with GI_{50} of 2.36–9.96 μM. Compound **6** exhibited weak cytotoxicity against solid cancer cells with GI_{50} values of 21.84–29.75 μM. Compound **7** showed weak activity against NALM6 (GI_{50} = 26.76 μM). Compound **8** was not active against all the tested cell lines (GI_{50} > 30 μM). From the activity results, it is noteworthy that rifamycin derivatives showed moderate or weak cytotoxicity, and the aromatic moiety is important for their cytotoxicity (**1** and **6**). Compounds **7** and **8** are composed of only an ansa-chain and showed weak or no cytotoxicity. The lack of a hydroxy group at the C-8 position (**6**) may reduce the activity. The results of this study were consistent with previous reports that naturally occurring rifamycins are generally not effective enough for new drug development. However, further research should be conducted to semi-synthesize their derivatives with lower toxicity against normal cells and better pharmacological properties.

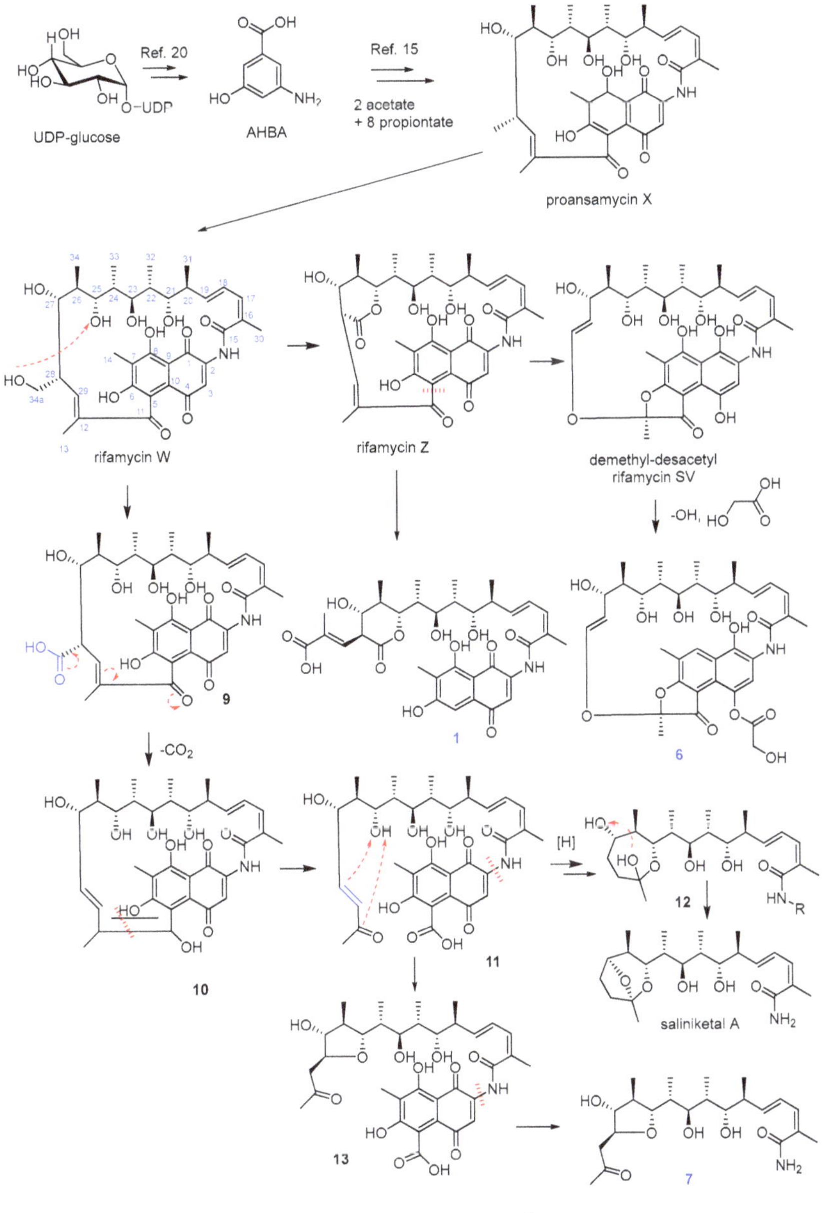

Figure 4. Plausible biosynthetic pathway of the new compounds.

Table 3. Growth inhibition (GI_{50}, μM) of **1** and **6-8** against cancer cell lines.

	1	**6**	**7**	**8**	**Adr.**
ACHN	8.45	>30	>30	>30	0.168
MDA-MB-231	8.79	>30	>30	>30	0.159
HCT-15	9.25	24.20	>30	>30	0.137
PC-3	8.46	26.59	>30	>30	0.144
NUGC-3	7.41	29.75	>30	>30	0.136
NCI-H23	8.05	21.84	>30	>30	0.151
HL-60	9.96	4.79	>30	>30	0.021
Raji	5.37	12.05	>30	>30	0.003
K562	7.17	9.53	>30	>30	0.057
RPMI-8402	4.75	2.45	>30	>30	0.014
NALM6	4.28	4.76	26.76	>30	0.002
U266	2.63	2.30	>30	>30	0.034
WSU-DLCL2	2.36	5.40	>30	>30	0.002
RPMI-1788	8.47	4.93	nt	nt	0.014

Adr.: Adriamycin as a positive control. nt: not tested. Six solid [ACHN (renal), MDA-MB-231 (breast), HCT-15 (colon), PC-3 (prostate), NUGC-3 (stomach), and NCI-H23 (lung)], seven blood [(HL-60 (acute myelogenous leukemia, AML), Raji (Burkitt's lymphoma), K562 (chronic myelogenous leukemia, CML), RPMI-8402 (T cell acute lymphocytic leukemia, T ALL), NALM6 (B cell acute lymphocytic leukemia, B ALL), U266 (multiple myeloma), WSU-DLCL2 (diffuse large B cell lymphoma, DLBCL) cells lines and a normal [RPMI-1788 (B lymphocytes)] cell line.

3. Materials and Methods

3.1. General Experimental Procedures

The 1D and 2D NMR spectra were measured by a Bruker 600 MHz spectrometer (Bruker BioSpin GmbH, Rheinstetten, Germany). UV–Vis spectra were obtained using a Shimadzu UV-1650PC spectrophotometer (Shimadzu Corporation, Kyoto, Japan). A JASCO FT/IR-4100 spectrophotometer (JASCO Corporation, Tokyo, Japan) was used to record IR spectra. A hybrid ion trap time-of-flight mass spectrometer (Shimadzu LC/MS-IT-TOF, Kyoto, Japan) was used for measuring high-resolution ESIMS experiments. HPLC was performed with a PrimeLine Binary pump (Analytical Scientific Instruments, Inc., El Sobrante, CA, USA) and a RI-101 detector (Shoko Scientific Co., Ltd., Yokohama, Japan). Semi-preparative HPLC was conducted using an ODS column (YMC-Pack-ODS-A, 250 × 10 mm i.d., 5 μM, Kyoto, Japan). A Rudolph Research Analytical Autopol III polarimeter (Rudolph Research Analytical, Hackettstown, NJ, USA) was used to record optical rotations. Mass culture was carried out using a 100 L fermenter (Fermentec Co., Ltd., Cheongju, Republic of Korea). All solvents were either HPLC grade or distilled prior to use.

3.2. Isolation of the Microorganisms from Marine Sediment Samples

Marine sediment samples were obtained off the coast of Dokdo Island in the Republic of Korea during expeditions in May 2022. The sediment samples were obtained using a grab sampler at a depth of approximately 200 m below the water's surface. The sediments were collected and stored at 5 °C upon return to the laboratory in sterile 50 mL conical tubes. *Actinomycetes* are spore-forming bacteria that can endure harsh environments and high temperatures. As a result, pretreatment with selective heating was employed to reduce non-spore-forming unwanted microorganisms. Each sample was weighed to 1.0 g, placed on a sterile plate, and kept at 60 °C for 30 min in a dry oven. The samples were then successively diluted to 10^{-1}, 10^{-2}, and 10^{-3} by sterile seawater, and each aliquot (100 μL) was spread on humic acid–vitamin agar (HV), actinomycetes isolation agar (AIA), and Bennett's agar (BN) media. The plates were kept in a BOD (bio-oxygen demand) incubator at 28 °C for

1~4 weeks until colonies could be seen with the naked eye. Colonies that could be seen were picked up and transferred onto new BN agar plates. The purification procedure was carried out repeatedly several times until single pure colonies were obtained.

3.3. Isolation and Identification of the Strain 225DD-027

The strain 225DD-027 was isolated from humic acid–vitamin agar after being incubated for 12 days. It was identified as *Salinispora arenicola* according to its morphological characteristics and results of 16S-rRNA gene sequence analysis by Macrogen Inc. (Seoul, Republic of Korea). The sequence of 225DD-027 was submitted to GenBank under accession number OR084782. The strain is currently preserved in the Microbial Culture Collection, Korea Institute of Ocean Science and Technology (KIOST), with an accession number of 225DD-027, under the curatorship of Hee Jae Shin.

3.4. Fermentation of the Strain 225DD-027 and Extraction and Isolation of Metabolites

Bennett's medium (BN, 1% glucose, 0.2% tryptone, 0.1% yeast extract, 0.1% beef extract, 0.5% glycerol, sea salts 32 g/L, and agar 17 g/L for agar medium) was used to conduct the seed and mass cultures of the strain 225DD-027. Firstly, the strain was cultured on Bennett's agar medium in a Petri dish for 14 days. The actively grown colonies were transferred aseptically into a 100 mL conical flask containing 50 mL of Bennett's broth medium and incubated on a rotary shaker (140 rpm) at 28 °C for 9 days. An aliquot (10 mL) was aseptically inoculated into a 2.0 L flask containing 1.0 L of BN broth. The strain was incubated at 28 °C for 7 days on a rotary shaker at 140 rpm, and then the culture broth was inoculated into a 100 L fermenter filled with 70 L of BN broth. The mass culture was carried out at 28 °C for 16 days and then harvested. The culture was separated into supernatant and mycelium by continuous centrifugation at 60,000 rpm, and the supernatant was extracted twice with an equal volume of EtOAc (70 L × 2). The EtOAc layer was evaporated under reduced pressure to obtain a crude extract (8.0 g). The extract was then fractionated into 15 fractions (fractions 1 to 15) by vacuum liquid chromatography on an ODS column using a stepwise elution with 3 × 300 mL each of 20%, 40%, 60%, and 80% MeOH in H_2O and 100% MeOH. The F7 fraction was subjected to a semi-preparative HPLC (YMC-Pack ODS-A, 250 × 10 mm i.d., 5 μm, flow rate 2.0 mL/min) with an isocratic elution of 45% MeOH in H_2O to obtain compound **7** (2.0 mg, t_R = 42 min). The F9 fraction was purified using semi-preparative HPLC (YMC-Pack ODS-A, 250 × 10 mm i.d., 5 μm, flow rate 2.0 mL/min) with an isocratic elution of 30% MeCN in H_2O to yield compounds **4** (3.0 mg, t_R = 40 min) and **8** (3.5 mg, t_R = 52 min). Compounds **5** (5.0 mg, t_R = 65 min) and **6** (3.3 mg, t_R = 75 min) were isolated from the F10 fraction using a semi-preparative HPLC (YMC-Pack ODS-A, 250 × 10 mm i.d., 5 μm, flow rate 2.0 mL/min) with an isocratic elution of 30% MeCN in H_2O. The F11 fraction was purified using a semi-preparative HPLC (YMC-Pack ODS-A, 250 × 10 mm i.d., 5 μm, flow rate 2.0 mL/min) with an isocratic elution of 54% MeCN in H_2O to yield compounds **1** (1.2 mg, t_R = 32 min), **2** (1.5 mg, t_R = 26 min), and **3** (1.5 mg, t_R = 22 min).

Salinisporamycin C (**1**): orange powder, $[\alpha]_D^{20}$ − 30.5 (*c* 0.1, MeOH); UV (MeOH) λ_{max} (log ε) 218 (4.65), 273 (4.30) nm; IR ν_{max} 3364, 2976, 2880, 1632, 1600, 1496, 1374, 1062, 1021 cm^{-1}; HRESIMS *m/z* 670.2852, calculated for $[C_{35}H_{44}NO_{12}]^+$, 670.2858; for ^1H NMR (CD_3OD, 600 MHz), see Table 1; for ^{13}C NMR (CD_3OD, 150 MHz), see Table 1.

Salinisporamycin D (**6**): orange powder, $[\alpha]_D^{20}$ + 35.0 (*c* 0.1, MeOH); UV (MeOH) λ_{max} (log ε) 222 (4.50), nm; IR ν_{max} 3364, 2966, 2851, 1759, 1643, 1590, 1222, 1099 cm^{-1}; HRESIMS *m/z* 706.2809, calculated for $[C_{36}H_{45}NO_{12}Na]^+$, 706.2834; for ^1H NMR (CD_3OD, 600 MHz), see Table 1; for ^{13}C NMR (CD_3OD, 150 MHz), see Table 1.

Salinifuran A (**7**): colorless solid, $[\alpha]_D^{20}$ − 50.0 (*c* 0.1, MeOH); UV (MeOH) λ_{max} (log ε) 204 (5.10), nm; IR ν_{max} 3339, 2961, 2922, 1706, 1660, 1596, 1458, 1024 cm^{-1}; HRESIMS *m/z* 434.2496, calculated for $[C_{22}H_{37}NO_6Na]^+$, 434.2513; for ^1H NMR (CD_3OD, 600 MHz), see Table 2; for ^{13}C NMR (CD_3OD, 150 MHz), see Table 2.

3.5. Cytotoxicity Assay

The cytotoxic activities of **1** and **6–8** against adherent cells and suspension cells were conducted by SRB (sulforhodamine B) assay [22] and CellTiter-Glo assay [23], respectively, as described earlier. The compounds were dissolved and serially diluted in dimethyl sulfoxide. GraphPad Prism 8 (GraphPad Software Inc., San Diego, CA, USA) was used to determine GI_{50} values. Cancer and normal cell lines were purchased from the Japanese Cancer Research Resources Bank (JCRB) (NUGC-3, JCRB Cell Bank/Cat. # JCRB0822), the DSMZ-German Collection of Microorganisms and Cell Cultures (RPMI-8402, DSMZ/Cat # ACC 290; WSU-DLCL2, DSMZ/Cat # ACC 575), and the American Type Culture Collection (ATCC) (PC-3, ATCC/Cat. # CRL-1435; MDA-MB-231, ATCC/Cat. # HTB-26; ACHN, ATCC/Cat. # CRL-1611; NCI-H23, ATCC/Cat. # CRL-5800; HCT-15, ATCC/Cat. # CCL-225; HL-60, ATCC/Cat. # CCL-240; Raji, ATCC/Cat # CCL-86; K562, ATCC/Cat # CCL-243; NALM6, ATCC/Cat # CRL-3273; U266, ATCC/Cat # TIB-196); RPMI-1788, ATCC/Cat # TIB-156). Cells were cultured in Dulbecco's Modified Eagles medium (ACHN, MDA-MB-231), RPMI-1640 medium (HCT-15, PC-3, NUGC-3, NCI-H23, Raji, NALM6, U266, WSU-DLCL2, RPMI-1788) or Improved Minimum Essential Medium (K562, HL-60), supplemented with fetal bovine serum and penicillin-streptomycin.

4. Conclusions

In conclusion, we have isolated eight rifamycin-related polyketides from the marine-derived actinomycetal strain *Salinispora arenicola* 225DD-027, including three new compounds (**1**, **6**, and **7**). The gross structures of the new compounds were elucidated by detailed analysis of their spectroscopic data (HRESIMS, 1D, and 2D NMR). Their absolute configuration was established by consideration of their biosynthetic relationship and comparison of their NMR chemical shifts, ^1H-^1H coupling constants, and ECD spectra with those of the co-isolated derivatives. The new compounds were evaluated for their cytotoxicity against one normal, six solid, and seven blood cancer cell lines, and **1** displayed moderate cytotoxicity against all the tested cancer cell lines with GI_{50} ranging from 2.36 to 9.96 μM. Further investigations should be performed to comprehend the mechanism of action of the active metabolites. The findings of this report have enriched the biological and chemical diversities of naturally occurring polyketides from the genus *Salinispora*.

Supplementary Materials: The following supporting information can be downloaded at https://www.mdpi.com/article/10.3390/md21090494/s1. Figure S1. Structures of some analogs of the isolated compounds. Figure S2. ^1H NMR spectrum of **1**. Figure S3. ^{13}C NMR spectrum of **1**. Figure S4. HSQC spectrum of **1**. Figure S5. ^1H-^1H COSY spectrum of **1**. Figure S6. HMBC spectrum of **1**. Figure S7. Selective 1D NOESY spectrum of **1** (irradiated at H-17). Figure S8. Selective 1D NOESY spectrum of **1** (irradiated at H-27). Figure S9. Selective 1D NOESY spectrum of **1** (irradiated at H-28). Figure S10. Selective 1D NOESY spectrum of **1** (irradiated at H-25). Figure S11. HRESIMS data of **1**. Figure S12. ^1H NMR spectrum of **6**. Figure S13. ^{13}C NMR spectrum of **6**. Figure S14. HSQC spectrum of **6**. Figure S15. ^1H-^1H COSY spectrum of **6**. Figure S16. HMBC spectrum of **6**. Figure S17. NOESY spectrum of **6**. Figure S18. HRESIMS data of **6**. Figure S19. ^1H NMR spectrum of **7**. Figure S20. ^{13}C NMR spectrum of **7**. Figure S21. HSQC spectrum of **7**. Figure S22. ^1H-^1H COSY spectrum of **7**. Figure S23. HMBC spectrum of **7**. Figure S24. Band selective HMBC of **7**. Figure S25. Selective 1D NOESY spectrum of **7** (irradiated at H-3). Figure S26. Selective 1D NOESY spectrum of **7** (irradiated at H-11). Figure S27. Selective 1D NOESY spectrum of **7** (irradiated at H-13). Figure S28. Selective 1D NOESY spectrum of **7** (irradiated at H-14). Figure S29. HRESIMS data of **7**. Figure S30. Comparison of ECD spectra of **7** and saliniketal A (**8**). Figure S31. Results of cytotoxicity test and dose–response curves for compounds **1** and **6–8**. Table S1. Comparison of chemical shifts of **1** and **2**. Table S2. Comparison of chemical shifts of **7** and **8**.

Author Contributions: Conceptualization, H.J.S.; investigation, C.V.A., J.-W.Y. and J.-H.K.; resources, H.-S.L. and C.-S.H.; writing—original draft preparation, C.V.A.; writing—review and editing, H.J.S.; visualization, J.S.K.; project administration, H.J.S.; funding acquisition, H.J.S. All authors have read and agreed to the published version of the manuscript.

Funding: This research was supported by the Korea Institute of Marine Science and Technology Promotion (KIMST) grants funded by the Ministry of Oceans and Fisheries, Korea [KIMST 20200610 (KIOST PM63560) and PG53501].

Institutional Review Board Statement: Not applicable.

Informed Consent Statement: Not applicable.

Data Availability Statement: The data presented in the article are available in the Supplementary Materials.

Acknowledgments: The authors thank Jung Hoon Choi, Korea Basic Science Institute, Ochang, Republic of Korea, for providing mass data.

Conflicts of Interest: The authors declare no conflict of interest.

References

1. Vitale, G.A.; Coppola, D.; Palma Esposito, F.; Buonocore, C.; Ausuri, J.; Tortorella, E.; de Pascale, D. Antioxidant Molecules from Marine Fungi: Methodologies and Perspectives. *Antioxidants* **2020**, *9*, 1183. [CrossRef]
2. De Simeis, D.; Serra, S. Actinomycetes: A Never-Ending Source of Bioactive Compounds-An Overview on Antibiotics Production. *Antibiotics* **2021**, *10*, 483. [CrossRef] [PubMed]
3. Jagannathan, S.V.; Manemann, E.M.; Rowe, S.E.; Callender, M.C.; Soto, W. Marine Actinomycetes, New Sources of Biotechnological Products. *Mar. Drugs* **2021**, *19*, 365. [CrossRef] [PubMed]
4. Kim, H.; Kim, S.; Kim, M.; Lee, C.; Yang, I.; Nam, S.J. Bioactive natural products from the genus *Salinospora*: A review. *Arch. Pharm. Res.* **2020**, *43*, 1230–1258. [CrossRef]
5. Bose, U.; Hewavitharana, A.K.; Ng, Y.K.; Shaw, P.N.; Fuerst, J.A.; Hodson, M.P. LC-MS-Based Metabolomics Study of Marine Bacterial Secondary Metabolite and Antibiotic Production in *Salinispora arenicola*. *Mar. Drugs* **2015**, *13*, 249–266. [CrossRef]
6. Jensen, P.R.; Moore, B.S.; Fenical, W. The marine actinomycete genus *Salinispora*: A model organism for secondary metabolite discovery. *Nat. Prod. Rep.* **2015**, *32*, 738–751. [CrossRef]
7. Lee, H.-S.; Jeong, G.-S. Salinosporamide A, a Marine-Derived Proteasome Inhibitor, Inhibits T Cell Activation through Regulating Proliferation and the Cell Cycle. *Molecules* **2020**, *25*, 5031. [CrossRef] [PubMed]
8. Feng, Y.; Liu, J.; Carrasco, Y.P.; MacMillan, J.B.; De Brabander, J.K. Rifamycin Biosynthetic Congeners: Isolation and Total Synthesis of Rifsaliniketal and Total Synthesis of Salinisporamycin and Saliniketals A and B. *J. Am. Chem. Soc.* **2016**, *138*, 7130–7142. [CrossRef]
9. Shi, Y.; Ye, F.; Song, Y.; Zhang, X.; Lu, C.; Shen, Y. Rifamycin W Analogues from *Amycolatopsis mediterranei* S699 Δrif-orf5 Strain. *Biomolecules* **2021**, *11*, 920. [CrossRef]
10. Bujnowski, K.; Synoradzki, L.; Darłak, R.C.; Zevaco, T.A.; Dinjus, E. Semi-synthetic zwitterionic rifamycins: A promising class of antibiotics; survey of their chemistry and biological activities. *RSC Adv.* **2016**, *6*, 114758–114772. [CrossRef]
11. Huang, H.; Wu, X.; Yi, S.; Zhou, Z.; Zhu, J.; Fang, Z.; Yue, J.; Bao, S. Rifamycin S and its geometric isomer produced by a newly found actinomycete, *Micromonospora rifamycinica*. *Antonie Van Leeuwenhoek* **2009**, *95*, 143–148. [CrossRef] [PubMed]
12. Grobbelaar, M.; Louw, G.E.; Sampson, S.L.; van Helden, P.D.; Donald, P.R.; Warren, R.M. Evolution of rifampicin treatment for tuberculosis. *Infect. Genet. Evol.* **2019**, *74*, 103937. [CrossRef] [PubMed]
13. Masamune, S.; Imperiali, B.; Garvey, D.S. Synthesis of ansamycins: The ansa chain of rifamycin S. *J. Am. Chem. Soc.* **1982**, *104*, 5528–5531. [CrossRef]
14. Brufani, M.; Fedeli, W.; Giacomello, G.; Vaciago, A. The x-ray analysis of the structure of rifamycin Y. *Experientia* **1967**, *23*, 508–512. [CrossRef]
15. Wilson, M.C.; Gulder, T.A.; Mahmud, T.; Moore, B.S. Shared biosynthesis of the saliniketals and rifamycins in *Salinispora arenicola* is controlled by the sare1259-encoded cytochrome P450. *J. Am. Chem. Soc.* **2010**, *132*, 12757–12765. [CrossRef]
16. Lancini, G.C.; Gallo, G.G.; Sartori, G.; Sensi, P. Isolation and structure of rifamycin L and its biogenetic relationship with other rifamycins. *J. Antibiot.* **1969**, *22*, 369–377. [CrossRef]
17. Nakata, M.; Akiyama, N.; Kamata, J.-I.; Kojima, K.; Masuda, H.; Kinoshita, M.; Tatsuta, K. The total synthesis of rifamycin W. *Tetrahedron* **1990**, *46*, 4629–4652. [CrossRef]
18. Ghisalba, O.; Traxler, P.; Nüesch, J. Early intermediates in the biosynthesis of ansamycins. I. Isolation and identification of protorifamycin I. *J. Antibiot.* **1978**, *31*, 1124–1131. [CrossRef]
19. Williams, P.G.; Asolkar, R.N.; Kondratyuk, T.; Pezzuto, J.M.; Jensen, P.R.; Fenical, W. Saliniketals A and B, Bicyclic Polyketides from the Marine Actinomycete *Salinispora arenicola*. *J. Nat. Prod.* **2007**, *70*, 83–88. [CrossRef]
20. Floss, H.G.; Yu, T.-W. RifamycinMode of Action, Resistance, and Biosynthesis. *Chem. Rev.* **2005**, *105*, 621–632. [CrossRef]
21. Suffness, M.; Pezzuto, J.M. Assays related to cancer drug discovery. In *Methods in Plant Biochemistry: Assays for Bioactivity*; Hostettmann, K., Ed.; Academic Press: London, UK, 1991; pp. 71–133.

22. Choi, B.K.; Trinh, P.T.H.; Lee, H.S.; Choi, B.W.; Kang, J.S.; Ngoc, N.T.D.; Van, T.T.T.; Shin, H.J. New Ophiobolin Derivatives from the Marine Fungus *Aspergillus flocculosus* and Their Cytotoxicities against Cancer Cells. *Mar. Drugs* **2019**, *17*, 346. [CrossRef] [PubMed]
23. Lee, E.; Cho, H.; Lee, D.K.; Ha, J.; Choi, B.J.; Jeong, J.H.; Ryu, J.H.; Kang, J.S.; Jeon, R. Discovery of 5-Phenoxy-2-aminopyridine Derivatives as Potent and Selective Irreversible Inhibitors of Bruton's Tyrosine Kinase. *Int. J. Mol. Sci.* **2020**, *21*, 8006. [CrossRef] [PubMed]

marine drugs

MDPI

Article

Actinoquinazolinone, a New Quinazolinone Derivative from a Marine Bacterium *Streptomyces* sp. CNQ-617, Suppresses the Motility of Gastric Cancer Cells

Sultan Pulat [1,†], Da-Ae Kim [2,†], Prima F. Hillman [2,†], Dong-Chan Oh [3], Hangun Kim [1,*], Sang-Jip Nam [2,*] and William Fenical [4,*]

1 College of Pharmacy and Research Institute of Life and Pharmaceutical Sciences, Sunchon National University, Suncheon 57922, Republic of Korea; sultanpulat@s.scnu.ac.kr
2 Department of Chemistry and Nanoscience, Ewha Womans University, Seoul 03760, Republic of Korea; 123rlaekdo@ewhain.net (D.-A.K.); primafitriah@gmail.com (P.F.H.)
3 Natural Products Research Institute, College of Pharmacy, Seoul National University, Seoul 08826, Republic of Korea; dongchanoh@snu.ac.kr
4 Center of Marine Biotechnology and Biomedicine, Scripps Institution of Oceanography, University of California San Diego, La Jolla, CA 92093-0204, USA
* Correspondence: hangunkim@sunchon.ac.kr (H.K.); sjnam@ewha.ac.kr (S.-J.N.); wfenical@ucsd.edu (W.F.)
† These authors contributed equally to this work.

Abstract: A HPLC-UV guided fractionation of the culture broth of *Streptomyces* sp. CNQ-617 has led to the isolation of a new quinazolinone derivative, actinoquinazolinone (**1**), as well as two known compounds, 7-hydroxy-6-methoxy-3,4-dihydroquinazolin-4-one (**2**) and 7-methoxy-8-hydroxy cycloanthranilylproline (**3**). The interpretation of 1D, 2D NMR, and MS spectroscopic data revealed the planar structure of **1**. Furthermore, compound **1** suppressed invasion ability by inhibiting epithelial–mesenchymal transition markers (EMT) in AGS cells at a concentration of 5 μM. In addition, compound **1** decreased the expression of seventeen genes related to human cell motility and slightly suppressed the signal transducer and activator of the transcription 3 (STAT3) signal pathway in AGS cells. Together, these results demonstrate that **1** is a potent inhibitor of gastric cancer cells.

Keywords: actinoquinazolinone; *Streptomyces* sp.; marine natural products; quinazolinone; gastric cancer; motility

1. Introduction

Cancer is the uncontrolled growth and division of cells in the body [1]. Gastric cancer, also known as stomach cancer, is responsible for an estimated 768,793 deaths, making it the fourth leading cause of cancer death in 2020 [2,3]. Suppressed metastasis may be a target in gastric cancer therapy [4]. During the epithelial—mesenchymal transition (EMT) process, cancer cells take on a mesenchymal cell phenotype to spread to a different part of the body. Therefore, EMT plays a significant role in metastatic cancers [5,6]. Furthermore, the signal transducer and activator of transcription 3 (STAT3) is a kind of oncogene that can promote the invasion and migration potential of cancer cells [7]. Thus, suppressing the EMT and STAT3 signal pathways is crucial for developing effective cancer therapies.

Marine microorganisms, including actinobacteria, have emerged as a promising source for the discovery of novel bioactive compounds with potential pharmacological properties [8,9]. Actinobacteria are Gram-positive bacteria that have been extensively studied for their ability to produce secondary metabolites with a wide range of biological activities. Many of these compounds have demonstrated promising activity against various diseases, including cancer, bacterial infections, and viral infections [10,11]. The high biodiversity of marine-derived actinobacteria provides a rich source of novel compounds, which is one of their main advantages [11]. Additionally, marine environments offer unique ecological niches, including extreme temperatures, pressures, and salinity, which can produce unique compounds not found in terrestrial environments. Thus, marine-derived actinobacteria are considered a valuable resource for drug discovery and development [10–12].

Streptomyces sp. strain CNQ-617 is a marine-derived actinobacterium isolated from sediment samples collected from La Jolla Submarine Canyon in California. This strain has been shown to produce several bioactive compounds with potential therapeutic applications [10]. *Streptomyces* is a well-known genus of actinobacteria known for producing a large number of secondary metabolites, including many clinically important antibiotics. Indeed, *Streptomyces* species are thought to have produced approximately two-thirds of all known antibiotics [11,13,14]. Researchers have also discovered several novel bioactive compounds derived from marine-derived *Streptomyces* species in recent years.

Therefore, marine derived *Streptomyces* and other actinobacteria are regarded as a valuable resource for the discovery of novel bioactive compounds with potential therapeutic applications [15–26]. Marineosins A and B are two structurally related compounds that were first discovered from this strain. They are analogs of the natural product prodigiosin and have been shown to possess strong and selective anticancer activity against a variety of cancer cell lines by inducing apoptosis, inhibiting angiogenesis, and disrupting microtubule assembly [26,27].

In addition to marineosins A and B, this strain has also been shown to produce deoxyvasicinone, a compound with potential anti-melanogenic properties. Deoxyvasicinone has been shown to inhibit melanin production in murine and human melanoma cells, suggesting that it could be a promising agent for treating hyperpigmentation disorders [10]. Moreover, further extensive investigation of crude extracts from *Streptomyces* sp. strain CNQ-617 has resulted in the isolation of a novel quinazolinone derivative, actinoquinazolinone (**1**). This study reported the isolation of actinoquinazolinone (**1**) along with two known compounds, 7-hydroxy-6-methoxy-3,4-dihydroquinazolin-4-one (**2**) and 7-methoxy-8-hydroxy cycloanthranilylproline (**3**) (Figure 1), as well as the structural characterization and bioactivity of **1**.

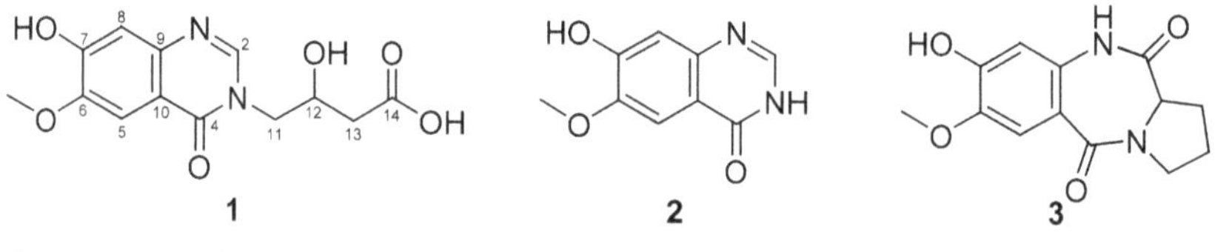

Figure 1. Chemical Structures of actinoquinazolione (**1**), 7-hydroxy-6-methoxy-3,4-dihydroquinazolin-4-one (**2**), and 7-methoxy-8-hydroxy cycloanthranilylproline (**3**).

2. Results and Discussion

Actinoquinazolinone (**1**) was isolated as a yellowish brown oil with a molecular formula of $C_{13}H_{14}N_2O_6$ based on the HR-FAB-MS ion at m/z 295.0924 $[M + H]^+$ (calcd for $C_{13}H_{15}N_2O_6$, 295.0930). The ^1H NMR spectrum of **1** (Table 1, Figures S1–S5) displayed one hetero-aromatic proton at δ_H 8.07 (^1H, s, H-2), two aromatic protons at δ_H 7.46 (1H, s, H-5) and 6.98 (1H, s, H-8), one methoxy group at δ_H 3.88 (3H, s, 6-Ome), and one exchangeable proton at δ_H 10.35 (1H, s, OH). Based on spectroscopic data from ^{13}C NMR and HSQC, six quaternary carbons were assigned at δ_C 159.7 (C-4), 148.2 (C-6), 153.0 (C-7), 143.9 (C-9), 113.8 (C-10), and 172.2 (C-14), two methylene carbons at δ_C 51.2 (C-11) and 39.8 (C-13), four methine carbons at δ_C 147.1 (C-2), 105.7 (C-5), 110.9 (C-8), and 65.0 (C-12), and one methoxy carbon at δ_C 55.7 (6-Ome).

Table 1. NMR Spectral Data for Compounds **1** (DMSO-d_6) [a].

No.	1			
	d_C, mult. [b]	d_H (*J* in Hz)	COSY	HMBC
2	147.1, CH	8.07, s		4, 9, 10, 11
4	159.7, qC			
5	105.7, CH	7.46, s		4, 6, 7, 8, 9, 10
6	148.2, qC			
7	153.0, qC			
8	110.9, CH	6.98, s		4, 6, 7, 9, 10
9	143.9, qC			
10	113.8, qC			
11a	51.2, CH_2	3.74, dd (13.4, 8.2)	12	2, 4, 12, 13
11b		4.12, dd (13.4, 3.9)		
12	65.0, CH	4.18, m	13	
13a	39.8, CH_2	2.29, dd (15.5, 8.2)		11, 12, 14
13b		2.45, dd (15.5, 4.7)		
14	172.2, qC			
6-Ome	55.7, CH_3	3.88, s		6
7-OH		10.35, s		
12-OH				
14-OH				
14-Ome				

[a] 400 MHz for ^{1}H NMR and 100 MHz for ^{13}C NMR. [b] Numbers of attached protons were determined by analysis of 2D spectra.

Additional 2D NMR analyses allowed the structure of **1** to be constructed. The quinazolin-4-one unit was assigned by the NMR signals of six aromatic carbons at δ_C 105.7 (C-5), 148.2 (C-6), 153.0 (C-7), 110.9 (C-8), 143.9 (C-9), and 113.8 (C-10), and two hetero-aromatic carbons at δ_C 147.1 (C-2) and 159.7 (C-4), along with the HMBC correlations from H-2 to C-4, C-9 and C-10; from H-5 to C-4, C-6, C-7 and C-10; and from H-8 to C-7, C-9 and C-10. In addition, HMBC correlations from 6-Ome to C-6 provided the attachment of the methoxy group at C-6. Furthermore, COSY cross peaks [H-11/H-12 and H-12/H-13] and long-range HMBC correlations of H-12 and H-13 with C-14 (δ_C 172.2) as well as the carbon chemical shift of C-12 (δ_C 65.0) allowed the construction of the 3-hydroxybutanoic acid moiety. This moiety was linked to the quinazolinone moiety through the nitrogen atom between C-2 and C-4 from the consideration of the carbon chemical shift of C-11 (δ_C 51.2) and from the observation of the long-range HMBC correlation from H-12 to C-2 and C-4. Additionally, the unassigned hydroxy group was determined to be located at C-7 based on the carbon chemical shift of C-7 (δ_C 153.0) and the molecular formula of the compound. Therefore, the final structure of actinoquinazolione (**1**) was determined to be 7-hydroxy-6-methoxy quinazolinone with a 3-hydroxy butanoic acid moiety, as shown in Figure 2.

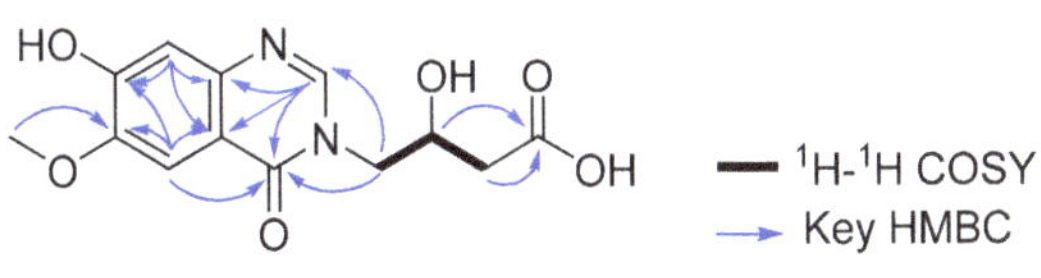

Figure 2. COSY and key HMBC correlations of **1**.

The ^{1}H NMR (400 MHz, DMSO-d_6) spectrum of **2** revealed one hetero-aromatic proton at δ_H 7.90 (1H, d, *J* = 3.47, H-2), two aromatic protons at δ_H 7.43 (1H, s, H-5) and 6.98 (1H, s, H-8), one methoxyl group at δ_H 3.87 (3H, s, 6-Ome), and two exchangeable protons at δ_H 11.93 (1H, s, OH) and 10.27 (1H, br s, NH) (Figure S6). The interpretation of ^{13}C NMR spectral data revealed nine carbons at δ_C 160.1 (C-4), 153.0 (C-7), 148.0 (C-2), 144.9 (C-6), 143.6 (C-9), 114.7 (C-10), 111.3 (C-8), 105.5 (C-5), and 55.7 (6-Ome) (Figure S7).

Compound **2** was identified as 7 hydroxy-6-methoxy-3,4-dihydroquinazolin-4-one based on a comparison of its NMR data to that of a previously reported synthetic compound [28]. However, it was the first report of the compound being isolated from a natural source.

Compound (**3**) was isolated as yellowish oil and its molecular formula was determined to be $C_{13}H_{14}N_2O_4$ by HR-FAB-MS $[M+H]^+$ ion at m/z 263.1029. The ^{1}H NMR spectrum of compound **3** displayed *para*-coupled aromatic protons at δ_H 7.36 (1H, s, H-1) and 6.58 (1H, s, H-4) (Figure S8). The ^{13}C NMR spectrum of **3** showed twelve carbons at δ_C 171.2 (C-11), 166.6 (C-5), 151.1 (C-8), 145.4 (C-7), 131.4 (C-9a), 117.9 (C-5a), 111.8 (C-6), 107.7 (C-9), 57.2 (C-11a), 47.1 (C-3), 25.8 (C-1), 23.4 (C-2), and one methoxy group at δ_C 55.4 (7-Ome) (Figure S9). The chemical structure of **3** was determined as 7-methoxy-8-hydroxy cycloanthranilylproline based on the comparison of NMR data to those of previously reported ones [25].

Compounds **1** and **2** are quinazolinone derivatives with an *N*-containing heterocyclic scaffold. Quinazolinones are a class of nitrogen containing heterocyclic compounds found in nature which are produced by plants and microorganisms [29,30]. Quinazolinones have sparked considerable interest in the fields of medicinal chemistry and drug discovery. The chemical structure of quinazolinones has been shown to possess a wide range of pharmacological properties [31]. Furthermore, quinazolinones are considered as a significant scaffold of various therapeutic and biological activities, including anticancer [32], anticonvulsant [33], anti-cholinesterase [34], anti-diabetic [35], antimalarial [36], antimicrobial [37,38], antitubercular [39], antihypertensive [40], anti-HIV [41], anti-inflammatory [42], and antipsychotic [43]. Other therapeutic and biological activities include cellular phosphorylation inhibition [44], kinase inhibitory [45], dihydrofolate reductase inhibition [46], inhibitors of tubuline polymerization [47], dopamine agonists, and diuretic activities [48,49]. Reported microbial-derived quinazolinones, penicamide A, penoxazolones A and B, aspertoryadins A–J, nortryptoquivaline, 2-(4-hydroxybenzyl)quinazolin-4(3H)-one, and penipanoids B and C, are isolated from the ascidian-derived fungus *Penicillium* sp. 4829 [50], the cold-seep-derived fungus *Penicillium oxalicum* [51], the marine-derived fungus *Aspergillus* sp. HNMF114 [52,53], the sea fan-derived fungus *Neosartorya siamensis* [54], the entomopathogenic fungus *Isaria farinose* [55], and the sediment-derived fungus *Penicillium paneum* SD-44 [56], respectively. In addition, several quinazolinones from *Streptomyces* have been reported, including 2-(1H-indol-3-yl)quinazolin-4-(3H)-one, quinazolin-4(3H)-one, 2-methylquinazolin-4(3H)-one [57], 2-(4-hydroxyphenyl) quinazolin-4(3H)-one [50], quinazolinones A and B, 4(3H)-quinazolinone [58], 2-(2-carboxyethyl)-8-hydroxyquinazolin-4(3H)-one, 2-(2-carboxyethyl)-6-hydroxyquinazolin-4(3H)-one, 2-(4-hydroxyphenyl)quinazolin-4(3H)-one [59], farinamycin [60], 2-Methyl-3H-quinazolin-4-one and 1H-quinazoline-2,4-dione and arborine [61,62]. Moreover, these quinazolinones have been reported to have various biological activities, such as cytotoxicity to Vero cells [63], antifungal activity against *P. litchi* [64], and cytotoxicity against KB and HL-60 cell lines [65].

Additionally, compounds **1** and **2** share structural similarities with previously reported compound 4-(7,8-dihydroxy-4-oxoquinazolin-3(4H)-yl) butanoic acid, which was isolated from the leather coral-derived fungus *Xylaria* sp. FM1005 [66]. However, the structures of compounds **1** and **2** differ from that of the previously reported compound. In the quinazolinone moiety, compound **1** has a substituted methoxy group at C-6 and an additional hydroxy group attached at C-12, but no 8-OH group. Meanwhile, compound **2** has a similar structure to compound **1**, except for the absence of the 3-hydroxybutanoic acid substituent on the amide moiety. In addition, **1–3** have been tested for their viability of cancer cell lines. The relative cell viability of cancer cell lines A549 (lung cancer), AGS (gastric cancer), and Caco-2 (colorectal cancer) was measured by an MTT assay after treatment with various concentrations of **1–3** for 48 h. The result showed that treatment with 100 μM of compound **1** significantly decreased the cell viability of A549, AGS, and Caco-2. However, 100 μM of compound **2** did not affect the cell viability of A549 and AGS, while suppressing the cell viability of Caco-2. Moreover, 100 μM of compound **3** suppressed the cell viability of AGS and Caco-2 while having no significant effect on the cell viability of A549 (Figure 3). Therefore, these results showed that compound **1** is more effective in reducing the cell viability of A549, AGS, and Caco-2 than the other two compounds. However, it should be noted that the observed cell viability reduction by **1–3** is modest even at 100 μM.

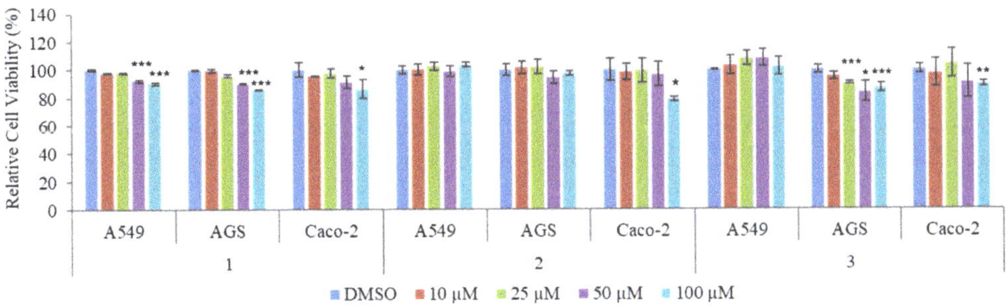

Figure 3. The effect of different concentrations of actinoquinazolione (**1**), 7-hydroxy-6-methoxy-3,4-dihydroquinazolin-4-one (**2**), and 7-methoxy-8-hydroxy cycloanthranilylproline (**3**) on cell viability of AGS, A549, and Caco-2. Cell viability was measured by using MTT assays. Data are presented as mean ± SD and analysis was performed by Student's *t*-test ($n = 3$). * $p < 0.05$; ** $p < 0.01$; *** $p < 0.001$.

To confirm the concentration-dependent inhibitory effect of compound **1** on cancer motility, we evaluated invasion assays in A549, AGS, and Caco-2 cells. From the results (Figure 4A,B), **1** displayed a dose-dependent inhibitory effect on the invasion ability of AGS at concentrations from 1 to 5 μM, whereas the invasion ability of A549 and Caco-2 cells were not affected by treatment of **1**. The results indicated that **1** has a higher suppression activity on the AGS invasion ability than A549 and Caco-2.

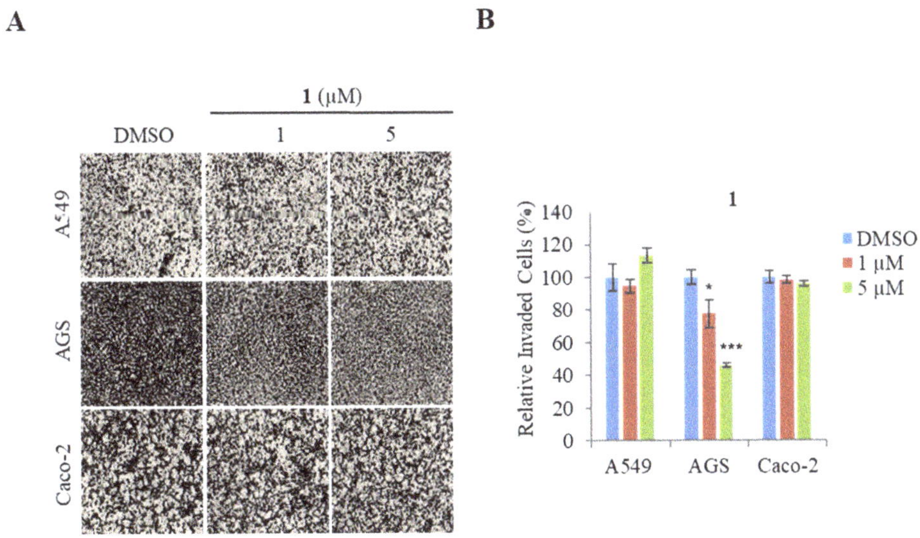

Figure 4. Effect of actinoquinazolione (**1**) on the invasion ability of AGS, A549, and Caco2 cells. (**A**) representative images of each insertion in the invasion assay. (**B**) relative percentage of invaded cells. Data are presented as the mean ± SD and analysis was performed by Student's *t*-test ($n = 5$). * $p < 0.05$, *** $p < 0.001$.

Cancer metastasis accounts for approximately 90% of cancer deaths [67,68]. A poor prognosis can be caused by the EMT, which is linked to metastasis [69]. E-cadherin is known to suppress cancer metastasis; the loss of its expression promotes the EMT markers

E-cadherin, Snail, Slug, and Twist [69]. We assessed whether compound **1** decreased the motility associated with EMT by using qPCR assays and Western blot assays (Figure 5A). Based on the result, treatment with 5 μM of **1** significantly promoted the protein and mRNA expression level of E-cadherin in AGS cells (Figure 5B,C). Furthermore, the protein and mRNA expression levels of the EMT effector N-cadherin and the EMT transcription factors Snail, Slug, and Twist were decreased in AGS by treatment with 5 μM of **1** (Figure 5B,C).

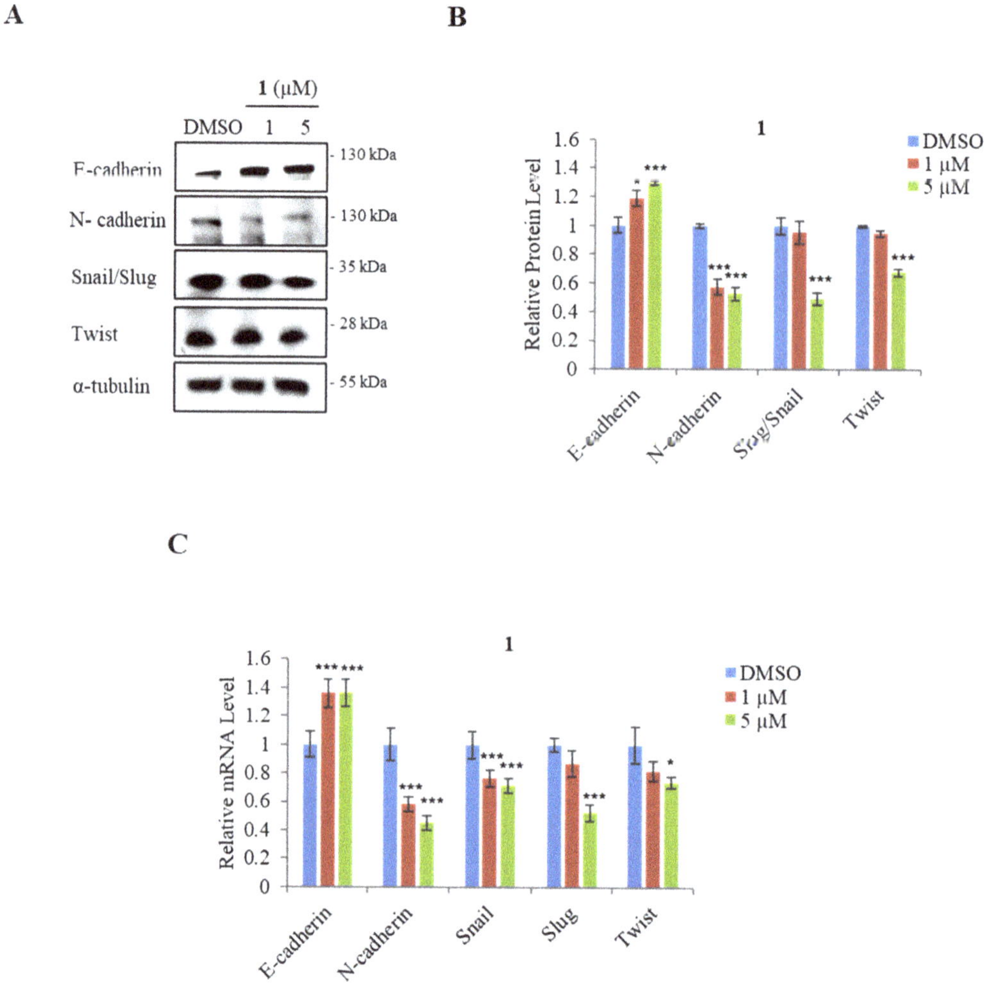

Figure 5. Effect of actinoquinazolione (**1**) on EMT markers in AGS cells. (**A**) Western blot analysis of E-cadherin, N-cadherin Snail/Slug, and Twist. (**B**) relative protein levels of E-cadherin, N-cadherin Snail/Slug, and Twist. (**C**) relative mRNA expression levels of E-cadherin, N-cadherin Snail, Slug, and Twist. mRNA expression levels were normalized against the glyceraldehyde 3-phosphate dehydrogenase (GAPDH) housekeeping gene. Data are presented as mean ± SD and analysis was performed by Student's *t*-test ($n = 3$).* $p < 0.05$; *** $p < 0.001$.

Previous studies have shown that STAT3 and EMT interact with each other to promote cancer metastasis. EMT is the downstream mediator of STAT3 and, therefore, the upregulation of the positive effect of STAT3 on the EMT process [70]. Western blot assays were performed to assess whether treatment with **1** affects the STAT3 protein level. The results (Figure 6A,B) indicate that **1** did not affect the total STAT3 protein level, whereas 5 μM of **1** slightly decreased the protein level of phosphorylated STAT3 (p- STAT3) in AGS cells.

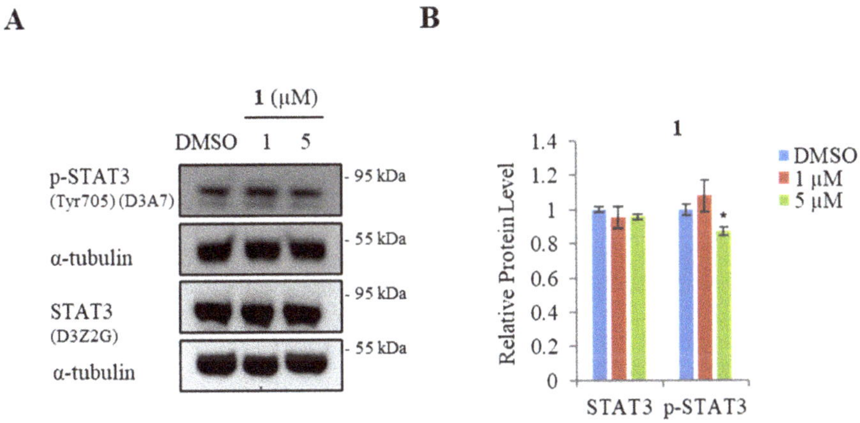

Figure 6. Effect of actinoquinazolione (**1**) on STAT3 in AGS cells. (**A**) Western blot analysis of STAT3 and p-STAT3. (**B**) relative protein levels of STAT3 and p-STAT3. Data are presented as mean ± SD and analysis was performed by Student's *t*-test ($n = 3$). * $p < 0.05$.

Finally, the Human Cell Motility RT2 Profiler PCR Array was used to examine the effect of compound **1** on the mRNA expression level of cell motility-related genes. The results (Figure 7) showed that treatment with 5 μM of **1** decreased the expression of ARP2/3 actin-related protein 2/3 (ACTR2/3), rho guanine nucleotide exchange factor (GEF) 7 (ARHGEF7), cell division cycle 42 (CDC42), V-crk sarcoma virus CT10 oncogene homolog (CRK), cortactin (CTTN), enabled homolog (ENAH), insulin-like growth factor 1 (IGF-1), insulin-like growth factor 1 receptor (IGF1R), mitogen-activated protein kinase 1 (MAPK1), Met proto-oncogene (hepatocyte growth factor receptor (MET), Phosphoinositide-3-kinase, catalytic (PIK3CA), rho family GTPase 3 (RND3), rho-associated, coiled-coil containing protein kinase 1 (ROCK1), Vimentin (VIM), WAS protein family 1 (WASF1), and walkout-Aldrich syndrome protein-like (WASL). These genes are related to cancer cell motility and could be used to treat cancer. ACTR2/3 regulates cell motility by playing an important role in actin dynamics and cytoskeleton organization [71]. The ARHGEF7 gene stimulates cancer cell motility and invasiveness by modifying the cytoskeleton [72]. CDC42 is as known a structural homolog of the Rho GTPase family; inhibition of CDC42 can reduce cancer progression by suppressing distinct GEFs [73]. CRK is a regulator of kinase and overexpression of CRK is associated with adenocarcinomas of the stomach [74]. CTTN is a regulator of actin polymerization by binding the actin-regulated protein complex ACTR2/3 [75]. ENAH includes a member of the ENAH/VASP family which can modify cell morphology and adhesion in the metastasis process [76]. IGF1 promotes cell proliferation by suppressing apoptosis in cancer [77]. MAPK1 is closely related to invasion and metastasis via modulated EMT [78]. The invasiveness and metastasis of aggressive cancer cells link to the overexpression of oncogene MET [79]. PIK3CA has been related to cancer cell motility, which is the second most frequent mutant oncogene. A statistical analysis showed that mutation of PIK3CA is the reason for more than 10% of cancer cases [80]. RND3 may serve as a predictor of EMT upregulation [81]. ROCK1 is a small GTPase Rho downstream effector that is crucial in cancer metastasis [82]. VIM has been related to cancer metastasis by promoting the EMT process [83]. WASF1, also known as WAVE1 (WASP family verprolin homologous protein 1), is associated with regulating actin cytoskeleton dynamics for cancer cell invasion and migration [84].

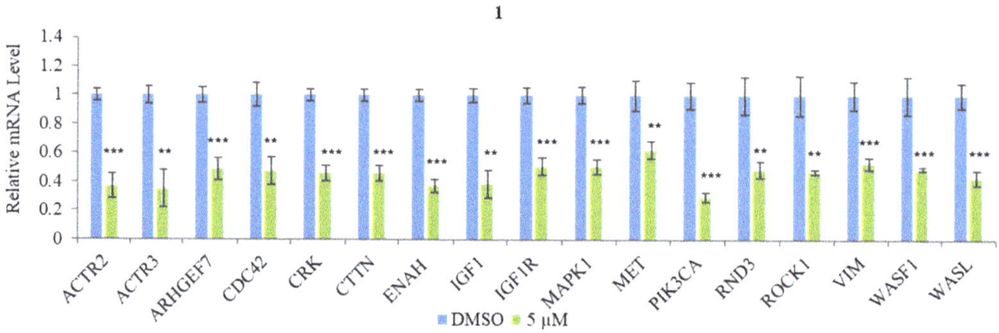

Figure 7. Effect of actinoquinazolione (**1**) on cell motility-related genes in AGS cells Relative mRNA expression levels of ACTR2/3, ARHGEF7, CDC42, CRK, CTTN, ENAH, IGF-1, IGF1R, MAPK1, MET, PIK3CA, RND3, ROCK1, VIM, WASF1, and WASL in AGS cells treated with 5μM of **1**. Data are presented as mean ± SD and analysis was performed by Student's *t*-test (n = 3). ** $p < 0.01$; *** $p < 0.001$.

3. Materials and Methods

3.1. General Experimental Procedures

Optical rotations were measured using a Kruss Optronic P-8000 polarimeter with a 5 cm cell. Infrared spectra were measured with a Varian Scimitar Series FT-IR spectrometer in methanol (MeOH). The NMR spectra were established by an Agilent NMR spectrometer (Agilent, Santa Clara, CA, USA, at 400 MHz for ^{1}H and at 100 MHz for ^{13}C) equipped at the Drug Development Research Core Center using the signals of the residual solvent as internal references (δ_H 2.50 ppm and δ_C 39.5 ppm for dimethyl sulfoxide-d_6 (DMSO-d_6) and δ_H 3.31 ppm and δ_C 4.91 ppm for deuterated methanol (CD_3OD). The low-resolution LC/MS measurements were recorded on the Agilent Technologies 1260 quadrupole and Waters Micromass ZQ LC/MS system using a reversed-phase column (Phenomenex Luna C18 (2) 100 Å, 50 mm × 4.6 mm, 5 μm) at a flow rate of 1.0 mL/min at the National Research Facilities and Equipment Center (NanoBioEnergy Materials Center) at Ewha Womans University. Open column chromatography was performed using silica (40–63 μm, Merck silica gel 60, Kenilworth, NJ, USA) eluting with a gradient solvent of dichloromethane (CH_2Cl_2) and methanol (MeOH). The fractions were purified via semi-preparative HPLC using a Waters 996 Photodiode Array Detector HPLC coupled with a reversed-phase Phenomenex Luna C18 (2) (100 Å, 250 nm × 10 mm, 5 μm) column with a mixture of acetonitrile and H_2O at a flow rate of 2.0 mL/min. High-resolution mass spectra were recorded on a JMS-700 mass spectrometer (JEOL Ltd., Tokyo, Japan) at Seoul National University.

3.2. Collection and Phylogenetic Analysis of the CNQ-617 Strain

The marine actinomycete strain CNQ-617 was isolated from a marine sediment sample collected offshore of La Jolla, California. The strain was specified as the MAR3 clade based on 16S rDNA analysis. The phylogenetic analysis revealed that this strain showed 99.7% similarity to *Streptomyces cacaoi* based upon the result of NCBI blast analysis of the partial 16S rDNA. The gene sequence data are available from GenBank (deposit #EU161093).

3.3. Cultivation and Extraction

Streptomyces strain CNQ-617 was cultured in 160 of 2.5-L Ultra Yield Flasks each containing 1 L of the medium (10 g/L of soluble starch, 2 g/L of yeast, 4 g/L of peptone, 10 g/L of $CaCO_3$, 20 g/L of KBr, 8 g/L $Fe_2(SO_4)_3 \cdot 4H_2O$ dissolved in 750 mL of natural seawater and 250 mL of distilled water) at 27 °C with constant shaking at 120 rpm. After

15 days, the culture broth was extracted with ethyl acetate (EtOAc; 160 L in total) to obtain 16.0 g of EtOAc extract.

3.4. Isolation of Compounds

The crude extract (16.0 g) of the CNQ-617 strain was fractionated by medium-pressure liquid chromatography (MPLC) eluting with a step gradient of CH_2Cl_2 and MeOH (100/0, 99/1, 98/2, 96/4, 95/5, 90/10, 80/20, 50/50, 0/100, *v/v*, 600 mL for each gradient) to afford fractions M1–M9. The fourth fraction M4 was purified by HPLC (Phenomenex Luna C18(2) 100 Å, 250 mm × 10 mm, 5 μm) with 15% acetonitrile in H_2O with 0.1% trifluoroacetic acid (TFA) at a flow rate of 2.0 mL/min to yield 19.0 mg actinoquinazolinone (**1**, t_R 14.5 min) and 7-methoxy-8-hydroxy cycloanthranilylproline (**3**, t_R 27.0 min). Fraction M8 was also purified by reversed phase HPLC (Phenomenex 100 Å, 250 mm × 10 mm, 5 μm,) under isocratic conditions with 11% acetonitrile in H_2O with 0.1% TFA at flow rate 2.0 mL/min to yield 7-hydroxy-6-methoxy-3,4-dihydroquinazolin-4-one (**2**, t_R 15.9 min).

Actinoquinazolinone (**1**): yellowish brown oil; $[\alpha]_D^{25}$ = +62.4 (*c* 0.19, MeOH); UV (MeOH) λ_{max} (log ε) 202 (2.4), 243 (2.7), 309 (1.9), 322 (1.9) nm; IR (KBr) ν_{max} 3188, 2956, 2925, 1658, 1457 cm^{-1} (Figure S10), ^1H and ^{13}C NMR data, Table 1, Figures S1–S5; HR-FAB-MS *m/z* 295.0924 $[M + H]^+$ (Figure S11, calcd for $C_{13}H_{15}N_2O_6$, 296.0930).

7-Hydroxy-6-methoxy-3,4-dihydroquinazolin-4-one (**2**): ^1H (400 MHz, DMSO-d_6, Figure S6); δ_H 7.91 (s, H-2), 7.43 (s, H-5), 6.98 (s, H-8), 3.87 (s, 6-OMe), ^{13}C (100 MHz, DMSO-d_6, Figure S7); δ_C 160.1 (C-4), 153.0 (C-7), 148.0 (C-2), 144.9 (C-6), 143.6 (C-9), 114.7 (C-10), 111.3 (C-8), 105.5 (C-5), 55.7 (6-OMe), LR-ESI-MS *m/z* 193.1 $[M + H]^+$.

7-methoxy-8-hydroxy cycloanthranilylproline (**3**): $[\alpha]_D^{25}$ = +275 (c 0.22, MeOH); IR (KBr) ν_{max} 3214, 1693, 1607, 1519, 1437, 1274, 1201, 1179, 786 cm^{-1}; UV (MeOH) λ_{max} (log ε) 220 (7.76), 260 (3.79), 300 (3.31) nm, ^1H (500 MHz, CD_3OD, Figure S8); δ_H 7.36 (s, H-6), 6.58 (s, H-9), 4.16 (m. H-11a), 3.91 (s, 7-OCH_3), 3.72 (m, H-3), 3.57 (m, H-3), 2.67 (m, H-1), 2.05 (m, H-1), 2.02 (m, H-2), ^{13}C (125 MHz, CD_3OD, Figure S9); δ_C 171.2 (C-11), 166.6 (C-5), 151.1 (C-8), 145.4 (C-7), 131.4 (C-9a), 117.9 (C-5a), 111.8 (C-6), 107.7 (C-9), 57.2 (C-11a), 55.4 (7-OCH_3), 47.1 (C-3), 25.8 (C-1), 23.4 (C-2), HR-FAB-MS *m/z* 263.1029 $[M + H]^+$ (calcd for $C_{13}H_{14}N_2O_4$, 263.1029).

3.5. Cell Culture

Cell lines A549 (lung cancer), AGS (gastric cancer), and Caco-2 (colorectal cancer) were cultured in Roswell Park Memorial Institute (RPMI) 1640 Medium or Dulbecco's Modified Eagle Medium (DMEM) (Gen Depot, Barker, TX, USA), supplemented with 10% FBS and 1% penicillin–streptomycin solution C in a humid environment with 5% CO_2 [85].

3.6. MTT Assay

A549 (3 × 10^3 cells/well), AGS (3 × 10^3 cells/well), and Caco-2 (2.5 × 10^3 cells/well) were seeded on 96-well plates for gown overnight, and then treated with DMSO (Sigma-Aldrich) or various concentrations of actinoquinazolione (**1**), 7-hydroxy-6-methoxy-3,4-dihydroquinazolin-4-one (**2**), and 7-methoxy-8-hydroxy cycloanthranilylproline (**3**) for 48 h. MTT was added to the cultures for 4 h after treatment. In the final step of MTT, the cells were lysed with 150 μL of DMSO and the absorbance was measured using a spectrophotometer (Bio Tek Instruments, Winooski, VT, USA) [86,87].

3.7. Invasion Assay

Transwell containing polycarbonate membranes with 8 μm pores coated with 1% gelatin-coated polycarbonate was used to measure the invasion ability of AGS cells. The AGS cells were seeded in media containing 0.2% bovine serum albumin (BSA), then treated with 1 and 5 μM concentrations of compound **1** for 24 h and DMSO as a control. The lower chamber was filled with 600 μL RPMI containing 0.2% BSA and 6 μg/mL fibronectin (EMD Millipore Corp., Billerica, MA, USA) as a chemoattractant. Diff-Quik kit (Sysmex, Kobe, Japan) was used for the fixation and dying of AGS cells after 24 h treatment, the cells in the upper chambers were quantified using a *K1-Fluo* Confocal *Microscope* (Nanoscope Systems, Republic of Korea) and i-Solution FL Auto Software (IMT i-Solution Inc., Vancouver, QC, Canada) [88,89].

3.8. qPCR

Total RNA of AGS cells was extracted by RNAiso Plus (Takara, Otsu, Japan) according to the manufacturer's suggestions. Using a Moloney Murine Leukemia Virus (M-MLV) kit, total RNA (1 μg) from DMSO as well as 1 and 5 μM of treatment with compound **1** groups were converted to cDNA. SYBR Green (Enzynomics, Seoul, Republic of Korea) was used to evaluate relative gene expression and CFX (Bio-Rad, Hercules, CA, USA) was applied for analysis [90,91].

3.9. Western Blots

The AGS cells were seeded in 6 well plates for gown overnight, and then treated with DMSO as well as 1 and 5 μM concentrations of **1**. After 24 h treatment, rinsed with PBS, then extracted using lysis buffer. The extracted protein was separated by SDS-PAGE. The membranes were incubated in blocking buffer (20 mmol/l Tris-HCl, 137 mmol/l NaCl, pH 7.6, 492 containing 0.1% Tween and 3% nonfat dry milk) for one hour and antibodies against E-cadherin and N-cadherin (BD Bioscience, San Jose, CA, USA); Snail/Slug and Twist (Abcam, London, UK); α-tubulin, STAT3, and p-STAT3 (Cell Signaling Technology, Danvers, MA, USA) were detected by horseradish peroxidase-conjugated secondary antibodies (Thermo Fisher Scientific, Waltham, MA, USA) using the Immobilon Western Chemiluminescent HRP Substrate Kit (Millipore, Billerica, MA, USA). The Multi Gauge 3.0 (Fujifilm, Tokyo, Japan) software was used for analyzing the density of the bands [92,93].

3.10. Statistical Analysis

Data is represented as means ± standard deviation. All statistical analyses were carried out using the Sigma Plot software. Student's t-test was used to compare statistically significant differences between two groups. A p-value less than 0.05 was considered statistically significant.

4. Conclusions

In summary, the exploration of marine natural products from marine sediment-derived *Streptomyces* sp. CNQ-617 has led to the discovery of a novel compound, actinoquinazolinone (**1**), along with two previously reported compounds, 7-hydroxy-6-methoxy-3,4-dihydroquinazolin-4-one (**2**) and 7-methoxy-8-hydroxy cycloanthranilylproline (**3**). Furthermore, compound **1** exhibited moderate antibacterial activity against the Gram-positive bacteria *K. rhizophila* KCTC 1915 and weak inhibitory activities against *B. subtilis* KCTC 1021 and *S. aureus* KCTC 1927. In addition, compound **1** showed higher activity than compounds **2** and **3** in decreasing the cell viability of cancer cells. Moreover, compound **1** suppressed the invasion ability of the EMT and STAT3 signal pathways, and some of the cell motility-related genes. These findings highlight the potential of marine sediment-derived *Streptomyces* sp. CNQ-617 as a source of novel bioactive compounds that may have therapeutic applications. Further studies are required to determine the potential therapeutic effect and the potential side effect of **1**.

Supplementary Materials: The following are available online at https://www.mdpi.com/article/10.3390/md21090489/s1, Figures S1–S5 NMR spectra of actinoquinazolinone (**1**) in DMSO-d_6; Figures S6 and S7 NMR spectra of 7-hydroxy-6-methoxy-3,4-dihydroquinazolin-4-one (**2**) in DMSO-d_6; Figures S8 and S9 NMR spectra of 7-methoxy-8-hydroxy cycloanthranilylproline (**3**) in CD_3OD; Figures S10 and S11 IR and HRMS spectra actinoquinazolinone (**1**).

Author Contributions: S.P.: Data curation, Investigation, Writing—Original draft; D.-A.K.: Data curation, Investigation, Writing—Original draft; P.F.H.: Data curation, Investigation, Writing—Original draft; D.-C.O.: Writing—Review and editing; H.K.: Conceptualization, Methodology, Writing—

Review and editing; S.-J.N.: Conceptualization, Methodology, Writing—Review and editing, Supervision; W.F.: Writing—Review and editing, Resources. All authors have read and agreed to the published version of the manuscript.

Funding: This research was supported by the National Research Foundation of Korea, grant funded by the Korean Government (Ministry of Science and ICT; no. 2021R1A4A2001251 to S.-J.N.). Isolation of the bacterium was a result of the financial support from the US National Cancer Institute (grant CA R37044848 to W.F.).

Institutional Review Board Statement: Not applicable.

Data Availability Statement: The data presented in this study are available on request from the corresponding author.

Conflicts of Interest: The authors declare no conflict of interest.

References

1. Gerstberger, S.; Jiang, Q.; Ganesh, K. Metastasis. *Cell* **2023**, *186*, 1564–1579. [CrossRef]
2. World Health Organisation. Cancer. 2022. Available online: http://www.who.int/news-room/fact-sheets/detail/cancer (accessed on 7 July 2023).
3. Le, T.C.; Pulat, S.; Lee, J.; Kim, G.J.; Kim, H.; Lee, E.-Y.; Hillman, P.F.; Choi, H.; Yang, I.; Oh, D.-C.; et al. Marine Depsipeptide Nobilamide I Inhibits Cancer Cell Motility and Tumorigenicity via Suppressing Epithelial–Mesenchymal Transition and MMP2/9 Expression. *ACS Omega* **2022**, *7*, 1722–1732. [CrossRef]
4. Jiang, J.; Cao, B.; Chen, Y.; Luo, H.; Xue, J.; Xiong, X.; Zou, T. Alkylgold(III) Complexes Undergo Unprecedented Photo-Induced β-Hydride Elimination and Reduction for Targeted Cancer Therapy. *Angew. Chem. Int. Ed.* **2022**, *61*, e202201103. [CrossRef]
5. Hashimoto, I.; Oshima, T. Claudins and Gastric Cancer: An Overview. *Cancers* **2022**, *14*, 290. [CrossRef]
6. Huang, Y.; Guo, Y.; Xu, Y.; Liu, F.; Dai, S. Flotillin-1 promotes EMT of gastric cancer *via* stabilizing Snail. *PeerJ* **2022**, *10*, e13901. [CrossRef]
7. Ouyang, S.; Li, H.; Lou, L.; Huang, Q.; Zhang, Z.; Mo, J.; Li, M.; Lu, J.; Zhu, K.; Chu, Y.; et al. Inhibition of STAT3-ferroptosis negative regulatory axis suppresses tumor growth and alleviates chemoresistance in gastric cancer. *Redox Biol.* **2022**, *52*, 102317. [CrossRef]
8. Wei, Q.; Guo, J.-S. Developing natural marine products for treating liver diseases. *World J. Clin. Cases* **2022**, *10*, 2369–2381. [CrossRef]
9. Karthikeyan, A.; Joseph, A.; Nair, B.G. Promising bioactive compounds from the marine environment and their potential effects on various diseases. *J. Genet. Eng. Biotechnol.* **2022**, *20*, 14. [CrossRef]
10. Lee, S.-E.; Kim, M.-J.; Hillman, P.F.; Oh, D.-C.; Fenical, W.; Nam, S.-J.; Lim, K.-M. Deoxyvasicinone with anti-melanogenic activity from marine-derived *Streptomyces* sp. CNQ-617. *Mar. Drugs* **2022**, *20*, 155. [CrossRef]
11. Fenical, W.; Jensen, P.R. Developing a new resource for drug discovery: Marine actinomycete bacteria. *Nat. Chem. Biol.* **2006**, *2*, 666–673. [CrossRef]
12. Kala, R.R.; Chandrika, V. Effect of different media for isolation, growth and maintenance of actinomycetes from mangrove sediments. *Indian J. Mar. Sci.* **1993**, *22*, 297–299.
13. Mast, Y.; Stegmann, E. Actinomycetes: The antibiotics producers. *Antibiotics* **2019**, *8*, 105. [CrossRef]
14. Jensen, P.R.; Mincer, T.J.; Williams, P.G.; Fenical, W. Marine actinomycete diversity and natural product discovery. *Antonie Van Leeuwenhoek* **2005**, *87*, 43–48. [CrossRef]
15. Song, F.; Hu, J.; Zhang, X.; Xu, W.; Yang, J.; Li, S.; Xu, X. Unique cyclized thiolopyrrolones from the marine-derived *Streptomyces* sp. BTBU20218885. *Mar. Drugs* **2022**, *20*, 214. [CrossRef]
16. Shaaban, M.; Shaaban, K.A.; Kelter, G.; Fiebig, H.H.; Laatsch, H. Mansouramycins E–G, cytotoxic isoquinolinequinones from marine streptomycetes. *Mar. Drugs* **2021**, *19*, 715. [CrossRef]
17. Shen, X.; Wang, X.; Huang, T.; Deng, Z.; Lin, S. Naphthoquinone-based meroterpenoids from marine-derived *Streptomyces* sp. B9173. *Biomolecules* **2020**, *10*, 1187. [CrossRef]
18. Wu, J.; Zhu, Y.; Zhang, M.; Li, H.; Sun, P. Micaryolanes A and B, Two new caryolane-type sesquiterpenoids from marine *Streptomyces* sp. AH25. *Chem. Biodivers.* **2020**, *17*, e2000769. [CrossRef]
19. Chang, Y.; Xing, L.; Sun, C.; Liang, S.; Liu, T.; Zhang, X.; Zhu, T.; Pfeifer, B.A.; Che, Q.; Zhang, G.; et al. Monacycliones G–K and *ent*-gephyromycin A, angucycline derivatives from the marine-derived *Streptomyces* sp. HDN15129. *J. Nat. Prod.* **2020**, *83*, 2749–2755. [CrossRef]
20. Liu, M.; Yang, Y.; Gong, G.; Li, Z.; Zhang, L.; Guo, L.; Xu, B.; Zhang, S.; Xie, Z. Angucycline and angucyclinone derivatives from the marine-derived *Streptomyces* sp. *Chirality* **2022**, *34*, 421–427. [CrossRef]
21. Guo, L.; Yang, Q.; Wang, G.; Zhang, S.; Liu, M.; Pan, X.; Pescitelli, G.; Xie, Z. Ring D-modified and highly reduced angucyclinones from marine sediment-derived *Streptomyces* sp. *Front. Chem.* **2021**, *9*, 756962. [CrossRef]
22. Guo, Z.; Ma, S.; Khan, S.; Zhu, H.; Zhang, B.; Zhang, S.; Jiao, R. Zhaoshumycins A and B, Two unprecedented antimycin-type depsipeptides produced by the marine-derived *Streptomyces* sp. ITBB-ZKa6. *Mar. Drugs* **2021**, *19*, 624. [CrossRef] [PubMed]

23. Cho, E.; Kwon, O.-S.; Chung, B.; Lee, J.; Sun, J.; Shin, J.; Oh, K.-B. Antibacterial activity of chromomycins from a marine-derived *Streptomyces microflavus*. *Mar. Drugs* **2020**, *18*, 522. [CrossRef] [PubMed]
24. Karim, R.U.; In, Y.; Zhou, T.; Harunari, E.; Oku, N.; Igarashi, Y. Nyuzenamides A and B: Bicyclic peptides with antifungal and cytotoxic activity from a marine-derived *Streptomyces* sp. *Org. Lett.* **2021**, *23*, 2109–2113. [CrossRef]
25. Aksoy, S.; Küçüksolak, M.; Uze, A.; Bedir, E. Benzodiazepine Derivatives from Marine-Derived Streptomyces cacaoi 14CM034. *Rec. Nat. Prod.* **2021**, *15*, 602–607. [CrossRef]
26. Peng, J.; Zhang, Q.; Jiang, X.; Ma, L.; Long, T.; Cheng, Z.; Zhang, C.; Zhu, Y. New piericidin derivatives from the marine-derived *streptomyces* sp. SCSIO 40063 with cytotoxic activity. *Nat. Prod. Res.* **2022**, *36*, 2458–2464. [CrossRef]
27. Salem, S.M.; Kancharla, P.; Florova, G.; Gupta, S.; Lu, W.; Reynolds, K.A. Elucidation of Final Steps of the Marineosins Biosynthetic Pathway through Identification and Characterization of the Corresponding Gene Cluster. *J. Am. Chem. Soc.* **2014**, *136*, 4565–4574. [CrossRef]
28. Perera, B.G.K.; Maly, D.J. Design, synthesis and characterization of "clickable" 4-anilinoquinazoline kinase inhibitors. *Mol. Biosyst.* **2008**, *4*, 542–550. [CrossRef]
29. Zhang, J.; Liu, J.; Ma, Y.; Ren, D.; Cheng, P.; Zhao, J.; Zhang, F.; Yao, Y. One-pot synthesis and antifungal activity against plant pathogens of quinazolinone derivatives containing an amide moiety. *Bioorg. Med. Chem. Lett.* **2016**, *26*, 2273–2277. [CrossRef]
30. Wattanapiromsakul, C.; Forster, P.; Waterman, P. Alkaloids and limonoids from Bouchardatia neurococca: Systematic significance. *Phytochemistry* **2003**, *64*, 609–615. [CrossRef]
31. Rakesh, K.; Manukumar, H.; Gowda, D.C. Schiff's bases of quinazolinone derivatives: Synthesis and SAR studies of a novel series of potential anti-inflammatory and antioxidants. *Bioorg. Med. Chem. Lett.* **2015**, *25*, 1072–1077. [CrossRef]
32. Radwan, A.A.; Alanazi, F.K.; Al-Dhfyan, A. Synthesis, and docking studies of some fused-quinazolines and quinazolines carrying biological active isatin moiety as cell-cycle inhibitors of breast cancer cell lines. *Drug Res.* **2013**, *63*, 129–136. [CrossRef]
33. El-Azab, A.S.; ElTahir, K.E. Design and synthesis of novel 7-aminoquinazoline derivatives: Antitumor and anticonvulsant activities. *Bioorg. Med. Chem. Lett.* **2012**, *22*, 1879–1885. [CrossRef] [PubMed]
34. Yousefi, B.; Azimi, A.; Majidinia, M.; Shafiei-Irannejad, V.; Badalzadeh, R.; Baradaran, B.; Zarghami, N.; Samadi, N. Balaglitazone reverses P-glycoprotein-mediated multidrug resistance via upregulation of PTEN in a PPARγ-dependent manner in leukemia cells. *Tumor Biol.* **2017**, *39*, 1010428317716501. [CrossRef] [PubMed]
35. Malamas, M.S.; Millen, J. Quinazolineacetic acids and related analogs as aldose reductase inhibitors. *J. Med. Chem.* **1991**, *34*, 1492–1503. [CrossRef] [PubMed]
36. Jiang, S.; Zeng, Q.; Gettayacamin, M.; Tungtaeng, A.; Wannaying, S.; Lim, A.; Hansukjariya, P.; Okunji, C.O.; Zhu, S.; Fang, D. Antimalarial activities and therapeutic properties of febrifugine analogs. *Antimicrob. Agents Chemother.* **2005**, *49*, 1169–1176. [CrossRef]
37. Ghorab, M.M.; Ismail, Z.H.; Abdalla, M.; Radwan, A.A. Synthesis, antimicrobial evaluation and molecular modelling of novel sulfonamides carrying a biologically active quinazoline nucleus. *Arch. Pharm. Res.* **2013**, *36*, 660–670. [CrossRef]
38. Ghorab, M.M.; Ismail, Z.H.; Radwan, A.A.; Abdalla, M. Synthesis and pharmacophore modeling of novel quinazolines bearing a biologically active sulfonamide moiety. *Acta Pharm.* **2013**, *63*, 1–18. [CrossRef]
39. Devi, K.; Kachroo, M. Synthesis and antitubercular activity of some new 2,3-disubstituted quinazolinones. *Der. Pharm. Chem.* **2014**, *6*, 353–359.
40. Khan, I.; Zaib, S.; Batool, S.; Abbas, N.; Ashraf, Z.; Iqbal, J.; Saeed, A. Quinazolines and quinazolinones as ubiquitous structural fragments in medicinal chemistry: An update on the development of synthetic methods and pharmacological diversification. *Bioorg. Med. Chem.* **2016**, *24*, 2361–2381. [CrossRef]
41. Mohamed, Y.A.; Amr, A.E.-G.E.; Mohamed, S.F.; Abdalla, M.M.; Al-Omar, M.A.; Shfik, S.H. Cytotoxicity and anti-HIV evaluations of some new synthesized quinazoline and thioxopyrimidine derivatives using 4-(thiophen-2-yl)-3,4,5,6-tetrahydrobenzo[h]quinazoline-2(1H)-thione as synthon. *J. Chem. Sci.* **2012**, *124*, 693–702. [CrossRef]
42. Priya, M.G.R.; Girija, K.; Ravichandran, N. In vitro study of anti-inflammatory and antioxidant activity of 4-(3H)-quinazolinone derivatives. *Rasayan J. Chem.* **2011**, *4*, 418–424.
43. Bojarski, A.J.; Kowalski, P.; Kowalska, T.; Duszyńska, B.; Charakchieva-Minol, S.; Tatarczyńska, E.; Kłodzińska, A.; Chojnacka-Wójcik, E. Synthesis and pharmacological evaluation of new Arylpiperazines. 3-{4-[4-(3-chlorophenyl)-1-piperazinyl]butyl}-quinazolidin-4-one—A dual serotonin 5-HT1A/5-HT2A receptor ligand with an anxiolytic-like activity. *Bioorg. Med. Chem.* **2002**, *10*, 3817–3827. [CrossRef] [PubMed]
44. Traxler, P.; Green, J.; Mett, H.; Séquin, U.; Furet, P. Use of a Pharmacophore Model for the Design of EGFR Tyrosine Kinase Inhibitors: Isoflavones and 3-Phenyl-4(1*H*)-quinolones. *J. Med. Chem.* **1999**, *42*, 1018–1026. [CrossRef] [PubMed]
45. Ôrfi, L.; Kökösi, J.; Szász, G.; Kövesdi, I.; Mák, M.; Teplán, I.; Kéri, G. Heterocondensed quinazolones: Synthesis and protein-tyrosine kinase inhibitory activity of 3,4-dihydro-1H,6H-[1,4]oxazino-[3,4-b]quinazolin-6-one derivatives. *Bioorg. Med. Chem.* **1996**, *4*, 547–551. [CrossRef] [PubMed]
46. Nerkar, A.G.; Saxena, A.K.; Ghone, S.A.; Thaker, A.K. In silico screening, synthesis and in vitro evaluation of some quinazolinone and pyridine derivatives as dihydrofolate reductase inhibitors for anticancer activity. *J. Chem.* **2009**, *6*, S97–S102. [CrossRef]
47. Hour, M.-J.; Huang, L.-J.; Kuo, S.-C.; Xia, Y.; Bastow, K.; Nakanishi, Y.; Hamel, E.; Lee, K.-H. 6-Alkylamino- and 2,3-Dihydro-3′-methoxy-2-phenyl-4-quinazolinones and Related Compounds: Their Synthesis, Cytotoxicity, and Inhibition of Tubulin Polymerization. *J. Med. Chem.* **2000**, *43*, 4479–4487. [CrossRef]

48. Grosso, J.A.; Nichols, D.E.; Kohli, J.D.; Glock, D. Synthesis of 2-(alkylamino)-5,6- and -6,7-dihydroxy-3,4-dihydroquinazolines and evaluation as potential dopamine agonists. *J. Med. Chem.* **1982**, *25*, 703–708. [CrossRef]
49. Bouley, R.; Ding, D.; Peng, Z.; Bastian, M.; Lastochkin, E.; Song, W.; Suckow, M.A.; Schroeder, V.A.; Wolter, W.R.; Mobashery, S.; et al. Structure–Activity Relationship for the 4(3*H*)-Quinazolinone Antibacterials. *J. Med. Chem.* **2016**, *59*, 5011–5021. [CrossRef]
50. Chen, J.; Wu, D.; He, F.; Liu, M.; Wu, H.; Ding, J.; Su, W. Gallium(III) triflate-catalyzed one-pot selective synthesis of 2,3-dihydroquinazolin-4(1H)-ones and quinazolin-4(3H)-ones. *Tetrahedron Lett.* **2008**, *49*, 3814–3818. [CrossRef]
51. Liu, Y.-P.; Fang, S.-T.; Shi, Z.-Z.; Wang, B.-G.; Li, X.-N.; Ji, N.-Y. Phenylhydrazone and Quinazoline Derivatives from the Cold-Seep-Derived Fungus *Penicillium oxalicum*. *Mar. Drugs* **2020**, *19*, 9. [CrossRef]
52. Liu, S.-S.; Yang, L.; Kong, F.-D.; Zhao, J.-H.; Yao, L.; Yuchi, Z.-G.; Ma, Q.-Y.; Xie, Q.-Y.; Zhou, L.-M.; Guo, M.-F.; et al. Three New Quinazoline-Containing Indole Alkaloids From the Marine-Derived Fungus *Aspergillus* sp. HNMF114. *Front. Microbiol.* **2021**, *12*, 680879. [CrossRef] [PubMed]
53. Kong, F.-D.; Zhang, S.-L.; Zhou, S.-Q.; Ma, Q.-Y.; Xie, Q.-Y.; Chen, J.-P.; Li, J.-H.; Zhou, L.-M.; Yuan, J.-Z.; Hu, Z.; et al. Quinazoline-Containing Indole Alkaloids from the Marine-Derived Fungus *Aspergillus* sp. HNMF114. *J. Nat. Prod.* **2019**, *82*, 3456–3463. [CrossRef] [PubMed]
54. Prata-Sena, M.; Ramos, A.; Buttachon, S.; Castro-Carvalho, B.; Marques, P.; Dethoup, T.; Kijjoa, A.; Rocha, E. Cytotoxic activity of Secondary Metabolites from Marine-derived Fungus *Neosartorya siamensis* in Human Cancer Cells. *Phytother. Res.* **2016**, *30*, 1862–1871. [CrossRef] [PubMed]
55. Ma, C.; Li, Y.; Niu, S.; Zhang, H.; Liu, X.; Che, Y. *N*-Hydroxypyridones, Phenylhydrazones, and a Quinazolinone from *Isaria farinosa*. *J. Nat. Prod.* **2011**, *74*, 32–37. [CrossRef] [PubMed]
56. Li, C.-S.; An, C.-Y.; Li, X.-M.; Gao, S.-S.; Cui, C.-M.; Sun, H.-F.; Wang, B.-G. Triazole and Dihydroimidazole Alkaloids from the Marine Sediment-Derived Fungus *Penicillium paneum* SD-44. *J. Nat. Prod.* **2011**, *74*, 1331–1334. [CrossRef]
57. Chang, F.-R.; Wu, C.-C.; Hwang, T.-L.; Patnam, R.; Kuo, R.-Y.; Wang, W.-Y.; Lan, Y.-H.; Wu, Y.-C. Effect of active synthetic 2-substituted quinazolinones on anti-platelet aggregation and the inhibition of superoxide anion generation by neutrophils. *Arch. Pharm. Res.* **2003**, *26*, 511–515. [CrossRef]
58. Machushynets, N.V.; Wu, C.; Elsayed, S.S.; Hankemeier, T.; van Wezel, G.P. Discovery of novel glycerolated quinazolinones from *Streptomyces* sp. MBT27. *J. Ind. Microbiol. Biotechnol.* **2019**, *46*, 483–492. [CrossRef]
59. Xue, J.H.; Xu, L.X.; Jiang, Z.-H.; Wei, X. Quinazoline Alkaloids from Streptomyces michiganensis. *Chem. Nat. Compd.* **2012**, *48*, 839–841. [CrossRef]
60. Nett, M.; Hertweck, C. Farinamycin, a Quinazoline from *Streptomyces griseus*. *J. Nat. Prod.* **2011**, *74*, 2265–2268. [CrossRef]
61. Maskey, R.P.; Shaaban, M.; Grün-Wollny, I.; Laatsch, H. Quinazolin-4-one Derivatives from *Streptomyces* Isolates. *J. Nat. Prod.* **2004**, *67*, 1131–1134. [CrossRef]
62. Vollmar, D.; Thorn, A.; Schuberth, I.; Grond, S. A comprehensive view on 4-methyl-2-quinazolinamine, a new microbial alkaloid from Streptomyces of TCM plant origin. *J. Antibiot.* **2009**, *62*, 439–444. [CrossRef] [PubMed]
63. Kornsakulkarn, J.; Saepua, S.; Srijomthong, K.; Rachtawee, P.; Thongpanchang, C. Quinazolinone alkaloids from actinomycete Streptomyces sp. BCC 21795. *Phytochem. Lett.* **2015**, *12*, 6–8. [CrossRef]
64. Feng, N.; Ye, W.; Wu, P.; Huang, Y.; Xie, H.; Wei, X. Two New Antifungal Alkaloids Produced by Streptoverticillium morookaense. *J. Antibiot.* **2007**, *60*, 179–183. [CrossRef] [PubMed]
65. Carmichael, J.; Degraff, W.G.; Gazdar, A.F.; Minna, J.D.; Mitchell, J.B. Evaluation of a Tetrazolium-based Semiautomated Colorimetric Assay: Assessment of Chemosensitivity testing. *Cancer Res.* **1987**, *47*, 936–942.
66. Zaman, K.A.U.; Park, J.H.; DeVine, L.; Hu, Z.; Wu, X.; Kim, H.S.; Cao, S. Secondary Metabolites from the Leather Coral-Derived Fungal Strain *Xylaria* sp. FM1005 and Their Glycoprotein IIb/IIIa Inhibitory Activity. *J. Nat. Prod.* **2021**, *84*, 466–473. [CrossRef]
67. Dillekås, H.; Rogers, M.S.; Straume, O. Are 90% of deaths from cancer caused by metastases? *Cancer Med.* **2019**, *8*, 5574–5576. [CrossRef]
68. Dou, R.; Liu, K.; Yang, C.; Zheng, J.; Shi, D.; Lin, X.; Wei, C.; Zhang, C.; Fang, Y.; Huang, S.; et al. EMT-cancer cells-derived exosomal miR-27b-3p promotes circulating tumour cells-mediated metastasis by modulating vascular permeability in colorectal cancer. *Clin. Transl. Med.* **2021**, *11*, e595. [CrossRef]
69. Padmanaban, V.; Krol, I.; Suhail, Y.; Szczerba, B.M.; Aceto, N.; Bader, J.S.; Ewald, A.J. E-cadherin is required for metastasis in multiple models of breast cancer. *Nature* **2019**, *573*, 439–444. [CrossRef]
70. Sadrkhanloo, M.; Entezari, M.; Orouei, S.; Ghollasi, M.; Fathi, N.; Rezaei, S.; Hejazi, E.S.; Kakavand, A.; Saebfar, H.; Hashemi, M.; et al. STAT3-EMT axis in tumors: Modulation of cancer metastasis, stemness and therapy response. *Pharmacol. Res.* **2022**, *182*, 106311. [CrossRef]
71. Goley, E.D.; Welch, M.D. The ARP2/3 complex: An actin nucleator comes of age. *Nat. Rev. Mol. Cell Biol.* **2006**, *7*, 713–726. [CrossRef]
72. Lei, X.; Deng, L.; Liu, D.; Liao, S.; Dai, H.; Li, J.; Rong, J.; Wang, Z.; Huang, G.; Tang, C.; et al. ARHGEF7 promotes metastasis of colorectal adenocarcinoma by regulating the motility of cancer cells. *Int. J. Oncol.* **2018**, *53*, 1980–1996. [CrossRef] [PubMed]
73. Maldonado, M.d.M.; Medina, J.I.; Velazquez, L.; Dharmawardhane, S. Targeting Rac and Cdc42 GEFs in Metastatic Cancer. *Front. Cell Dev. Biol.* **2020**, *8*, 201. [CrossRef] [PubMed]
74. Tsuda, M.; Tanaka, S. Roles for Crk in Cancer Metastasis and Invasion. *Genes Cancer* **2012**, *3*, 334–340. [CrossRef] [PubMed]

75. Dedes, K.J.; Lopez-Garcia, M.-A.; Geyer, F.C.; Lambros, M.B.K.; Savage, K.; Vatcheva, R.; Wilkerson, P.; Wetterskog, D.; Lacroix-Triki, M.; Natrajan, R.; et al. Cortactin gene amplification and expression in breast cancer: A chromogenic in situ hybridisation and immunohistochemical study. *Breast Cancer Res. Treat.* **2010**, *124*, 653–666. [CrossRef] [PubMed]
76. Urbanelli, L.; Massini, C.; Emiliani, C.; Orlacchio, A.; Bernardi, G.; Orlacchio, A. Characterization of human Enah gene. *Biochim. Biophys. Acta (BBA)—Gene Struct. Expr.* **2006**, *1759*, 99–107. [CrossRef] [PubMed]
77. Costa-Silva, D.R.; Barros-Oliveira, M.D.C.; Borges, R.S.; Campos-Verdes, L.M.; Da Silva-Sampaio, J.P.; Escorcio-Dourado, C.S.; Martins, L.M.; Alencar, A.P.; Baracat, E.C.; Silva, V.C.; et al. Insulin-like growth factor 1 gene polymorphism in women with breast cancer. *Med. Oncol.* **2017**, *34*, 59. [CrossRef]
78. Li, X.-W.; Tuergan, M.; Abulizi, G. Expression of MAPK1 in cervical cancer and effect of MAPK1 gene silencing on epithelial-mesenchymal transition, invasion and metastasis. *Asian Pac. J. Trop. Med.* **2015**, *8*, 937–943. [CrossRef]
79. Galeazzi, E.; Olivero, M.; Gervasio, F.C.; De Stefani, A.; Valente, G.; Comoglio, P.M.; Di Renzo, M.F.; Cortesina, G. Detection ofMET oncogene/hepatocyte growth factor receptor in lymph node metastases from head and neck squamous cell carcinomas. *Eur. Arch. Oto-Rhino-Laryngol.* **1997**, *254*, S138–S143. [CrossRef]
80. Arafeh, R.; Samuels, Y. PIK3CA in cancer: The past 30 years. *Semin. Cancer Biol.* **2019**, *59*, 36–49. [CrossRef]
81. Paysan, L.; Piquet, L.; Saltel, F.; Moreau, V. Rnd3 in Cancer: A Review of the Evidence for Tumor Promoter or Suppressor. *Mol. Cancer Res.* **2016**, *14*, 1033–1044. [CrossRef]
82. Li, X.; Cheng, Y.; Wang, Z.; Zhou, J.; Jia, Y.; He, X.; Zhao, L.; Dong, Y.; Fan, Y.; Yang, X.; et al. Calcium and TRPV4 promote metastasis by regulating cytoskeleton through the RhoA/ROCK1 pathway in endometrial cancer. *Cell Death Dis.* **2020**, *11*, 1009. [CrossRef] [PubMed]
83. Taş, İ.; Han, J.; Park, S.-Y.; Yang, Y.; Zhou, R.; Gamage, C.D.; Van Nguyen, T.; Lee, J.-Y.; Choi, Y.J.; Yu, Y.H.; et al. Physciosporin suppresses the proliferation, motility and tumourigenesis of colorectal cancer cells. *Phytomedicine* **2019**, *56*, 10–20. [CrossRef] [PubMed]
84. Marchesin, V.; Montagnac, G.; Chavrier, P. ARF6 Promotes the Formation of Rac1 and WAVE-Dependent Ventral F-Actin Rosettes in Breast Cancer Cells in Response to Epidermal Growth Factor. *PLoS ONE* **2015**, *10*, e0121747. [CrossRef] [PubMed]
85. Zhou, R.; Yang, Y.; Park, S.-Y.; Nguyen, T.T.; Seo, Y.-W.; Lee, K.H.; Lee, J.H.; Kim, K.K.; Hur, J.-S.; Kim, H. The lichen secondary metabolite atranorin suppresses lung cancer cell motility and tumorigenesis. *Sci. Rep.* **2017**, *7*, 8136. [CrossRef] [PubMed]
86. Vardar, D.; Aydin, S.; Hocaoğlu, I.; Acar, H.Y.; Başaran, N. An In Vitro Study on the Cytotoxicity and Genotoxicity of Silver Sulfide Quantum Dots Coated with Meso-2,3-dimercaptosuccinic Acid. *Turk. J. Pharm. Sci.* **2019**, *16*, 282–291. [CrossRef]
87. Varlı, M.; Pham, H.T.; Kim, S.-M.; Taş, İ.; Gamage, C.D.B.; Zhou, R.; Pulat, S.; Park, S.-Y.; Sesal, N.C.; Hur, J.-S.; et al. An acetonic extract and secondary metabolites from the endolichenic fungus Nemania sp. EL006872 exhibit immune checkpoint inhibitory activity in lung cancer cell. *Front. Pharmacol.* **2022**, *13*, 986946. [CrossRef]
88. Yang, Y.; Park, S.-Y.; Nguyen, T.T.; Yu, Y.H.; Van Nguyen, T.; Sun, E.G.; Udeni, J.; Jeong, M.-H.; Pereira, I.; Moon, C.; et al. Lichen Secondary Metabolite, Physciosporin, Inhibits Lung Cancer Cell Motility. *PLoS ONE* **2015**, *10*, e0137889. [CrossRef]
89. Lian, S.; Park, J.S.; Xia, Y.; Nguyen, T.T.; Joo, Y.E.; Kim, K.K.; Kim, H.K.; Jung, Y.D. *MicroRNA-375* Functions as a Tumor-Suppressor Gene in Gastric Cancer by Targeting Recepteur d'Origine Nantais. *Int. J. Mol. Sci.* **2016**, *17*, 1633. [CrossRef]
90. Suhail, Y.; Cain, M.P.; Vanaja, K.; Kurywchak, P.A.; Levchenko, A.; Kalluri, R.; Kshitiz. Systems Biology of Cancer Metastasis. *Cell Syst.* **2019**, *9*, 109–127. [CrossRef]
91. Gamage, C.D.B.; Kim, J.-H.; Yang, Y.; Taş, İ.; Park, S.-Y.; Zhou, R.; Pulat, S.; Varlı, M.; Hur, J.-S.; Nam, S.-J.; et al. Libertellenone T, a Novel Compound Isolated from Endolichenic Fungus, Induces G2/M Phase Arrest, Apoptosis, and Autophagy by Activating the ROS/JNK Pathway in Colorectal Cancer Cells. *Cancers* **2023**, *15*, 489. [CrossRef]
92. Ouhtit, A.; Thouta, R.; Zayed, H.; Gaur, R.L.; Fernando, A.; Rahman, M.; Welsh, D.A. CD44 mediates stem cell mobilization to damaged lung *via* its novel transcriptional targets, Cortactin and Survivin. *Int. J. Med Sci.* **2020**, *17*, 103–111. [CrossRef] [PubMed]
93. Pulat, S.; Hillman, P.F.; Kim, S.; Asolkar, R.N.; Kim, H.; Zhou, R.; Taş, İ.; Gamage, C.D.B.; Varlı, M.; Park, S.-Y.; et al. Marinobazzanan, a Bazzanane-Type Sesquiterpenoid, Suppresses the Cell Motility and Tumorigenesis in Cancer Cells. *Mar. Drugs* **2023**, *21*, 153. [CrossRef] [PubMed]

marine drugs

Article

Marine Polyether Phycotoxin Palytoxin Induces Apoptotic Cell Death via Mcl-1 and Bcl-2 Downregulation

Jaemyun Kim [1,†], Seungwon Ji [1,†,‡], Jin-Young Lee [1,§], Jean Lorquin [2], Barbora Orlikova-Boyer [1,3], Claudia Cerella [1,3], Aloran Mazumder [1,‖], Florian Muller [3,¶], Mario Dicato [3], Olivier Detournay [4,*] and Marc Diederich [1,*]

1 Department of Pharmacy, College of Pharmacy, Seoul National University, 1 Gwanak-ro, Gwanak-gu, Seoul 08626, Republic of Korea; vankim36@naver.com (J.K.); jsw0525@gmail.com (S.J.); barbora.orlikova@lbmcc.lu (B.O.-B.); claudia.cerella@lbmcc.lu (C.C.); aloran.mazumder@gmail.com (A.M.)
2 Institut Méditerranéen d'Océanologie, 163 Avenue de Luminy, CEDEX 09, 13288 Marseille, France
3 Laboratoire de Biologie Moléculaire et Cellulaire du Cancer (LBMCC), BAM3 Pavillon 2, 6A Rue Nicolas-Ernest Barblé, L-1210 Luxembourg, Luxembourg
4 Planktovie SAS, 45 Rue Frédéric Joliot Curie, CEDEX 13, 13013 Marseille, France
* Correspondence: olivier@planktovie.biz (O.D.); marcdiederich@snu.ac.kr (M.D.); Tel.: +33-6727-69688 (O.D.); +82-2-880-8919 (M.D.)
† These authors contributed equally to this work.
‡ Current address: Life Sciences, LGChem, Ltd., E8 Block LG Science Park, 30 Magokjungang 10-ro, Gangseo-gu, Seoul 07795, Republic of Korea.
§ Current address: Department of Biological Sciences, Keimyung University, 1095 Dalgubeol-daero, Dalseo-gu, Daegu 42601, Republic of Korea.
‖ Current address: Aging and Cancer Immuno-Oncology, Sanford Burnham Prebys Medical Discovery Institute, La Jolla, CA 92037, USA.
¶ Current address: Laboratory of Molecular Angiogenesis, GIGA-Research, Avenue de l'Hôpital, 1, 4020 Liège, Belgium.

Abstract: Palytoxin is considered one of the most potent biotoxins. As palytoxin-induced cancer cell death mechanisms remain to be elucidated, we investigated this effect on various leukemia and solid tumor cell lines at low picomolar concentrations. As palytoxin did not affect the viability of peripheral blood mononuclear cells (PBMC) from healthy donors and did not create systemic toxicity in zebrafish, we confirmed excellent differential toxicity. Cell death was characterized by a multi-parametric approach involving the detection of nuclear condensation and caspase activation assays. zVAD-sensitive apoptotic cell death was concomitant with a dose-dependent downregulation of antiapoptotic Bcl-2 family proteins Mcl-1 and Bcl-xL. Proteasome inhibitor MG-132 prevented the proteolysis of Mcl-1, whereas the three major proteasomal enzymatic activities were upregulated by palytoxin. Palytoxin-induced dephosphorylation of Bcl-2 further exacerbated the proapoptotic effect of Mcl-1 and Bcl-xL degradation in a range of leukemia cell lines. As okadaic acid rescued cell death triggered by palytoxin, protein phosphatase (PP)2A was involved in Bcl-2 dephosphorylation and induction of apoptosis by palytoxin. At a translational level, palytoxin abrogated the colony formation capacity of leukemia cell types. Moreover, palytoxin abrogated tumor formation in a zebrafish xenograft assay at concentrations between 10 and 30 pM. Altogether, we provide evidence of the role of palytoxin as a very potent and promising anti-leukemic agent, acting at low picomolar concentrations in cellulo and in vivo.

Keywords: palytoxin; cell death; apoptosis; Bcl-2; Mcl-1; leukemia; solid tumors

1. Introduction

Palytoxin (Figure 1) was initially found in soft corals from tropical areas of the Pacific Ocean, for example, Hawaii; it was first discovered in the tropical soft coral Palythoa species, a zoanthid [1]. Palytoxin was first characterized by the chemist Moore in 1981.

This compound represents one of the largest polyether-type phycotoxins [1]. This non-peptidic toxin consists of a long polyhydroxylated and partially unsaturated chain of 129 carbon atoms, and the aliphatic backbone contains 64 chiral centers [2]. Eight double bonds can exhibit geometrical *cis/trans* isomerism so that palytoxin can present over 1021 stereoisomers [3]. Structural analogs of palytoxin were also discovered and included ostreocin [4], ovatoxin [5], and mascarenotoxin [6]. The molecular weight of palytoxin ranges from 2658 to 2680 g/mol, depending on the Palythoa species from which it was obtained [2]. Palytoxin features lipophilic and hydrophilic regions and is considered a super-carbon-chain compound with the longest chain of carbon atoms in any known natural product [7]. Palytoxin is heat-stable, resists boiling, and remains stable in neutral aqueous solutions. A rapid decomposition is observed under acid or alkaline conditions leading to the loss of its toxicity [2].

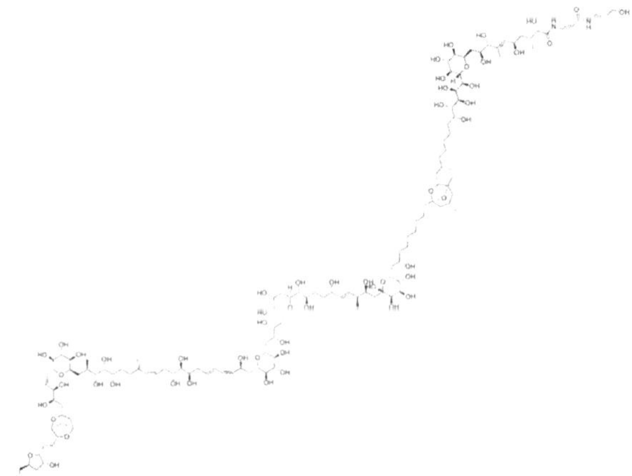

Figure 1. Structure of palytoxin.

The molecular action of palytoxin leads to the inhibition of the Na^+/K^+ adenosine triphosphatase (ATPase) channel [8,9]. This transmembrane protein exchanges three Na^+ ions and two K^+ ions using ATP hydrolysis as the driving force. The electrochemical gradient generated by the sodium pump for maintaining cell homeostasis is then inhibited by palytoxin. Palytoxin binds to the extracellular domain of the Na^+/K^+-ATPase to transform the pump into a non-specific, permanently open ion channel causing membrane depolarization, voltage-gated ion channel opening, and a massive increase of calcium ions (Ca^{2+}) into the cytosol [10] strongly interfering with vital functions of the cell. An alteration of intracellular cation concentration, in particular, a calcium increase, is associated with cell death as a modification in the distribution of these ions across the plasma membrane plays a crucial role in palytoxin-induced cell-type specific cytotoxic response [11]. Further characterization of the anticancer mode of action of this compound would allow a better understanding of cell death mechanisms triggered by palytoxin at the cellular level.

Here, we first focused on assessing differential cell toxicity and mechanisms involved in palytoxin-induced cell death in human leukemia cell lines. Palytoxin activates intrinsic and extrinsic apoptotic pathways triggered by alterations in the expression levels of the pro- and antiapoptotic Bcl-2 family proteins. Moreover, we provide evidence that palytoxin inhibits 3D tumor growth in colony formation assays and xenograft models. Altogether our results show that palytoxin acts as a potent and promising anti-leukemic agent at picomolar concentrations.

2. Results

2.1. Cytotoxic Effect of Palytoxin on Human Cancer Cells

Before investigating the cell death mechanisms, we first evaluated the antiproliferative and cytotoxic effects of palytoxin on various leukemia (Figure 2A–C) (Supplementary Figure S1) and solid tumor cell lines (Supplementary Figure S1). Cells were treated for 2, 4, 6, and 8 h at different concentrations of palytoxin, and viability was assessed by a Trypan Blue exclusion assay. Our results showed that solid tumor cell lines were more resistant to palytoxin under our experimental conditions than leukemia cell types. We also used PBMCs from healthy donors (Figure 2D) to evaluate the differential toxicity of palytoxin. We treated cells with palytoxin at various concentrations and conducted Trypan Blue staining to assess cell integrity and viability. At concentrations of 100 pM, palytoxin did not generate levels of toxicity comparable to cancer cells.

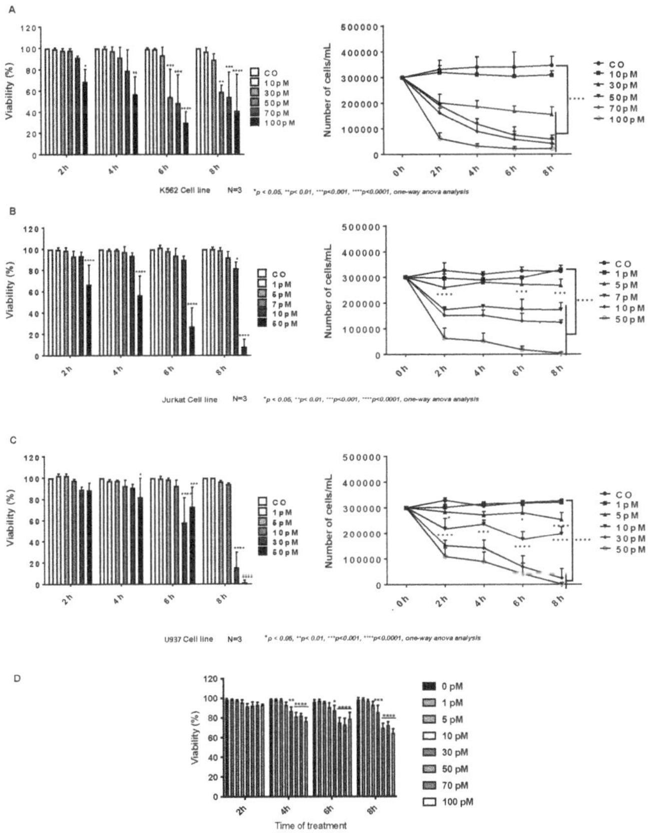

Figure 2. Differential cytotoxic effect of palytoxin on human leukemia cell lines. (**A**) Effects of Palytoxin on human chronic leukemia K562 cell viability and proliferation. (**B**) Effects of palytoxin on human T-cell leukemia Jurkat cell viability and proliferation. (**C**) Effects of Palytoxin on human histiocytic lymphoma U937 cell lines. (**D**) Time and concentration-dependent effect of palytoxin on the viability of healthy PBMCs from three buffy coats. Data are the mean of SD ± of three independent experiments. Statistical significance was assessed as * $p < 0.05$, ** $p < 0.01$, *** $p < 0.001$, **** $p < 0.0001$.

2.2. Effect of Palytoxin on Healthy Zebrafish Embryos

Palytoxin was used at various concentrations to treat zebrafish embryos and larvae for 24 h. Interestingly, we did not observe any toxicity nor alterations of the morphology of the yolk-sac nor axial/tail malformations (Figure 3A–C). Altogether this compound demonstrates a remarkable differential toxicity and selectively targets cancer cells.

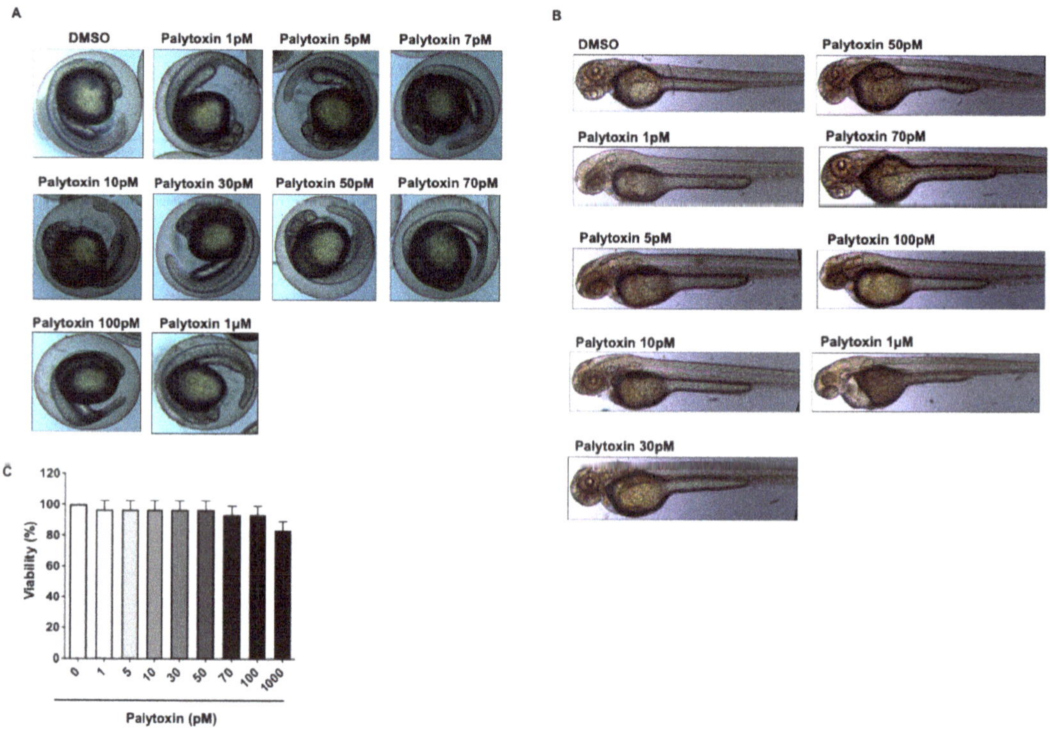

Figure 3. Differential effects of palytoxin on zebrafish embryos and healthy cells. (**A**) Effects of palytoxin on developmental defects in zebrafish embryos. Zebrafish embryos were incubated with palytoxin at concentrations from 1 pM to 1 μM for 24 h. (**B**) Effect of palytoxin exposure on zebrafish morphology scale bar: 20 μM. Zebrafish exposed to palytoxin did not exhibit moderate or severe defects of morphology. (**C**) Effect of palytoxin on the viability of healthy PBMCs. PBMCs from healthy donors were treated with indicated palytoxin concentrations for 24 h. Results correspond to the mean of ±SD of the quantification of three independent experiments.

2.3. Palytoxin-Induced Cell Death Leads to Caspase Activation in U937 Cells

We subsequently investigated whether palytoxin could trigger caspase-dependent apoptotic cell death. Palytoxin-induced cell death was identified by changes in the nuclear morphology typical of apoptotic cell death after staining with Hoechst and PI (Figure 4A). As caspase activation is sensitive to pan-caspase inhibitor zVAD, we concluded that palytoxin induces apoptosis (Figure 4B). Palytoxin induced the cleavage of the pro-caspases-8 and -9 and executor pro-caspases-3 and -7 after 6 h of treatment in a dose-dependent manner (Figure 4C). These results further confirmed by luminescent assays where palytoxin induced the enzymatic activity of caspase-3/7 in U937 cells (Figure 4D).

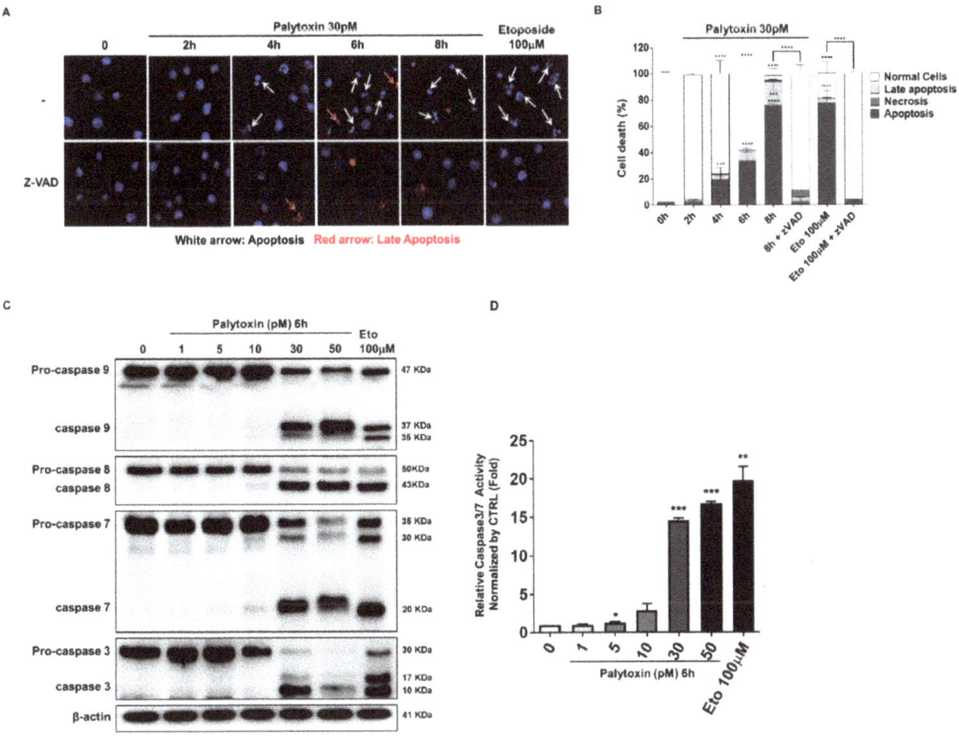

Figure 4. Palytoxin-induced cell death leads to caspase activation in U937 cells. (**A**) Hoechst/PI staining of palytoxin-treated cells. White arrows indicate cells displaying apoptotic features such as fragmented and condensed nuclei. Red arrows indicate PI-positive cells undergoing late apoptosis and presenting necrotic morphology. (**B**) The percentage of apoptotic cells was evaluated by counting cells corresponding to apoptosis, late apoptosis, and necrosis. At least 100 cells in three random fields were counted by fluorescence microscopy. (**C**) Palytoxin activation of pro-caspase-8, -9, -7, and -3 was investigated by Western blot analysis (left; one of three independent experiments). Enzymatic activity of caspases-3 and -7 was upregulated in a dose-dependent manner. (right; data representative of three independent experiments (mean ± SD). (**D**) Etoposide-treated cells (100 µM, 4 h) were positive controls for the induction of apoptosis. * $p < 0.05$, ** $p < 0.01$, *** $p < 0.001$, **** $p < 0.0001$ versus control.

2.4. Palytoxin Downregulates Expression of Antiapoptotic Bcl-2 Family Proteins

As the induction of apoptosis can be triggered by the inhibition of antiapoptotic proteins or activation of proapoptotic mechanisms, we investigated the overall expression levels of the Bcl-2 family proteins after palytoxin treatment (Figure 5A). Myeloid cell leukemia-1 (Mcl-1) and B-cell lymphoma-extra large (Bcl-xL) expression are downregulated in a dose-dependent manner. In contrast, B-cell lymphoma 2 (Bcl-2) is affected to a lesser extent. Moreover, proapoptotic Bcl-2 interacting domain death agonist (BID) was truncated by palytoxin treatment (Figure 5B), which implied that the amplification of intrinsic and extrinsic cell death pathways could be expected [12]. We generalized our finding by investigating the effect of palytoxin on a range of leukemia cell types (Figure 5C–E). Our results show a consistent decrease in Mcl-1 expression before the execution of cell death and before any other Bcl-2 family protein. We further generalized our findings by validating the modulation of Bcl-2 family proteins in solid tumor cell lines (Supplementary Figure S2).

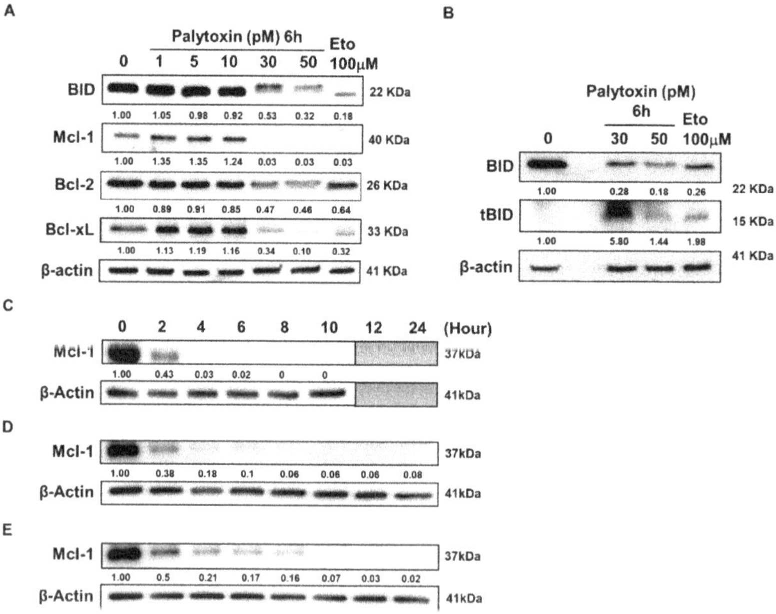

Figure 5. Palytoxin downregulates the expression of antiapoptotic Bcl-2 family proteins. (**A**) Western blot analysis of antiapoptotic Bcl-2 family protein expression levels inhibited by palytoxin after 6 h of treatment in U937. (**B**) Western blot analysis of the truncation of proapoptotic protein BID induced by palytoxin in U937. Western blot analysis of the Mcl-1 protein expression inhibited by palytoxin in a kinetic approach in K562 (**C**), Jurkat (**D**), and Raji (**E**). Western blot results are representative of three independent experiments.

2.5. Mcl-1 Is Downregulated by Palytoxin in a Proteasome-Dependent Manner

It is well established that antiapoptotic Mcl-1 can be downregulated by several mechanisms [13], including caspase-mediated- or proteasome-dependent degradation [14]. Accordingly, we assessed palytoxin-induced Mcl-1 degradation in the presence of two prototypical inhibitors, zVAD and MG-132. Our results show that palytoxin-induced Mcl-1 degradation is completely abolished in the presence of MG-132, underlining the essential role of proteasome degradation in the effect of palytoxin (Figure 6A). Unexpectedly, the three major proteasomal enzymatic activities, including trypsin, chymotrypsin, and caspase-like, were upregulated after palytoxin treatment, most likely further exacerbating the degradation of Mcl-1 (Figure 6B).

To get a deeper insight into the chronology of the molecular events triggered by palytoxin, we attempted to identify drivers of cell death rather than investigate the consequence of ongoing cellular demise. We used a kinetic approach to compare proteasomal activation, Mcl-1 degradation, and caspase activation. We obtained a rapid and significant activation of proteasomal activities before Mcl-1 degradation and caspase cleavage (Figure 6C). In parallel, ATP levels were quantified in the cells. We also observed a rapid decline in ATP levels (Figure 6D). BID was cleaved at early steps, which is in line with our hypothesis, as BID requires polyubiquitination and proteasomal activation for its processing (Figure 6D). Altogether, we concluded that palytoxin selectively targets essential cell death regulators before activation of the executioner caspase 3 and overall cellular degradation.

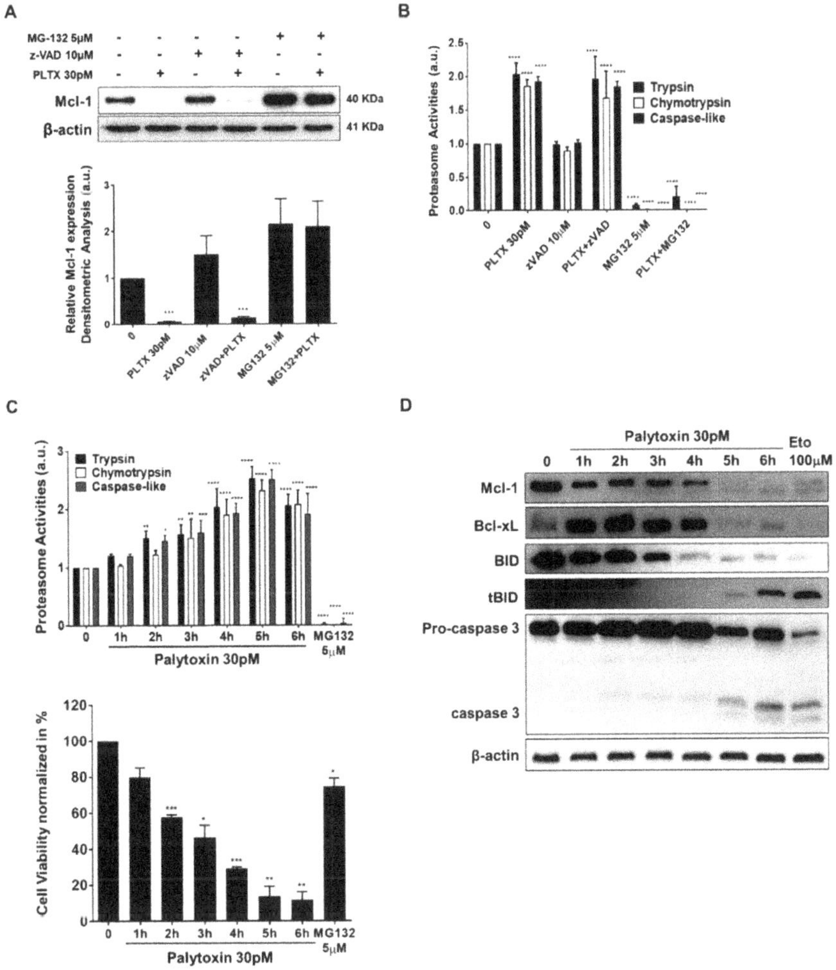

Figure 6. Mcl-1 is ubiquitously downregulated by palytoxin in a proteasome-dependent manner. (**A**) Palytoxin-induced proteasome-dependent degradation of Mcl-1 in U937 cells. Band intensities were quantified using ImageJ software. Values represent the mean of ±SD for three independent experiments. (**B**) The three major proteolytic activities of the 26S proteasome were assessed under the same conditions as the Western blots. MG-132 at 5 μM was used as a positive control for proteasomal inhibition in U937 cells. The asterisk indicates significant differences between treated versus control, **** $p < 0.0001$. (**C**) Kinetic analysis of the assessment of three major proteasome activities in U937 cells. Cell viability was determined to normalize the three major proteasome activities induced by palytoxin. (**D**) Expression of Mcl-1 and Bcl-xL degradation, BID truncation, and Caspase 3 cleavage was evaluated by Western blot analysis under the same conditions. Data representative of three independent experiments is shown as mean ± SD. * $p < 0.05$, ** $p < 0.01$, *** $p < 0.001$, **** $p < 0.0001$ versus control.

2.6. Bcl-2 Serine 70 Dephosphorylation Induced by Palytoxin Is Mediated through Protein Phosphatase 2A Activation

Our results also show that palytoxin affects Bcl-2 expression and phosphorylation levels witnessed by a discrete upshift of the band [15] (Figure 7A). We investigated phosphorylation levels of Bcl-2 as it is well known that serine 70 phosphorylation is required for the pro-survival function of this protein [16]. Our results show a dose-dependent dephosphorylation of Bcl-2, potentially contributing to a loss of its pro-survival function (Figure 7A). Serine 70 phosphorylation of Bcl-2 can be abrogated by phosphatase activation, mainly by protein phosphatase 2A (PP2A) activity [17]. Accordingly, in the next step, we used chemical inhibitors of selected cell signaling pathways, including okadaic acid used at a concentration inhibiting specifically PP2A. Our results show that PP2A inhibition partially rescues U937 cells from palytoxin-induced cell death, whereas other kinase pathways do not seem to be involved. (Figure 7B).

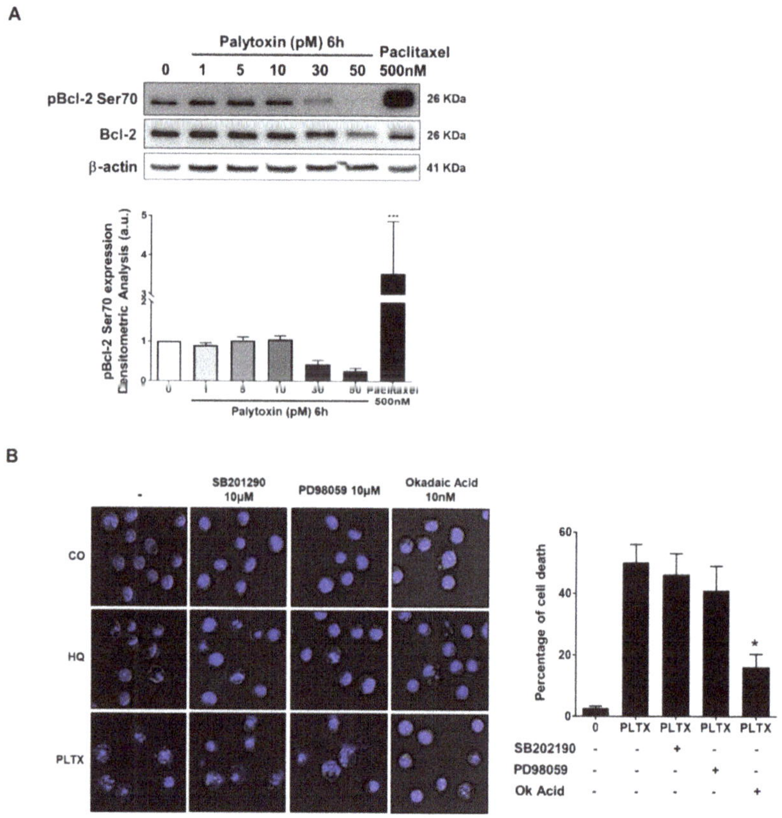

Figure 7. Bcl-2 serine70 dephosphorylation induced by palytoxin is mediated through protein phosphatase 2 activation in U937 cells. (**A**) Palytoxin induces a dose-dependent dephosphorylation of Bcl-2 at serine70 in U937 cells. Western blot is representative of three independent experiments. Band intensities were quantified using ImageJ software. Paclitaxel (500 nM, 8 h) is used as a positive control for multisite phosphorylation of Bcl-2. *** $p < 0.005$ versus control. (**B**) Okadaic acid, a protein phosphatase 2A (PP2A) inhibitor, rescues U937 cells from palytoxin-induced cell death. Hydroquinone (10 μM, 24 h) was used as a positive control for PP2A activation. Cells were stained with Hoechst to analyze the nuclear morphology merged with phase contrast images using ImageJ. The percentage of cell death was evaluated by counting the number of cells undergoing various types of cellular death. Three independent fields of 100 cells were quantified. SB202190 and PD98059 were used as MAP kinase inhibitors. Data representative of three independent experiments is shown as mean ± SD. * $p < 0.05$.

Altogether, we concluded that palytoxin-induced dephosphorylation of Bcl-2 by PP2A exacerbates the proapoptotic effect of Mcl-1 and Bcl-xL degradation and that okadaic acid could rescue in part palytoxin-induced cell death.

2.7. Anticancer Effect of Palytoxin in 3D Cell Culture and Zebrafish Xenografts

We investigated the colony formation ability of cancer cells in the presence of increasing concentrations of palytoxin to confirm its potential to impair the replicative capacity of cancer cells. After 10 days of treatment, colony formation in AML cell lines was strongly reduced by palytoxin at concentrations from 0.4 pM. Concentrations beyond 1 pM completely abrogated colony formation capacity (Figure 8A–D). Besides AML cells, palytoxin significantly inhibited colony formation in CML cell lines, K562 and imatinib-resistant K562 (K562IR) (Figure 8E,F). Moreover, we generalized our findings with the solid prostate cancer cell line PC3. Concentrations between 0.5 and 1 pM abrogated colony formation (Supplementary Figure S3) and prevented spheroid formation in a dose-dependent manner (Supplementary Figure S4).

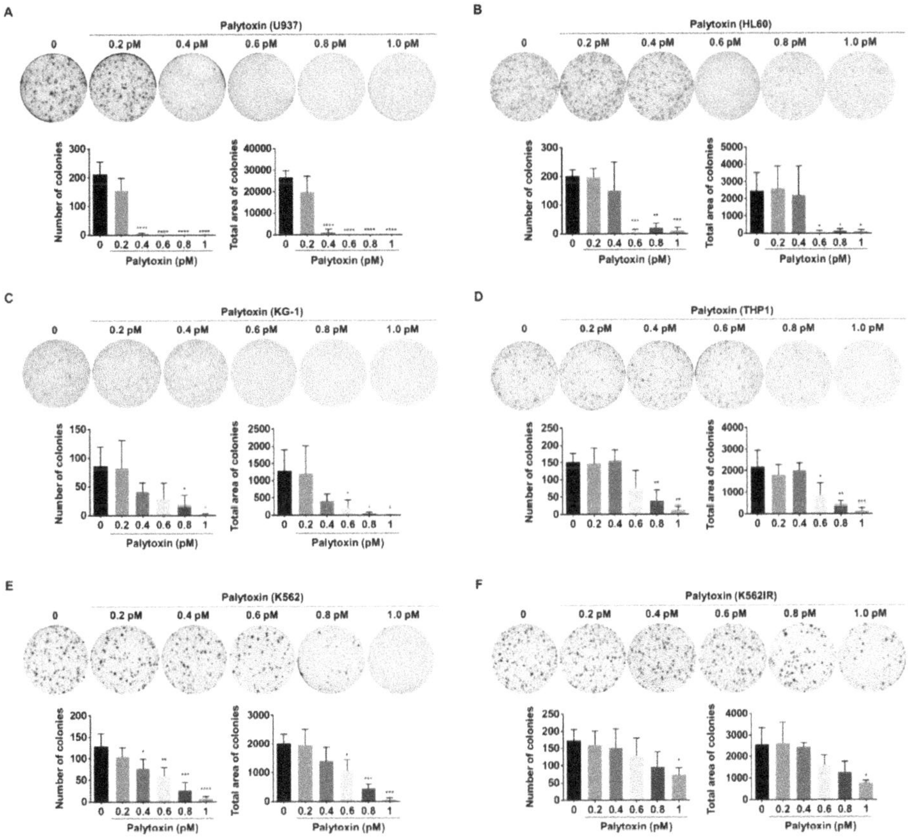

Figure 8. Palytoxin reduces the colony-forming ability in leukemia cell lines. Palytoxin showed an inhibitory effect on colony formation in a dose-dependent manner in U937 (**A**), HL60 (**B**), KG-1 (**C**), THP1 (**D**), K562 (**E**), and K562IR (**F**). All data represent the mean ± SD. of three independent experiments. Statistical significance was assessed as * $p < 0.05$, ** $p < 0.01$, *** $p < 0.001$, **** $p < 0.0001$ versus control.

To further extend our evaluation of the anticancer potential of palytoxin, we examined the ability of palytoxin to abrogate tumor development in an ex vivo zebrafish xenotransplantation model. Fluorescently labeled leukemia cells were pre-treated for 6 hours with palytoxin at 5, 10, and 30 pM and then injected into the yolk sac of zebrafish embryos. Results revealed that the tumor-associated fluorescence intensity signal was drastically lowered in the palytoxin-treated zebrafish group compared to the untreated controls as early as 5 pM (Figure 9A–F for a representative overview; Supplementary Figure S5 shows all nine fish for each group).

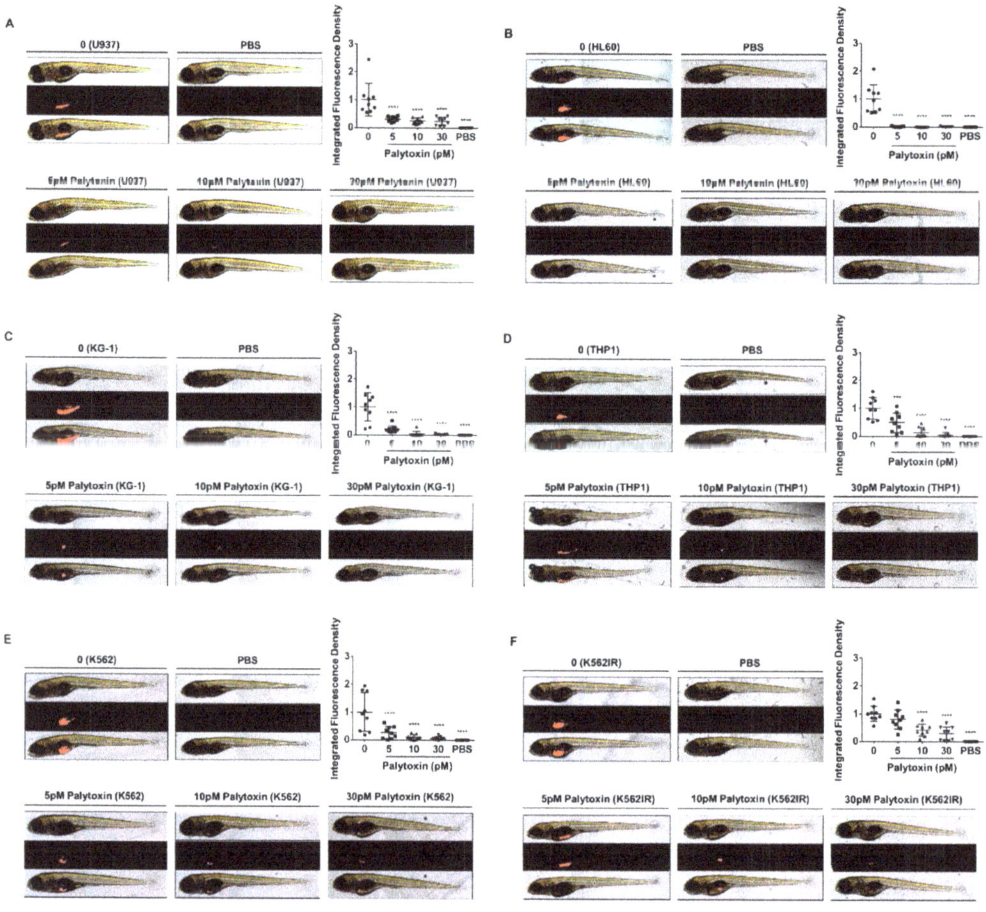

Figure 9. Palytoxin inhibits colony-forming ability in in vivo zebrafish xenografts. In vivo antitumor forming ability by palytoxin was evaluated by zebrafish xenografts. Top: bright field, middle: CM-Dil, bottom: merge. (**A**) U937, (**B**) HL60, (**C**) KG-1, (**D**) THP1, (**E**) K562, (**F**) K562IR cells were used for generating zebrafish xenograft and nine zebrafishes were assessed per condition (Supplementary Figure S5). Statistical significance was assessed as *** $p < 0.001$, **** $p < 0.0001$.

3. Discussion

We demonstrated that palytoxin, one of the most toxic marine biotoxins known [18], can significantly induce apoptotic cell death at low picomolar concentrations in different cancer cell types. We focused on cell death mechanisms, especially in acute myeloid leukemia (AML) U937 cells.

So far, palytoxins have essentially been investigated at high nanomolar doses. Palytoxins act as a skin tumor promoter when combined with a carcinogenic agent. It can modulate critical signal transduction pathways involved in carcinogenesis and inflammation [19].

It has been shown that palytoxin stimulates prostaglandin production from arachidonic acid and activates mitogen-activated protein kinases (MAPKs), including extracellular signal-regulated kinase (ERK), c-Jun N-terminal kinase (JNK) and p38 mitogen-activated protein kinase (p38) [20].

In contrast, this manuscript shows that palytoxin induced apoptosis at lower pM concentrations in a caspase-dependent manner. Apoptosis is the most common and well-defined form of programmed cell death, a physiological process of cellular suicide [21]. However, as we observed a small measurable amount of non apoptotic cell death after caspase inhibition by zVAD, it is essential to determine in the future which type of secondary cell death mechanism the cell activates in the absence of apoptotic capacity [22]. In that sense, investigating the activation of non-caspase proteases inducing calpains or cathepsins could be interesting [23,24].

Among Bcl-2 family proteins, Mcl-1 and Bcl-xL were found to be strongly downregulated by palytoxin, even at low picomolar concentrations. As we observed a consistent and early onset of BID truncation, the differential effect of extrinsic versus intrinsic cell death pathway is interesting and will be investigated by pathway-specific caspase inhibitors [12].

We demonstrated that palytoxin rapidly reduces Mcl-1 protein levels without involving caspase-dependent modulation. Palytoxin instead induced proteasome-dependent degradation of Mcl-1. Three major proteasome activities are upregulated by palytoxin. Ubiquitin E3 ligases Skp Cullin F-box containing F-box WD repeat domain containing 7 (SCFFbw7), β-transducin repeat-containing protein 1 (SCFβ-TrCP), and Mcl-1 ubiquitin ligase E3 (Mule) [25,26] could then promote Usp9x (ubiquitin-specific peptidase 9, X-linked) which is required for Mcl-1 deubiquitination [27]. Moreover, Bcl-2 homology domain-3 (BH-3) only proteins, including p53 upregulated modulator of apoptosis (PUMA) or Phorbol-12-myristate-13-acetate-induced protein 1 (NOXA), induce the degradation of Mcl-1 at the mitochondrial level, which also requires the E3 ligase Mule [28]. The implication of NOXA in regulating Mcl-1 proteasomal degradation will support our hypothesis as the disruption of the 26S proteasome function by different mechanisms triggers the rapid accumulation of proteasome-dependent BH-3-only family proteins and subsequent cell death induced by apoptosis [28].

It will be interesting to investigate the overexpression of Mcl-1 with plasmid constructs, specifically wild-type and proteasome-resistant isoforms of Mcl-1 [29]. Overexpression of these proteins will further allow the strengthening of the hypothesis of proteasomal degradation. Similarly, stably-transfected Jurkat T cells expressing mutated Bcl-2 (serine70, serine87, and threonine 69) will allow us to understand the role of Bcl-2 expression regulated by palytoxin in various models [30,31].

This study also showed that inhibition of PP2A activity rescued palytoxin-induced cell death, which implies that phosphatases play a significant role in cellular mechanisms activated by palytoxin [32]. PP2A has been suggested as a therapeutic target in Philadelphia chromosome-positive chronic or acute myeloid leukemia, where PP2A inactivation is a recurrent event [32]. Palytoxin could restore PP2A or related phosphatases to induce caspase-dependent apoptosis mediated through AKT and ERK1/2 pathways [33]. PP2A exerts inhibitory and stimulatory effects on MAP kinase signaling pathways [34]. Previous findings suggested that palytoxin activates the mitogen-activated protein kinase (MAPK) cascade (including extracellular signal-regulated protein kinases 1 and 2 (ERK1/2), c-Jun N-terminal kinases/stress-activated protein kinase (JNK) and p38 protein kinase) in response to heat shock protein 27 (HSP27) phosphorylation in human breast adenocarcinoma (MCF-7) cells [35]. In monocyte-derived human macrophages, palytoxin phosphorylates p38 MAPK. It activates nuclear factor kappa B (NF-κB) pathways by increasing the mRNA levels of inflammation-related genes like interleukin 8 (IL-8), an inhibitor of kappa alpha (IκB-α), leading to NF-κB nuclear translocation [6]. These observations allow us to hypothesize that palytoxin may activate a proinflammatory signaling cascade in leukemia cell lines by regulating kinases and phosphatases [36].

This manuscript is the first step in the preclinical evaluation of palytoxin. We are aware that there might be a long way to derive this high molecular weight compound into a druggable formulation. However, the potential of Na^+/K^+ ATPase modulating agents was clinically investigated and exploited by cardiac glycosides so that the molecular target of palytoxin is of clear clinical relevance. In the future, the potent cytotoxicity, combined with the described proinflammatory potential, could find clinical applications in targeted antibody-drug conjugate (ADC) compounds like brentuximab vedotin or trastuzumab emtansine. Despite the limited success of first-generation ADCs, palytoxin could provide a cytotoxic, likely immunogenic warhead able to kill difficult-to-target cancer cells.

One of the future outcomes of this study is to validate the Na^+/K^+-ATPase inhibition by palytoxin as the possible cancer target. In this context, functional studies (i.e., silencing or overexpressing the pump subunits) and the future design of simplified analogs based on essential pharmacophores of palytoxin might be considered. Palytoxin inhibited tumor formation in a zebrafish xenograft model at concentrations between 10 and 30 pM. We plan to extend our investigation to animal models other than zebrafish to exclude any intrinsic evolutionary resistance developed by aquatic animal models. Furthermore, studies on primary cells will consolidate the documented differential cytotoxicity.

4. Materials and Methods

4.1. Cells and Medium

K562 (human chronic myelogenous leukemia), Jurkat (human T-lymphocyte), Raji (Burkitt lymphoma), and U937 (human histiocytic lymphoma) were purchased from DSMZ (Braunschweig, Germany). THP1, promyeloblast HL60 and bone marrow acute myelogenous leukemia KG-1 were obtained from the Korean cell line bank (KCLB, Seoul, Republic of Korea). All cells were cultured in Roswell Park Memorial Institute (RPMI) 1640 medium (Bio-Whittaker, Lonza, Rockland, ME, USA) containing a 1% (*v*/*v*) antibiotic/antimycotic mixture of 100 U/mL penicillin, 100 μg/mL streptomycin, and 0.25 μg/mL amphotericin B (Bio-Whittaker, Lonza, Rockland, ME, USA) at 37 °C and 5% of CO_2 in a humidified atmosphere. The Imatinib-resistant K562 (K562IR) cell line was a gift from the Korea Leukemia Bank, Catholic University, Seoul, and cultured in RPMI medium with 25 mM HEPES (Lonza, Rockland, ME, USA) supplemented with 10% (*v*/*v*) FBS, 1% (*v*/*v*) antibiotic-antimycotic and 1 μM of imatinib. Cells were cultured and harvested every three days and treated with palytoxin in an exponential growth phase. Cells were regularly tested for mycoplasma infection (MycoalertTM, Lonza, Rockland, ME, USA) per the manufacturer's instructions.

4.2. Compounds

Palytoxin was extracted from Palythoa Aff. Clavata following an established procedure (patent publication EP3087172B1). The compound, with a molecular mass of 2680.14 g mol^{-1}, was received as a powder, solubilized in DMSO (Sigma-Aldrich, Saint Louis, MO, USA), and further diluted to get working aliquots at 1 mM. Stocks and aliquots were stored at 4 °C for up to 2 years without loss of activity and protected from light and were used directly before the experiments. Etoposide was purchased from Sigma-Aldrich, Saint Louis, MO, USA, and dissolved in DMSO at a stock concentration of 50 mM. Pan-caspase inhibitor, z-VAD FMK, was purchased from Calbiochem (San Diego, CA, USA), dissolved in DMSO, and added 1 h before at a concentration of 50 μM. Protein phosphatase 2A inhibitor okadaic acid was purchased from Calbiochem (San Diego, CA, USA) and dissolved in DMSO at a stock concentration of 1 mM. Proteasome inhibitor MG-132 was purchased from Sigma-Aldrich (Saint Louis, MO, USA) and dissolved in DMSO at a stock concentration of 10 mM. MAP kinase inhibitors, SB202190 and PD98059, were purchased from Calbiochem (San Diego, CA, USA) and dissolved in DMSO at a stock concentration of 100 mM. Hydroquinone was purchased from Sigma-Aldrich (Saint Louis, MO, USA) and dissolved in DMSO at 10 mM. Inhibitors were used for 1h before palytoxin treatment at the indicated working concentrations.

4.3. Cell Viability Assessment

Cell vitality was assessed in three leukemia cell lines, K562, Jurkat, and U937. Each cell line was treated with various concentrations of palytoxin for 2, 4, 6, and 8 h in a dose-dependent manner. The percentage of viability was evaluated using the Trypan Blue exclusion test (0.2% Trypan Blue), and the percentage of viability of cells without palytoxin treatment was considered to be 100%.

4.4. Caspase 3/7 Activity Assay

3×10^5 U937 cells/mL were seeded in 96-well plates in triplicate in 75 μL for palytoxin treatment. The enzymatic activities of caspases- 3 and -7 were determined using a luminescent Caspase-glo®3/7 Assay (Promega, Cosmogenetech, Seoul, Republic of Korea). The assay was performed per the manufacturer's instruction by adding 75 μL of the caspase-3/7 substrate to U937 cells in suspension. After one hour of incubation with DEVD-aminoluciferin substrate and luciferase, the luminescent signal was measured using a Centro LB 960 microplate luminometer (Berthold Technologies, JCBio Co. Ltd., Seoul, Republic of Korea).

4.5. Proteasome Activity Assay

The Proteasome-Glo®cell-based assay (Promega, Cosmogenetech, Seoul, Korea) was used to evaluate the three major proteolytic enzyme activities (chymotrypsin-like, caspase-like, trypsin-like). The assays were performed as indicated in the manufacturer's protocol. U937 cells were treated at a concentration of 10^6 cells/mL in RPMI 1640 medium containing 0.1% FCS at indicated concentrations of palytoxin. After an incubation period, 50 μL of U937 cellular suspension was mixed with 50 μL of the assay reagent. The luminescence signal was measured on the Centro LB 960 Microplate Luminometer (Berthold Technologies, JCBio Co., Ltd., Seoul, Republic of Korea). The proteasome signal was normalized to the number of viable cells performed in parallel using CellTiter-Glo®(Promega, Cosmogenetech, Seoul, Republic of Korea). MG-132 at 5 μM (Sigma, USA) was used as a control for proteasomal inhibition.

4.6. Cell Lysate Preparations and Western Blots

Ten million U937 cells were seeded in 30 mL of RPMI 1640 medium (Lonza, Rockland, ME, USA) with 10% fetal bovine serum (FBS) (Biowest, Riverside, MO, USA) and 1% antibiotics (Lonza, Rockland, ME, USA). Cells were treated with palytoxin in a dose- and time-dependent manner as indicated. Cellular lysates were centrifuged at 22 °C, 350 g, for 7 min. After removal of the supernatant, the pellets were washed in 1ml phosphate-buffered saline (PBS) and centrifuged again at 4 °C, 350 g for 7 min. Afterward, the supernatants were removed, and the pellets were stored at −80 °C until use. The extraction was performed on ice to avoid the denaturation of the proteins. Whole-cell extracts were prepared with 5 mL of mammalian protein Extraction reagent (M-PER), per the manufacturer's instructions (Pierce, Appleton, WI, USA). Extraction reagents include 40 μL/mL protease inhibitor (Sigma, USA), 1 mM phenylmethylsulphonyl fluoride (PMSF) (Roche, Seoul, Republic of Korea), 1 mM sodium orthovanadate (Saint Louis, MO, USA), 100 μL/mL Phosphostop inhibitor (Roche, Seoul, Republic of Korea) and M-PER in a final volume of 5 mL. Depending on the pellet size, 500 μL of reagents were used for control and 300 μL for treated cell pellets. Dissolved pellets were centrifuged for 25 min at 4 °C and 18,000 g speed. Aliquots were stored at −80 °C.

Proteins from total extracts were separated using a sodium dodecyl sulfate-polyacrylamide gel electrophoresis (SDS-Page). Proteins were transferred onto a polyvinylidene fluoride (PVDF) membrane (GE Healthcare, Pittsburgh, PA, USA) and blocked with 5% non-fat milk or 5% bovine serum albumin (BSA) in PBS-Tween overnight. Equal loading of samples was controlled by using β-actin. Blots were incubated with primary antibodies: anti-β-actin (1/10000, A5441, Sigma-Aldrich, Saint Louis, MO, USA), anti-Caspase-3 (1/1000, 56053, Santa Cruz, Koram Biotech Corporation, Seoul, Republic of Korea), anti-Bcl-2 (1/2000,

Merck Calbiochem, OP60, Seoul, Republic of Korea), anti-Bcl-xL (1/1000, BD Biosciences, 610212, Seoul, Republic of Korea), anti-Caspase-7 (1/1000, 9494) anti-Caspase-8 (1/1000, 9746), anti-Caspase-9 (1/1000, 9502), anti-Mcl-1 (1/1000, 4572), anti-BID (1/1000, 2002), anti-pBcl-2 ser70 (1/2000, 2827) (all Cell Signaling Technologies, Koram Biotech Corporation, Seoul, Republic of Korea). All antibodies were diluted in a PBS-Tween solution containing 5% BSA or 5% non-fat milk per the provider's protocols. After incubation with primary antibodies, membranes were washed for 3×10 min with PBS-Tween, followed by 1h at RT with the corresponding secondary (HRP-conjugated) antibodies. After washing 3×10 min with PBS-Tween, specific immunoreactive proteins were visualized by autoradiography using the ECL Plus Western Blotting Detection System Kit®(GE Healthcare, Seoul, Republic of Korea).

4.7. Fluorescent Microscopy Analysis

3×10^5 U937 cells/mL were seeded in 24-well plates before palytoxin treatment. Then, 300 µL of treated cells were transferred into another 24-well plate for double staining with (1) the DNA-specific dye Hoechst 33342 (Sigma, USA) at 1 µL/mg for 30 min of incubation and (2) propidium iodide (Sigma, USA) at 1.5 µL/mg, diluted in PBS for 15 min of incubation. Induction of apoptosis was assessed by fluorescent microscopy (Nikon TI-U, Seoul, Republic of Korea) and expressed as the percentage of cells presenting fragmented/condensed nuclei. Different stages of nuclear fragmentation were considered, and at least 300 cells were counted in three independent fields as previously described [37–42]. Microscopy images were analyzed using the ImageJ 1.54 software (http://rsb.info.nih.gov/ij/docs/index.html, accessed on 4 March 2023).

4.8. Systemic Toxicity in Zebrafish

Zebrafish (Danio rerio) were obtained from the "Zebrafish International Resource Center" (ZIRC) (University of Oregon, Eugene, OR, USA) and maintained according to the zebrafish guidelines [43]. Adult fish were kept at 28.5 °C on a 14-h light/10-h dark cycle comparable to natural conditions, and all embryos were collected from natural mating as a unit of hours-post fertilization (HPF). Then, 0.003% phenylthiourea (PTU) was added 14 h before palytoxin treatment to remove the pigmentation of zebrafish models. Embryos were then treated with the indicated concentration of palytoxin in 24 HPF. Photographs were taken under light microscopy (Carl Zeiss Stereo microscope DV4, Seoul, Republic of Korea) to quantify viable zebrafish.

4.9. Differential Toxicity Effects on Healthy Peripheral Blood Mononuclear Cells

Peripheral blood mononuclear cells (PBMC) were purified from three freshly collected buffy coats from healthy adult human donors (Red Cross, Luxembourg, Luxembourg) after ethical approval (see informed consent statement) and informed written consent from all the donors, using the standard Ficoll-Hypaque (GE Healthcare, Roosendaal, The Netherlands) density separation method as previously described [40]. After isolation and three washes in Dulbecco's Phosphate Buffered Saline (DPBS) (Lonza, Rockland, ME, USA), cells were counted and re-suspended in RPMI 1640 medium supplemented with 10% heat-inactivated fetal calf serum and 1% antibiotics-antimycotic at a cell density of 2×10^6 cells/mL. The day after, cell concentration was adjusted to 1×10^6 cells/mL, and PBMCs were treated with palytoxin at indicated concentrations. After 8 hours of incubation, a Trypan Blue assay was used to analyze PBMC cell viability.

4.10. Colony Formation Assay

For colony formation assays, cells (10^3 cells/mL) were seeded into a semisolid methylcellulose medium (Methocult H4230, StemCell Technologies Inc., Seoul, Republic of Korea) and treated with indicated concentrations of palytoxin. Colonies were detected after 10 days of culture by adding 1 mg/mL of 3-(4,5-dimethylthiazol-2-yl)-2,5-diphenyltetrazoliumbromide

(MTT) reagent (Sigma, Seoul, Republic of Korea) and were scored by ImageJ software (U.S. National Institute of Health, Bethesda, MD, USA) [44].

4.11. Zebrafish Xenograft Assays

The zebrafish (*Danio rerio*) xenograft assay followed a setup we previously published [45].

4.12. Statistical Analysis

Data are presented as the mean of three independent experiments with standard deviations. All statistical analyses were done with GraphPad Prism 9.0. *p*-values below 0.05 were considered significant. See figure legends for details.

5. Conclusions

We have demonstrated that the marine compound palytoxin rapidly induces cell death through apoptosis in human leukemia cell lines. While downregulating the expression of Mcl-1, palytoxin activates BID truncation, eventually leading to intrinsic apoptotic pathways are a caspase-dependent cell death mechanism. While additional analysis is required to elucidate the role of phosphatases that could be involved, these findings show for the first time that palytoxin acts as an apoptosis inducer affecting leukemia cells able to prevent tumor formation in vivo and makes palytoxin a promising candidate for new potential anticancer drug development.

Supplementary Materials: The following are available online at https://www.mdpi.com/article/10.3390/md21040233/s1, Figure S1: Calculated IC50 values of different human cancer cell lines incubated with palytoxin at various concentrations between 2 and 8 h. Data are the mean of SD ± of three independent experiments; Figure S2: Palytoxin down-regulates the expression of anti-apoptotic Bcl-2 family proteins in solid tumor cell lines. Western blot analysis of anti-apoptotic Bcl-2 family protein expression levels in A549 (lung cancer), PC3 (prostate cancer), MCF7 (breast cancer), and SH-SY5Y (neuroblastoma) cells; Figure S3: Palytoxin reduces the colony-forming ability in PC3 prostate cancer cells. Palytoxin showed an inhibitory effect on colony formation in a dose-dependent manner. All data represent the mean ± SD. of three independent experiments. Statistical significance was assessed as ** $p < 0.01$ versus control; Figure S4: Palytoxin inhibited PC3 prostate cancer spheroid formation in a dose-dependent manner. Statistical significance was assessed as * $p < 0.05$ and *** $p < 0.0001$ versus control; Figure S5: Palytoxin inhibits tumor-forming ability in in vivo zebrafish xenografts. Fluorescently-labeled leukemia cells were treated with palytoxin at 5, 10, and 30 Pm for 6 h and then injected into the zebrafish yolk sac. A total of nine fish were obtained per condition. Top: bright field, middle: CM-Dil, bottom: merge. PBS injection was used as a control for injection toxicity.

Author Contributions: All authors have read and agreed to the published version of the manuscript. J.K., S.J., J.-Y.L., J.L., B.O.-B., C.C., A.M., F.M. and M.D. (Marc Diederich): developed methodology; J.K., S.J., J.-Y.L., B.O.-B., C.C. and M.D. (Marc Diederich): performed experiments and curated the investigations; J.K., S.J., J.-Y.L. and M.D. (Marc Diederich): wrote the original draft; J.K.: curated data visualization; B.O.-B., C.C., A.M. and M.D. (Marc Diederich): performed data curation; B.O.-B., C.C., O.D. and M.D. (Marc Diederich): conceptualize the study; B.O.-B., A.M. and O.D.: performed the formal analysis; C.C.: validate experiment reproducibility; J.L., O.D. and M.D. (Marc Diederich): provided resources; B.O.-B., C.C., A.M., M.D. (Mario Dicato), O.D. and M.D. (Marc Diederich): reviewed and/or revised the manuscript; M.D. (Mario Dicato). and M.D. (Marc Diederich): administrated the project and coordinated the study and the research activities; O.D. and M.D. (Marc Diederich): supervised the study and were responsible for funding acquisition.

Funding: Jaemyun Kim, Seungwon Ji, Jin-Young Lee, Barbora Orlikova-Boyer, Claudia Cerella, and Aloran Mazumder were supported by the BK21 plus program. Jaemyun Kim, Seungwon Ji, Jin-Young Lee, Aloran Mazumder, and Marc Diederich were supported by the National Research Foundation (NRF) by the MEST of Korea for Tumor Microenvironment Global Core Research Center (GCRC) grant (grant number NRF 2011-0030001). This work was also supported by the Seoul National University Research Grant (Funding number: 800-20160150) and by the Creative-Pioneering

Researchers Program through Seoul National University (SNU) (Funding number: 370C-20160062). Research at SNU is also supported by the National Research Foundation (NRF) (Grant Number 2022R1A2C101314111). Support from the BrainKorea21 FOUR program is acknowledged. Barbora Orlikova-Boyer, Claudia Cerella, Florian Muller, and Marc Diederich are supported by the "Recherche Cancer et Sang" foundation, the "Recherches Scientifiques Luxembourg" association, the "Een Häerz fir kriibskrank Kanner" association, the Action LIONS "Vaincre le Cancer" association, and by Télévie Luxembourg. Claudia Cerella also thanks the 'Waxweiler grant for cancer prevention research' (Action LIONS 'Vaincre le Cancer').

Institutional Review Board Statement: The study was conducted in agreement with the guidelines of the Institutional Animal Care and Use Committee (IACUC) of Seoul National University (SNU-191218-5-1; date of approval 29 June 2022).

Informed Consent Statement: PBMCs were obtained from Red Cross Luxembourg with informed consent obtained from all subjects (donators of PBMC blood products) involved in the study (LBMCC-2019-0001: Assessment of differential toxicity of new drugs or drug combinations in preclinical development in ex-vivo proliferating peripheral blood mononuclear cells vs. proliferating cancer cells; LBMCC-2019-0002: Assessment of toxicity of new drugs or drug combinations in preclinical development in non-proliferating peripheral blood mononuclear cells (acute systemic toxicity)).

Data Availability Statement: The data presented in this study are available on request from the corresponding author.

Conflicts of Interest: The authors declare no conflict of interest.

References

1. Moore, R.E.; Scheuer, P.J. Palytoxin: A new marine toxin from a coelenterate. *Science* **1971**, *172*, 495–498. [CrossRef] [PubMed]
2. Ramos, V.; Vasconcelos, V. Palytoxin and analogs: Biological and ecological effects. *Mar. Drugs* **2010**, *8*, 2021–2037. [CrossRef] [PubMed]
3. Aligizaki, K.; Katikou, P.; Nikolaidis, G.; Panou, A. First episode of shellfish contamination by palytoxin-like compounds from Ostreopsis species (Aegean Sea, Greece). *Toxicon* **2008**, *51*, 418–427. [CrossRef]
4. Ukena, T.; Satake, M.; Usami, M.; Oshima, Y.; Naoki, H.; Fujita, T.; Kan, Y.; Yasumoto, T. Structure elucidation of ostreocin D, a palytoxin analog isolated from the dinoflagellate Ostreopsis siamensis. *Biosci. Biotechnol. Biochem.* **2001**, *65*, 2585–2588. [CrossRef]
5. Amzil, Z.; Sibat, M.; Chomerat, N.; Grossel, H.; Marco-Miralles, F.; Lemee, R.; Nezan, E.; Sechet, V. Ovatoxin-a and palytoxin accumulation in seafood in relation to Ostreopsis cf. ovata blooms on the French Mediterranean coast. *Mar. Drugs* **2012**, *10*, 477–496. [CrossRef] [PubMed]
6. Crinelli, R.; Carloni, E.; Giacomini, E.; Penna, A.; Dominici, S.; Battocchi, C.; Ciminiello, P.; Dell'Aversano, C.; Fattorusso, E.; Forino, M.; et al. Palytoxin and an Ostreopsis toxin extract increase the levels of mRNAs encoding inflammation-related proteins in human macrophages via p38 MAPK and NF-kappaB. *PLoS ONE* **2012**, *7*, e38139. [CrossRef] [PubMed]
7. Inuzuka, T.; Fujisawa, T.; Arimoto, H.; Uemura, D. Molecular shape of palytoxin in aqueous solution. *Org. Biomol. Chem.* **2007**, *5*, 897–899. [CrossRef]
8. Hilgemann, D.W. From a pump to a pore: How palytoxin opens the gates. *Proc. Natl. Acad. Sci. USA* **2003**, *100*, 386–388. [CrossRef]
9. Rodrigues, A.M.; Almeida, A.C.; Infantosi, A.F. Effect of palytoxin on the sodium-potassium pump: Model and simulation. *Phys. Biol.* **2008**, *5*, 036005. [CrossRef]
10. Satoh, E.; Ishii, T.; Nishimura, M. Palytoxin-induced increase in cytosolic-free Ca(2+) in mouse spleen cells. *Eur. J. Pharmacol.* **2003**, *465*, 9–13. [CrossRef]
11. Rossini, G.P.; Bigiani, A. Palytoxin action on the Na(+),K(+)-ATPase and the disruption of ion equilibria in biological systems. *Toxicon* **2011**, *57*, 429–439. [CrossRef]
12. Luo, X.; Budihardjo, I.; Zou, H.; Slaughter, C.; Wang, X. Bid, a Bcl2 interacting protein, mediates cytochrome c release from mitochondria in response to activation of cell surface death receptors. *Cell* **1998**, *94*, 481–490. [CrossRef] [PubMed]
13. Abdelmohsen, K.; Lal, A.; Kim, H.H.; Gorospe, M. Posttranscriptional orchestration of an anti-apoptotic program by HuR. *Cell Cycle* **2007**, *6*, 1288–1292. [CrossRef] [PubMed]
14. Awan, F.T.; Kay, N.E.; Davis, M.E.; Wu, W.; Geyer, S.M.; Leung, N.; Jelinek, D.F.; Tschumper, R.C.; Secreto, C.R.; Lin, T.S.; et al. Mcl-1 expression predicts progression-free survival in chronic lymphocytic leukemia patients treated with pentostatin, cyclophosphamide, and rituximab. *Blood* **2009**, *113*, 535–537. [CrossRef] [PubMed]
15. Yamamoto, K.; Ichijo, H.; Korsmeyer, S.J. BCL-2 is phosphorylated and inactivated by an ASK1/Jun N-terminal protein kinase pathway normally activated at G(2)/M. *Mol. Cell. Biol.* **1999**, *19*, 8469–8478. [CrossRef]
16. Ruvolo, P.P.; Deng, X.; May, W.S. Phosphorylation of Bcl2 and regulation of apoptosis. *Leukemia* **2001**, *15*, 515–522. [CrossRef]

17. Deng, X.; Gao, F.; May, W.S. Protein phosphatase 2A inactivates Bcl2's antiapoptotic function by dephosphorylation and up-regulation of Bcl2-p53 binding. *Blood* **2009**, *113*, 422–428. [CrossRef]
18. Pelin, M.; Sosa, S.; Pacor, S.; Tubaro, A.; Florio, C. The marine toxin palytoxin induces necrotic death in HaCaT cells through a rapid mitochondrial damage. *Toxicol. Lett.* **2014**, *229*, 440–450. [CrossRef]
19. Wattenberg, E.V. Palytoxin: Exploiting a novel skin tumor promoter to explore signal transduction and carcinogenesis. *Am. J. Physiol. Cell Physiol.* **2007**, *292*, C24-32. [CrossRef]
20. Wattenberg, E.V. Modulation of protein kinase signaling cascades by palytoxin. *Toxicon* **2011**, *57*, 440–448. [CrossRef]
21. Kroemer, G. Mitochondrial control of apoptosis: An introduction. *Biochem. Biophys. Res. Commun.* **2003**, *304*, 433–435. [CrossRef] [PubMed]
22. Galluzzi, L.; Maiuri, M.C.; Vitale, I.; Zischka, H.; Castedo, M.; Zitvogel, L.; Kroemer, G. Cell death modalities: Classification and pathophysiological implications. *Cell Death Differ.* **2007**, *14*, 1237–1243. [CrossRef] [PubMed]
23. McCall, K. Genetic control of necrosis—Another type of programmed cell death. *Curr. Opin. Cell Biol.* **2010**, *22*, 882–888. [CrossRef] [PubMed]
24. Reiser, J.; Adair, B.; Reinheckel, T. Specialized roles for cysteine cathepsins in health and disease. *J. Clin. Investig.* **2010**, *120*, 3421–3431. [CrossRef]
25. Inuzuka, H.; Shaik, S.; Onoyama, I.; Gao, D.; Tseng, A.; Maser, R.S.; Zhai, B.; Wan, L.; Gutierrez, A.; Lau, A.W.; et al. SCF(FBW7) regulates cellular apoptosis by targeting MCL1 for ubiquitylation and destruction. *Nature* **2011**, *471*, 104–109. [CrossRef]
26. Warr, M.R.; Acoca, S.; Liu, Z.; Germain, M.; Watson, M.; Blanchette, M.; Wing, S.S.; Shore, G.C. BH3-ligand regulates access of MCL-1 to its E3 ligase. *FEBS Lett.* **2005**, *579*, 5603–5608. [CrossRef]
27. Mojsa, B.; Lassot, I.; Desagher, S. Mcl-1 ubiquitination: Unique regulation of an essential survival protein. *Cells* **2014**, *3*, 418–437. [CrossRef]
28. Gomez-Bougie, P.; Menoret, E.; Juin, P.; Dousset, C.; Pellat-Deceunynck, C.; Amiot, M. Noxa controls Mule-dependent Mcl-1 ubiquitination through the regulation of the Mcl-1/USP9X interaction. *Biochem. Biophys. Res. Commun.* **2011**, *413*, 460–464. [CrossRef]
29. Liu, Q.; Moldoveanu, T.; Sprules, T.; Matta-Camacho, E.; Mansur-Azzam, N.; Gehring, K. Apoptotic regulation by MCL-1 through heterodimerization. *J. Biol. Chem.* **2010**, *285*, 19615–19624. [CrossRef]
30. Basu, A.; Haldar, S. Microtubule-damaging drugs triggered bcl2 phosphorylation-requirement of phosphorylation on both serine-70 and serine-87 residues of bcl2 protein. *Int. J. Oncol.* **1998**, *13*, 659–664. [CrossRef]
31. Deng, X.; Gao, F.; Flagg, T.; May, W.S., Jr. Mono- and multisite phosphorylation enhances Bcl2's antiapoptotic function and inhibition of cell cycle entry functions. *Proc. Natl. Acad. Sci. USA* **2004**, *101*, 153–158. [CrossRef] [PubMed]
32. Cristobal, I.; Garcia-Orti, L.; Cirauqui, C.; Alonso, M.M.; Calasanz, M.J.; Odero, M.D. PP2A impaired activity is a common event in acute myeloid leukemia and its activation by forskolin has a potent anti-leukemic effect. *Leukemia* **2011**, *25*, 606–614. [CrossRef] [PubMed]
33. Perrotti, D.; Neviani, P. Protein phosphatase 2A: A target for anticancer therapy. *Lancet Oncol.* **2013**, *14*, e229–e238. [CrossRef] [PubMed]
34. Lee, T.; Kim, S.J.; Sumpio, B.E. Role of PP2A in the regulation of p38 MAPK activation in bovine aortic endothelial cells exposed to cyclic strain. *J. Cell. Physiol.* **2003**, *194*, 349–355. [CrossRef] [PubMed]
35. Berni, C.; Bellocci, M.; Sala, G.L.; Rossini, G.P. Palytoxin induces dissociation of HSP 27 oligomers through a p38 protein kinase pathway. *Chem. Res. Toxicol.* **2015**, *28*, 752–764. [CrossRef]
36. Shanley, T.P.; Vasi, N.; Denenberg, A.; Wong, H.R. The serine/threonine phosphatase, PP2A: Endogenous regulator of inflammatory cell signaling. *J. Immunol.* **2001**, *166*, 966–972. [CrossRef]
37. Song, S.; Kim, S.; El-Sawy, E.R.; Cerella, C.; Orlikova-Boyer, B.; Kirsch, G.; Christov, C.; Dicato, M.; Diederich, M. Anti-Leukemic Properties of Aplysinopsin Derivative EE-84 Alone and Combined to BH3 Mimetic A-1210477. *Mar. Drugs* **2021**, *19*, 285. [CrossRef]
38. Song, S.; Lee, J.Y.; Ermolenko, L.; Mazumder, A.; Ji, S.; Ryu, H.; Kim, H.; Kim, D.W.; Lee, J.W.; Dicato, M.; et al. Tetrahydrobenzimidazole TMQ0153 triggers apoptosis, autophagy and necroptosis crosstalk in chronic myeloid leukemia. *Cell Death Dis.* **2020**, *11*, 109. [CrossRef]
39. Ha, Y.N.; Song, S.; Orlikova-Boyer, B.; Cerella, C.; Christov, C.; Kijjoa, A.; Diederich, M. Petromurin C Induces Protective Autophagy and Apoptosis in FLT3-ITD-Positive AML: Synergy with Gilteritinib. *Mar. Drugs* **2020**, *18*, 57. [CrossRef]
40. Mazumder, A.; Lee, J.Y.; Talhi, O.; Cerella, C.; Chateauvieux, S.; Gaigneaux, A.; Hong, C.R.; Kang, H.J.; Lee, Y.; Kim, K.W.; et al. Hydroxycoumarin OT-55 kills CML cells alone or in synergy with imatinib or Synribo: Involvement of ER stress and DAMP release. *Cancer Lett.* **2018**, *438*, 197–218. [CrossRef]
41. Cerella, C.; Gaigneaux, A.; Mazumder, A.; Lee, J.Y.; Saland, E.; Radogna, F.; Farge, T.; Vergez, F.; Recher, C.; Sarry, J.E.; et al. Bcl-2 protein family expression pattern determines synergistic pro-apoptotic effects of BH3 mimetics with hemisynthetic cardiac glycoside UNBS1450 in acute myeloid leukemia. *Leukemia* **2017**, *31*, 755–759. [CrossRef] [PubMed]
42. Cerella, C.; Muller, F.; Gaigneaux, A.; Radogna, F.; Viry, E.; Chateauvieux, S.; Dicato, M.; Diederich, M. Early downregulation of Mcl-1 regulates apoptosis triggered by cardiac glycoside UNBS1450. *Cell Death Dis.* **2015**, *6*, e1782. [CrossRef] [PubMed]

43. Siccardi, A.J., 3rd; Garris, H.W.; Jones, W.T.; Moseley, D.B.; D'Abramo, L.R.; Watts, S.A. Growth and survival of zebrafish (Danio rerio) fed different commercial and laboratory diets. *Zebrafish* **2009**, *6*, 275–280. [CrossRef] [PubMed]
44. Florean, C.; Schnekenburger, M.; Lee, J.Y.; Kim, K.R.; Mazumder, A.; Song, S.; Kim, J.M.; Grandjenette, C.; Kim, J.G.; Yoon, A.Y.; et al. Discovery and characterization of Isofistularin-3, a marine brominated alkaloid, as a new DNA demethylating agent inducing cell cycle arrest and sensitization to TRAIL in cancer cells. *Oncotarget* **2016**, *7*, 24027–24049. [CrossRef] [PubMed]
45. Lee, J.Y.; Mazumder, A.; Diederich, M. Preclinical Assessment of the Bioactivity of the Anticancer Coumarin OT48 by Spheroids, Colony Formation Assays, and Zebrafish Xenografts. *J. Vis. Exp.* **2018**, *136*, e57490. [CrossRef]

marine drugs

MDPI

Article

The Blockade of Mitogen-Activated Protein Kinase 14 Activation by Marine Natural Product Crassolide Triggers ICD in Tumor Cells and Stimulates Anti-Tumor Immunity

Keng-Chang Tsai [1,2,†], Chia-Sheng Chen [3,†], Jui-Hsin Su [4,5], Yu-Ching Lee [2,6], Yu-Hwei Tseng [1] and Wen-Chi Wei [1,*]

1 National Research Institute of Chinese Medicine, Ministry of Health and Welfare, Taipei 112026, Taiwan
2 Ph.D. Program in Medical Biotechnology, College of Medical Science and Technology, Taipei Medical University, Taipei 110301, Taiwan
3 Department of Psychiatry, Kaohsiung Armed Forces General Hospital, Kaohsiung 80284, Taiwan
4 National Museum of Marine Biology and Aquarium, Pingtung 94450, Taiwan
5 Department of Marine Biotechnology and Resources, National Sun Yat-sen University, Kaohsiung 804201, Taiwan
6 TMU Research Center of Cancer Translational Medicine, Taipei Medical University, Taipei 110301, Taiwan
* Correspondence: jackwei@nricm.edu.tw; Tel.: +886-2-28201999 (ext. 3561)
† These authors contributed equally to this work.

Abstract: Immunogenic cell death (ICD) refers to a type of cell death that stimulates immune responses. It is characterized by the surface exposure of damage-associated molecular patterns (DAMPs), which can facilitate the uptake of antigens by dendritic cells (DCs) and stimulate DC activation, resulting in T cell immunity. The activation of immune responses through ICD has been proposed as a promising approach for cancer immunotherapy. The marine natural product crassolide, a cembranolide isolated from the Formosan soft coral *Lobophytum michaelae*, has been shown to have cytotoxic effects on cancer cells. In this study, we investigated the effects of crassolide on the induction of ICD, the expression of immune checkpoint molecules and cell adhesion molecules, as well as tumor growth in a murine 4T1 mammary carcinoma model. Immunofluorescence staining for DAMP ectolocalization, Western blotting for protein expression and Z′-LYTE kinase assay for kinase activity were performed. The results showed that crassolide significantly increased ICD and slightly decreased the expression level of CD24 on the surface of murine mammary carcinoma cells. An orthotopic tumor engraftment of 4T1 carcinoma cells indicated that crassolide-treated tumor cell lysates stimulate anti-tumor immunity against tumor growth. Crassolide was also found to be a blocker of mitogen activated protein kinase 14 activation. This study highlights the immunotherapeutic effects of crassolide on the activation of anticancer immune responses and suggests the potential clinical use of crassolide as a novel treatment for breast cancer.

Keywords: immunogenic cell death; damage-associated molecular patterns; mitogen-activated protein kinase 14; natural product; crassolide

1. Introduction

The World Health Organization recently estimated that in 2020, 2.3 million women were diagnosed with breast cancer and there were approximately 685,000 deaths worldwide. By the end of that year, 7.8 million women who had been diagnosed with breast cancer within the previous five years were still alive, making it the most common cancer globally [1,2].

Unlike conventional chemotherapy, which destroys malignant cells, cancer immunotherapy is a treatment that boosts the body's immune system to fight cancer. Immunotherapies that have shown sustained anticancer responses in several cancers hold promise for researchers and patients. Currently, identifying and developing potential targets to enhance anticancer responses is a key strategy in cancer immunotherapy. For example, immune checkpoint molecules like PD-1 and CTLA-4 have been identified as negative regulators of immune activation [3–5]. The binding of PD-L1 on cancer cells to PD-1 on T cells suppresses the activation and function of T cells [6,7]. In addition to immune checkpoints, cancer cells can also express other "don't eat me" signals, such as CD47 and CD24, on their surface to protect themselves from immune surveillance [8,9]. Despite the promising results of immunologic checkpoint blockade with antibodies, the objective response rate of clinical drugs still needs further improvement.

On the other hand, immunogenic cell death (ICD) refers to a type of cell death that stimulates immune responses. ICD is characterized by the surface exposure of damage-associated molecular patterns (DAMPs), a group of endogenous danger molecules that includes heat shock proteins (HSPs), glucose-related protein (GRP), HMGB1, calreticulin (CRT), and others [10,11]. These molecules can facilitate the uptake of antigens by dendritic cells (DCs) and stimulate DC activation, resulting in T cell immunity. Activation of immune responses through ICD has been proposed as a promising approach for cancer immunotherapy. Currently, a number of ICD-induced chemotherapeutic agents are being used clinically for cancer treatment [11].

Natural products from marine organisms are considered key sources for drug development [12]. For example, marine sponge natural products with anti-cancer activity have been developed into drugs [13]. However, research on the immunotherapeutic activity of marine natural products for cancer treatment is still limited. The marine natural product crassolide, a cembranolide isolated from the Formosan soft coral *Lobophytum michaelae*, has been shown to have cytotoxic effects on cancer cells [14]. Cytotoxic activities related to G2/M phase arrest and apoptosis were also reported [15]. In this study, we investigated the effects of crassolide on the induction of ICD, the expression of immune checkpoint molecules and cell adhesion molecules, as well as tumor growth in a murine 4T1 mammary carcinoma model. Additionally, we identified its target molecules. This study highlights the immunotherapeutic effects of crassolide on the activation of anti-cancer immune responses and suggests the potential clinical use of crassolide as a novel treatment for breast and other types of cancer.

2. Results

2.1. Crassolide Stimulated the Cytotoxicity against Human Breast Cancer Cells and Murine Mammary Carcinoma Cells

The structure of crassolide is shown in Figure 1. To determine the cytotoxic effects of crassolide on different types of mammary tumor cells, we used a methylthiazole tetrazolium (MTT) assay to measure the cell viability of test cells treated with crassolide at different concentrations for 24 h. The results showed that crassolide inhibits the cell viability of the four mammary carcinoma cells in a dose-dependent manner, as shown in Figure 2. The IC50 values of cell viability in MCF7, MDA-MB-231, 4T1-luc2, and TS/A cells were 9.35, 6.69, 24.6, and 3.74 μM, respectively (Table 1).

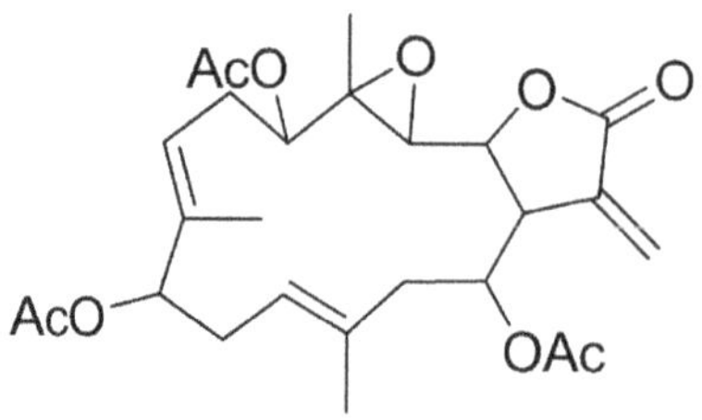

Crassolide

Figure 1. The chemical structure of crassolide.

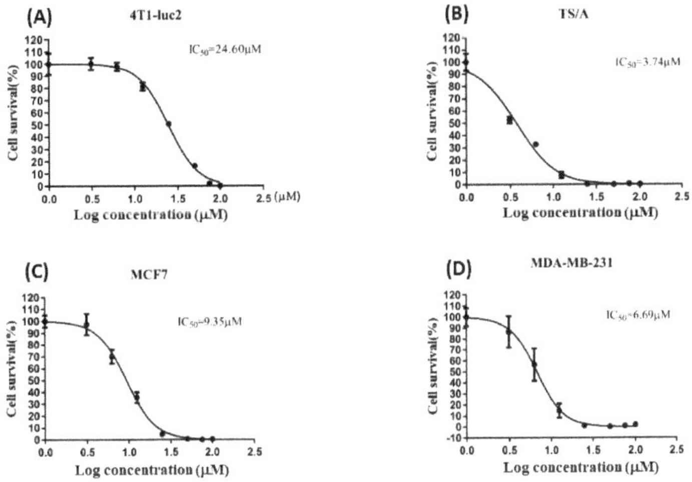

Figure 2. The cytotoxicity of crassolide in human breast cancer cells and murine mammary carcinoma cells. Cell lines 4T1-luc2 (**A**), TS/A (**B**), MCF7 (**C**) and MDA-MB-231 (**D**) were treated with increasing concentrations of crassolide for 24 h and cell survival was determined by MTT assay. Data are represented as the mean ± SD. The IC50 values of cell viability in MCF7, MDA-MB-231, 4T1-luc2, and TS/A cells were 9.35, 6.69, 24.6, and 3.74 μM, respectively.

Table 1. The IC50 values of cell viability in 4T1-luc2, TS/A, MCF7, and MDA-MB-231 cells.

Cell Line	IC_{50}
4T1-luc2	24.60
TS/A	3.74
MCF7	9.35
MDA-MB-231	6.69

2.2. Crassolide Significantly Increases the Expression of DAMPs on the Surface of 4T1-luc2 Murine Mammary Carcinoma Cells

Immunogenic cell death (ICD) of tumor cells, characterized by surface expression of damage-associated molecular patterns (DAMPs), stimulates antitumor immunity. HSP70, HSP90, HMGB1, and calreticulin (CRT) have been recognized as key DAMP molecules. Crassolide exhibited cytotoxicity in murine mammary carcinoma cells 4T1-luc2. We then investigated if crassolide can stimulate ICD in 4T1-luc2 cells by measuring the expression levels of HSP 70, HSP 90, HMGB1, and CRT on the surface of 4T1-luc2 cells that were incubated in different concentrations (50 to 3.125 μM) of crassolide for 24 h. The surface expression of HSP70, HSP90, HMGB1, and CRT were then measured by flow cytometry analysis. Figure 3A showed that the 4T1-luc2 cells' control group expressed 17.51% of HSP90, 9.16% of HSP70, 5.99% of HMGB1, and 19.56% of CRT. The 4T1-luc2 cells treated with crassolide had a substantial expression level of HSP90, reaching the highest peak at 25 μM treatment (50.08%). The highest expression level of HSP70 (29.10%) appeared with 12.5 μM treatment. Crassolide increased the expression of HMGB1 and CRT in a dose-dependent manner, with HMGB1 (96.48%) and CRT (78.68%) reaching the highest expression at 50 μM treatment, respectively. Crassolide-treated tumor cells were visualized for expression of ectoDAMPs by confocal microscopy through indirect immunofluorescent staining. The expression of HSP70, HSP90, HMGB1 and CRT was significantly increased in crassolide-treated tumor cells compared to untreated tumor cells (Figure 3B). These results indicate that crassolide significantly increases immunogenic cell death (ICD) in murine mammary carcinoma cells 4T1-luc2.

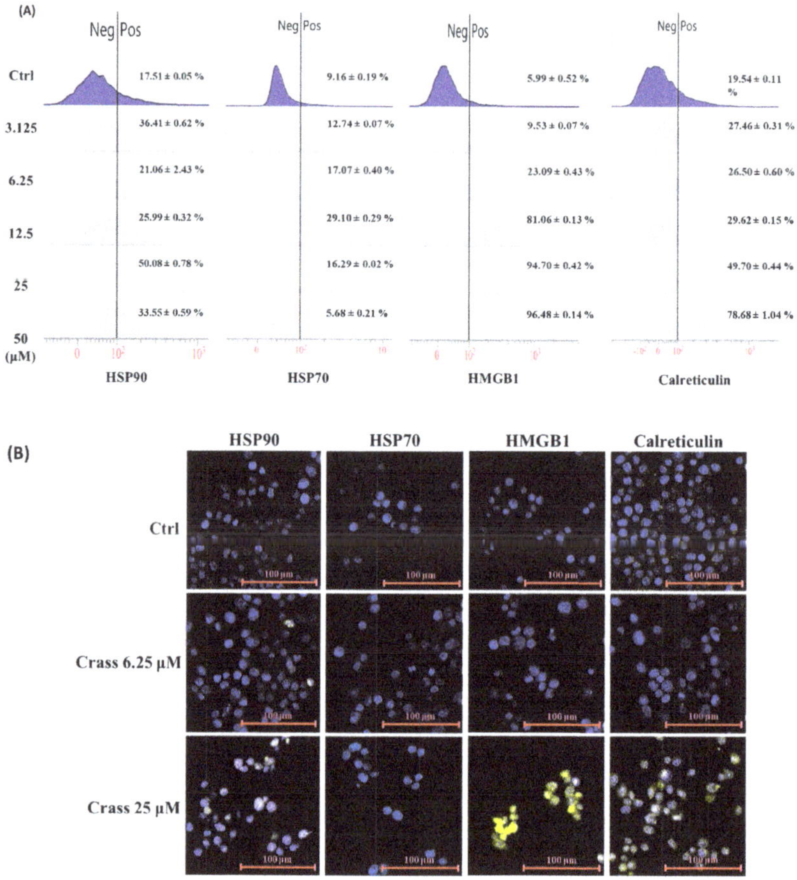

Figure 3. The effect of crassolide on the expression of DAMPs on the surface of 4T1-luc2 cells. The 4T1-luc2 cells were treated with increasing concentrations of crassolide for 24 h. (**A**) The expression level of DAMPs on the surface of 4T1-luc2 cells were determined by flow cytometry analysis. (**B**) Imaging of DAMP ectolocalization in crassolide-treated cells was examined under a confocal microscope. The HSP90, HSP70, HMGB1, and calreticulin proteins were stained with PE anti-HSP90, Alexa Fluor 488 anti-Hsp70, PE anti-HMGB1, and PE anti-calreticulin antibodies, respectively. The nuclei were stained with DAPI (shown in blue). The scale bar is 100 μm.

2.3. Crassolide Enhances Expression of Immune Checkpoint Molecule PD-L1 but Inhibits the Expression of Heat-Stable Antigen/CD24 on the Surface of 4T1-luc2

Our data showed that crassolide significantly induced immunogenic cell death (ICD) in 4T1-luc2 cells. We further examined the effect of crassolide on the regulation of "don't eat me signals" in these cells. The cells were treated with various concentrations of crassolide for 24 h, and we used flow cytometry analysis to measure the expression of PD-L1 and CD24 on the cell surface. Figure 4A illustrates that the control group of 4T1-luc2 cells expressed 48.94% PD-L1 and 74.56% CD24. Crassolide slightly decreased CD24 expression, but it significantly increased PD-L1 expression, with the highest peak at 50 μM treatment (86.71%). Additionally, the immunofluorescence image confirmed that crassolide enhances PD-L1 expression and suppresses CD24 expression on the surface of 4T1-luc2 cells (Figure 4B).

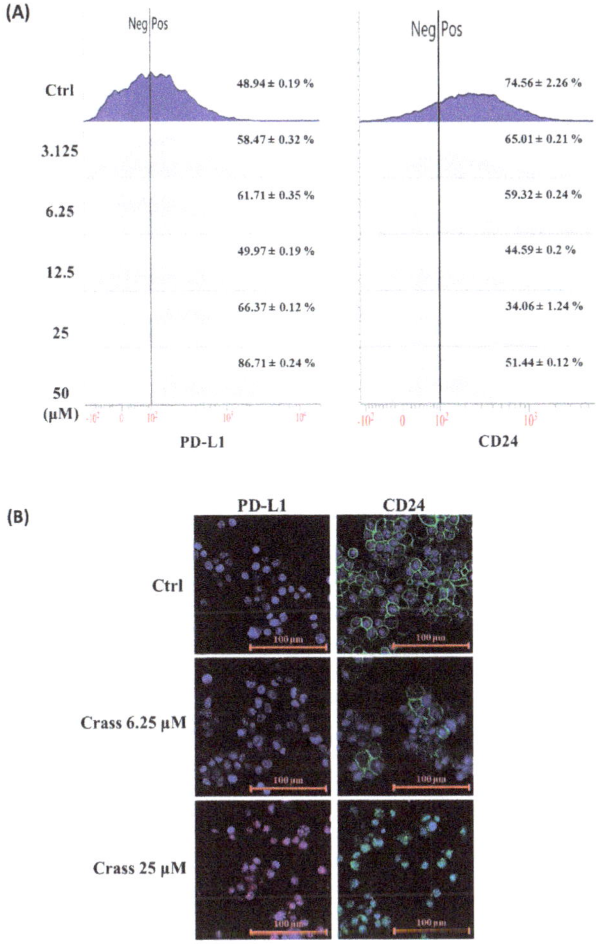

Figure 4. The effect of crassolide on the expression of DAMPs, PD-L1 and CD24 in 4T1-luc2 cells. The 4T1-luc2 cells were treated with increasing concentrations of crassolide for 24 h. (**A**) The expression level of PD-L1 and CD24 on the surface of 4T1-luc2 cells was determined by flow cytometry analysis. (**B**) Imaging of PD-L1 and CD24 ectolocalization in crassolide-treated cells was examined under a confocal microscope. The PD-L1 and CD24 proteins were stained with APC anti-PD-L1 and Alexa Fluor 488 anti-CD24 antibodies, respectively. The nuclei were stained with DAPI (shown in blue). The scale bar is 100 μm.

2.4. *Crassolide Significantly Induces the Translocation of DAMPs to the Surface of 4T1-luc2 Cells*

Crassolide significantly increased the expression levels of DAMPs and PD-L1 on the surface of 4T1-luc2 cells. To understand the molecular mechanisms underlying the regulatory effect of crassolide on the expression of DAMPs, CD24, and PD-L1, we evaluated whether crassolide can stimulate their expression in 4T1-luc2 cells. The 4T1-luc2 cells were incubated with different concentrations of crassolide for 24 h, and the total protein was collected for assessing the expression of HSP70, HSP90, CRT, and HMGB1 using Western blot assay. Figure 5A shows that crassolide suppressed the expression of HSP70, HSP90, and CRT, but had no effect on the expression of HMGB1 protein. Similarly, Figure 5B shows that crassolide suppressed the expression of CD24 and PD-L1. Taking into account the results from Figures 3–5, it can be inferred that crassolide suppressed the protein expression of DAMPs and PD-L1 but promoted the translocation of DAMPs and PD-L1 to the surface of 4T1-luc2 cells.

(A)

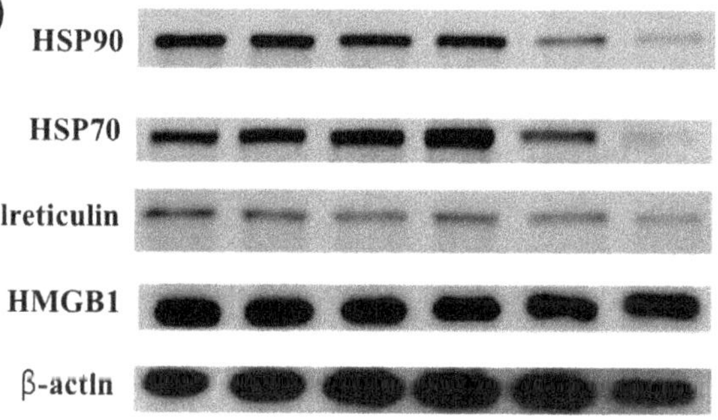

Crass(μM)	Mock	3.125	6.25	12.5	25	50
HSP90	1.00	0.90	0.84	0.85	0.35	0.11
HSP70	1.00	1.21	1.52	1.88	0.84	0.13
Calreticutin	1.00	0.79	0.65	0.71	0.57	0.31
HMGB1	1.00	0.96	0.89	0.74	0.76	1.08
β-actin	1.00	1.04	1.05	0.96	1.03	0.85

(B)

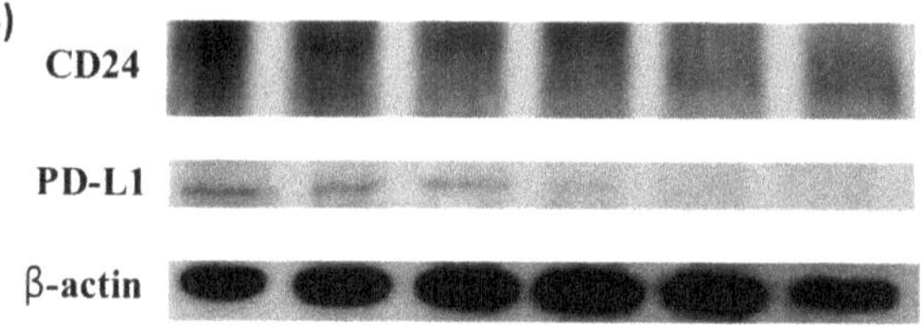

Crass(μM)	Mock	3.125	6.25	12.5	25	50
CD24	1.00	0.92	0.75	0.82	0.71	0.67
PD-L1	1.00	1.50	1.83	1.00	0.12	0.05
β-actin	1.00	1.04	1.05	0.96	1.03	0.85

Figure 5. The effect of crassolide on the protein expression of DAMPs, PD-L1 and CD24 in 4T1-luc2 cells. The 4T1-luc2 cells were treated with increasing concentrations of crassolide for 24 h and the total protein was collected for assessing the expression of DAMPs, PD-L1 and CD24. (**A**) The protein expression levels of HSP90, HSP70, calreticulin and HMGB1 in total protein extracts were measured using Western blot analysis and were normalized to the protein level of β-actin. Mock: DMSO as the vehicle control. (**B**) The protein expression levels of PD-L1 and CD24 in total protein extracts were measured using Western blot analysis and were normalized to the protein level of β-actin. Mock: DMSO as the vehicle control.

2.5. Crassolide-Treated 4T1-luc2 Cells Effectively Immunized Mice against Primary Tumors

To assess the ability of the ICD inducer to trigger antitumor immune responses, one method is to inject mice with in vitro killed tumor cells treated with the ICD inducer, followed by a challenge with untreated tumor cells [16]. To determine if crassolide-treated 4T1-luc2 cells can elicit antitumor immunity in mice with tumors, the mice were subcutaneously given 4T1-luc2 cells that underwent freeze-thaw cycles or treated with crassolide at 25 μM. The 4T1-luc2 tumor cells were implanted into the mammary fat pad orthotopically after 7 days of post-vaccination. The treatment of 4T1-luc2 cells with Crassolide seemed to suppress tumor growth, suggesting that it can induce anti-tumor immunity. (Figure 6A). Bioluminescence imaging (BLI) and quantitative data of BLI confirmed the effect, showing decreased activity in tumor cells. The p-value was less than 0.05 (Figure 6B,C). The body weight loss of treated mice was not impacted by the vaccine (Figure 6D).

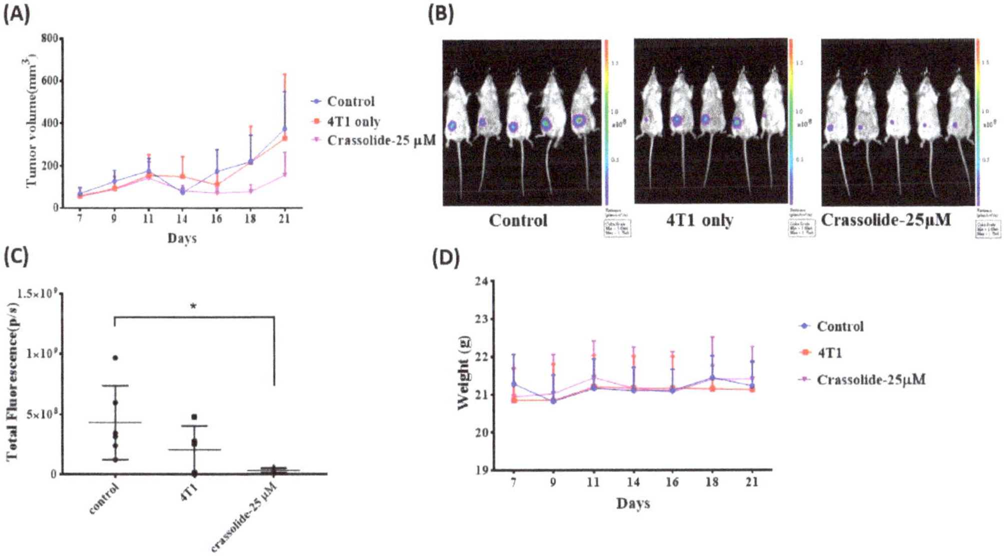

Figure 6. Crassolide-treated 4T1-luc2 cells effectively immunized mice against primary tumors. Test mice were vaccinated with 4T1-luc2 cells that underwent freeze-thaw cycles or were treated with crassolide at 25 μM for 24 h. At 7 d post-vaccination, live 4T1-luc2 tumor cells were implanted. Tumor progression in test mice was visualized by bioluminescence imaging (BLI). (**A**) Tumor volume was monitored until 21 d post tumor implantation. (**B**) BLI and (**C**) Quantitative data of BLI was determined at 16 d post tumor implantation. * $p < 0.05$ (**D**) Body weight of all test mice.

2.6. Crassolide Inhibited MAPK14 Kinase Activity

The target protein of crassolide was identified through a Discovery Studio pharmacophore reverse docking. The results showed MAPK14 kinase as a potential target protein. MAPK14, known as p38α kinase, is made up of two distinct parts, the smaller N-terminal lobe which is primarily composed of β-sheets, and the α-helical C-terminal lobe. The two lobes are connected by a flexible hinge that forms the ATP-binding site, and structural elements from both lobes contribute to this site. During the canonical activation pathway, MAP2Ks phosphorylate the TGY sequence in the activation loop, leading to significant structural changes and the creation of a distinctive β-sheet motif that is located away from both the ATP- and substrate-binding sites [17]. Figure 7A,B depicted crassolide docked with MAPK14 kinase. Crassolide established interactions with Thr106 and Lys53 through hydrogen bonds and with Leu167, Met109, Ile84, Ala51, and Val38 residues in the active site through hydrophobic interactions. The inhibitory effect of crassolide on MAPK14 kinase activity was confirmed in a cell-free system using a biochemical method (Z′-LYTE Kinase Assay). Results showed crassolide could concentration-dependently suppress MAPK14 kinase activity with an IC50 value of approximately 5.15 μM (Figure 7C).

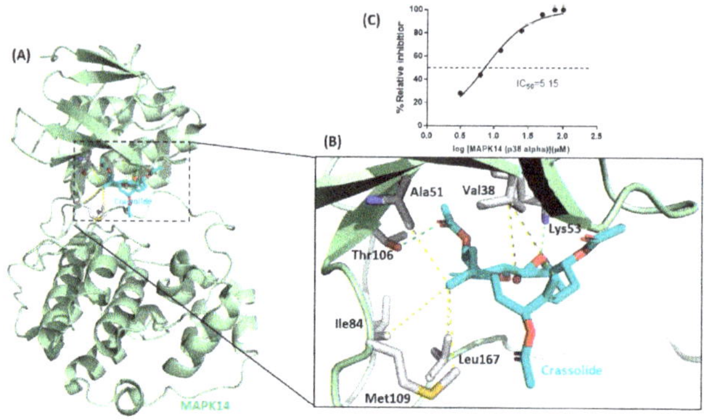

Figure 7. The blockade of mitogen-activated protein kinase 14 activation by crassolide. (**A**) Schematic representation of the molecular docking in the active site of MAPK14 (PDB 1DI9). The MAPK14 kinase is shown in light green cartoon. The key residues of kinase are shown in a stick representation. (**B**) The binding interactions between crassolide compound and MAPK14 are shown in hydrogen bonds (in green) and hydrophobic interactions (in yellow). (**C**) Dose–response curves of MAPK14 and its inhibitor crassolide in kinase inhibition assay.

2.7. Crassolide Up-Regulated Phosphorylation of MAPK14 and Its Downstream Targets in 4T1-luc2 Cells

The regulation of MAPK14 kinase activity is controlled by phosphorylation at two sites (Thr180/Tyr182) [17]. The effect of crassolide on the phosphorylation status of MAPK14 at Thr180 and Tyr182 was assessed in 4T1-luc2 cells. Results showed that crassolide upregulated the phosphorylation of Thr180 and Tyr182 in a dose-dependent manner (Figure 8). The effect of crassolide on the phosphorylation of downstream proteins of MAPK14 such as NF-κB, STAT1, and EIK-1 was also measured. Results showed that crassolide downregulated the phosphorylation of NF-κB, STAT1, and EIK-1 in 4T1-luc2 cells (Figure 8).

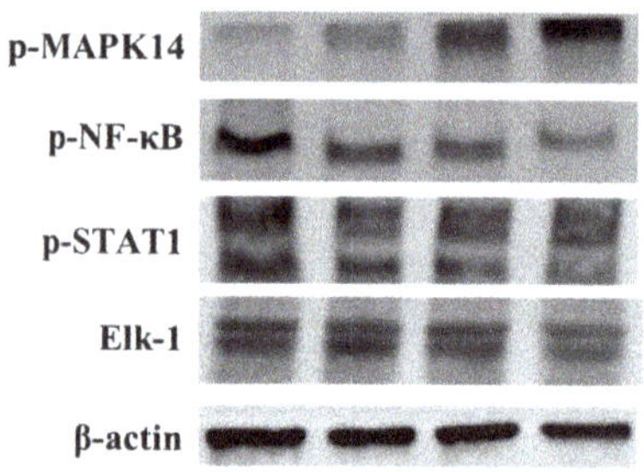

Crass(μM)	Mock	12.5	25	50
p-MAPK14	1.00	2.03	4.05	5.48
p-NFκB	1.00	0.63	0.53	0.37
p-STAT1	1.00	0.64	0.69	0.68
Elk-1	1.00	0.74	0.75	0.72
β-actin	1.00	0.80	0.75	0.62

Figure 8. The effect of crassolide on the phosphorylation of MAPK14, NF-κB and STAT1, and EIK-1 protein in 4T1-luc2 cells. The 4T1-luc2 cells were treated with increasing concentrations of crassolide for 24 h and the total protein was collected for assessing the phosphorylation of MAPK14, NF-κB and STAT1, and EIK-1 protein using Western blot analysis and were normalized to the protein level of β-actin. Mock: DMSO as the vehicle control.

3. Discussion

Immunogenic cell death (ICD) and damage-associated molecular patterns (DAMPs) are emerging as promising strategies in cancer therapy. ICD triggers an immune response against cancer cells, while DAMPs are molecules released by dying or damaged cells that activate the immune system. These mechanisms are being utilized to improve the efficacy of cancer immunotherapy. ICD and DAMPs have shown promising results in preclinical and clinical studies [11,18] and are being evaluated in combination with other immunotherapeutic approaches such as checkpoint inhibitors and vaccines [19–21]. ICD is triggered by different stressors, including endoplasmic reticulum (ER) stress and reactive oxygen species (ROS) production, and leads to the exposure of damage-associated molecular patterns (DAMPs) on the cell surface [22–24]. During the ICD process, immunogenic dead cells expose hallmarks on the cell surface and release substances that interact with immune cells and mediate immunogenicity. These hallmarks include calreticulin (CRT), ATP, and high mobility group B1 (HMGB1). ICD inducers, such as anthracyclines, PP1/GADD34 inhibitors, cardiac glycosides, oxaliplatin, bleomycin, cyclophosphamide, and shikonin, have been used to induce ICD and inhibit tumor growth [10,11]. Currently, only a few ICD inducers are being used in the clinic, but the development of new ICD inducers is expected to improve cancer treatment outcomes in the future.

The mitogen-activated protein kinases (MAPKs) are a highly conserved family of serine/threonine kinases that play a central role in a range of fundamental cellular processes such as cell growth, proliferation, death, and differentiation [25–27]. There are at least three distinct MAPK signaling modules in mammals that mediate extracellular signals into the nucleus to turn on responsive genes: ERK, JNK, and p38 kinase [26]. The MAPK pathway is essential in regulating many cellular processes, including inflammation, cell stress response, cell differentiation, and gene expression [27]. In the context of immunogenic cell death (ICD), the p38 MAPK pathway has been shown to be involved in the regulation of ER stress, which is a major causative agent of ICD [28]. In some cases, activation of p38 MAPK has been shown to promote ICD by inducing the release of danger signals and activating the immune system. The precise role of p38 MAPK in ICD is still not fully understood. There are four identified p38 MAP kinases: p38-α (MAPK14), p38-β (MAPK11), p38-γ (MAPK12/ERK6), and p38-δ (MAPK13/SAPK4) [27]. In this study, crassolide from marine soft coral was identified as a novel inhibitor of MAPK14. Crassolide not only significantly reduced the viability of human breast cancer cells and murine mammary carcinoma cells, but also increased ICD and decreased CD24 expression in the latter. Orthotopic tumor engraftment experiments showed that crassolide-treated tumors elicited anti-tumor immunity. These findings deepen our understanding of MAPK14's role in ICD and highlight crassolide's potential as a treatment for breast and other types of cancer by activating anti-cancer immune responses (Figure 9).

Crassolide was first found to have cytotoxicity in cancer cells [14]. Later, its ability to induce G2/M cell cycle arrest, apoptosis, and autophagy in cancer cells was investigated [15]. Based on observation of a crassolide-induced increase in phosphorylation of ERK, it was suggested that this capability was induced through ROS-mediated ER stress pathways [15]. Additionally, crassolide was also found to suppress dendritic cell maturation and attenuate experimental antiphospholipid syndrome. It was also found that, when applied at doses of only 10 and 20 mg/kg, crassolide produced hematotoxicity, hepatotoxicity, and renotoxicity, but these effects were not observed at a dose of 5 mg/kg [29]. In this study, we showed that crassolide inhibited p38α activity using a biochemical method (Figure 7C). Interestingly, crassolide upregulated the phosphorylation of p38α, known as its initial activation marker. In contrast, crassolide downregulated the phosphorylation of NF-κB, STAT1, and EIK-1, known as downstream effectors of p38α signaling transduction (Figure 8). Based on the research results and the similarity of their effects, we believe that crassolide is a novel p38 catalytic inhibitor (e.g., SB203580). Additionally, due to its structural similarity with ERK, we hypothesize that crassolide may also block ERK activity, resulting in an accumulation of ERK phosphorylation. However, further experiments are needed to confirm this hypothesis.

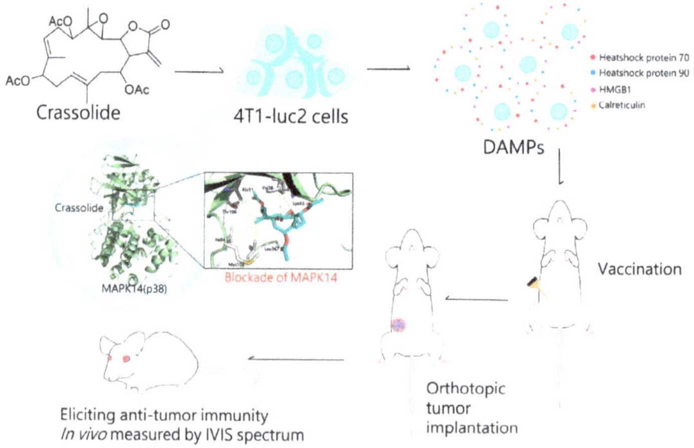

Figure 9. The schematic representation of crassolide triggers ICD in tumor cells and stimulates anti-tumor immunity.

The abundance of diverse marine life and their distinct biochemical profiles have led to the discovery of a multitude of biologically active natural products derived from marine organisms, making them a valuable source for the development of new drugs. Despite this potential, the process of discovering and utilizing these products can be challenging due to difficulties in cultivating marine organisms and the complex structure of their active compounds, leading to limited yields. Our study highlights a novel approach by showcasing the effectiveness of the marine compound crassolide in stimulating immunogenic cell death in tumor cells in vitro and eliciting anti-tumor immunity in vivo when used as a vaccine, demonstrating the potential of marine natural products for clinical applications. However, just as natural product research in the ocean may face limitations in its applications, the modification of crassolide to enhance its binding affinity with MPAK14 and the synthesis of crassolide through total or semi-synthesis may also face limitations due to the complexity of the compound's structure, which may restrict future applications and development.

4. Materials and Methods

4.1. Origin of Crassolide

Crassolide was obtained from Dr. Jui-Hsin Su at the National Museum of Marine Biology and Aquarium in Pingtung, Taiwan, and was isolated from the wild-type soft coral Lobophytum crissum.

4.2. Cell Lines

MCF7, MDA-MB-231 and TS/A cells were procured from the Food Industry Research and Development Institute (Hsinchu, Taiwan). The 4T1-luc2 cells, obtained from Dr. Pei-Wen Hsiao at Academia Sinica in Taipei, Taiwan, were developed from mouse mammary tumor 4T1 cells (ATCC, CRL-2539) and stably transfected with a luciferase transgene. These cells were cultured in RPMI-1640 (Invitrogen, 31800) supplemented with 10% fetal bovine serum (FBS) (GibcoTM, 10082147), 1 mM penicillin-streptomycin (GibcoTM, 15140122), MEM-Non-Essential Amino Acids Solution (NEAA) (ThermoFisher, 11140050), and 1 mM sodium pyruvate (GibcoTM, 11360070) at 37 °C in 5% CO_2 and 95% humidity.

4.3. Mice

Female 8-week-old BALB/c mice were purchased from the National Laboratory Animal Breeding and Research Center in Taipei, Taiwan. All mice were treated with standard environmental and food conditions, including a temperature of 22 ± 1 °C, 55 ± 5% humidity, and a 12-h light/dark cycle, and had unlimited access to food and water at the National Research Institute of Chinese Medicine (MOHW). The mice were randomly assigned to four groups to reduce experimental bias. The experimental procedures involving animals were conducted in accordance with the Guide for the Care and Use of Laboratory Animals (National Research Council, 2011) and were approved by the Animal Research Committee of the National Research Institute of Chinese Medicine (ref no: NRICM-IACUC-109-355-1).

4.4. Animal Model

For prophylactic vaccination, the mice (n = 15) were randomly assigned to 3 groups: Group 1 (n = 5) served as the control group and was injected with PBS. Group 2 (n = 5) was injected with 2×10^6 of 4T1-luc2 cells that had been put through freeze and thaw (F/T) cycles, where the cells were first frozen in liquid nitrogen for 90 s, then thawed at 4 °C for 4 min, and this process was repeated 4 times. Group 3 (n = 5) was injected with 2×10^6 of 4T1-luc2 cells that had been treated with crassolide (25 μM) for 24 h. Seven days post-vaccination, all four groups of mice were orthotopically implanted with 5×10^5 live 4T1-luc2 tumor cells in 100 μL of PBS into the mammary fat pad. The tumor size was observed and measured three times a week and bioluminescence imaging of tumors was monitored once a week. Tumor size was measured by caliper measurements, and tumor volume calculation was used following formula: 0.5 × length (mm) × width^2 (mm^2). Bioluminescence imaging of tumors was monitored using a noninvasive in vivo imaging system. The mice were injected intraperitoneally with 15 mg/kg of D-luciferin potassium (PerkinElmer, 122799) in PBS and were left for 5 min before imaging. The test mice were then anesthetized with 2.5% isoflurane using the XGI-8 Gas Anesthesia System (PerkinElmer, Boston, MA, USA), and the XENOGEN IVIS 50 (PerkinElmer, Boston, MA, USA) was applied.

4.5. Cell Viability Assay

MCF7, MDA-MB-231, and 4T1-luc2 tumor cells (1×10^4) were prepared and dispensed in vehicle or test compounds in 96-well plates. They were then washed with PBS and incubated in RPMI 1680, placed in a 5% CO_2 incubator for 24 h. After this, the cells were treated with crassolide (50 to 3.125 μM) for 24 h. All treatments were performed in triplicate cell cultures. Cell viability was assayed using the 3-(4, 5-dimethylthiazol-2-yl)-2,5-diphenyltetrazolium bromide (MTT) colorimetric method. The optical density at absorbance 570 nm (A570) was measured using a multi-wall scanning spectrophotometer.

4.6. Immunofluorescence

4T1-luc2 tumor cells were cultured in 24-well plates with 0.1% poly-L-lysine coated coverslips. These cells were grown in RPMI 1640 medium. The cells were washed with PBS and then treated with crassolide (50 to 3.125 μM) for 24 h. For fluorescent immunostaining, the cells were fixed with cold methanol (−20 °C) and blocked with 3% bovine serum albumin (BSA, Bionovas) in PBS. Primary antibodies for heat shock protein 90 (HSP90, 1:400, Cell signaling), heat shock protein 70 (HSP70, 1:400, Abcam), high mobility group box 1 (HMGB1, 1:400, Cell signaling), calreticulin (CRT, 1:400, Cell signaling) were added to the cells, diluted in 3% BSA, 0.1% tween-20 in PBS, and protected from light. Finally, the cells' nuclei were stained with 4,6-diamidino-2-phenylindole (DAPI, 5 μg/mL, Thermo Fisher Scientific, Inc.) for 5 min. To mount the expression of DAMPs on cells, the immunofluorescence staining protocol was applied, and then the cells were examined under a confocal microscope.

4.7. Detection of DAMPs Ectolocalization

The 4T1-luc2 tumor cells were treated with crassolide (50 to 3.125 μM) for 24 h. Aliquots of 1 × 10^6 4T1-luc2 tumor cells were harvested, washed with PBS, and stained with PE anti-HSP90 antibody (LSBio, LS-63265), Alexa Fluor 488 anti-Hsp70 antibody (BioLegend, #648004), PE anti-HMGB1 antibody (BioLegend, #651404), PE anti-calreticulin (Cell signaling, #62304), APC anti-PD-L1 (BioLegend, #124312), Alexa Fluor 488 anti-CD24 (BioLegend, #101816) in 0.5% bovine serum albumin (BSA, Bionovas) in PBS, and then analyzed using flow cytometry (BD FACSVerse, San Jose, CA, USA).

4.8. Western Blotting

To further investigate the effect of crassolide on tumor growth and the expression of immune checkpoint molecules, 4T1-luc2 tumor cells were treated with crassolide (at concentrations of 50 to 3.125 μM) for 1 h or 24 h. Aliquots of 1 × 10^6 cells were harvested and washed with PBS, then lysed with RIPA lysis and extraction buffer. Protein content was determined using the Coomassie (Bradford) Protein Assay Kit. Samples were then fractionated by 10% SDS-PAGE and proteins were transferred onto a nitrocellulose membrane filter paper sandwich (ThermoFisher, LC2001). The 1 h group was immunoblotted with antibodies specific for phospho-p44/42 MAPK (Erk1/2) (Cell Signaling Technology, #9101), phospho-NF-κB p65 (Ser536) (Cell Signaling Technology, #3033), phospho-p38 (Cell Signaling Technology, #4511), phospho-JNK (Cell Signaling Technology, #4668), anti-ELK1 (Abcam, ab218133), phospho-STAT1 (Cell Signaling Technology, #9167), and β-actin (Cell Signaling Technology, #8457). The 24-h group was immunoblotted with antibodies specific for HSP90 (Cell Signaling Technology, #4877), anti-HSP70 (Abcam, ab181606), anti-calreticulin (Abcam, ab2907), anti-PD-L1 (Abcam, ab213480), anti-CD24 (Abcam, ab290745), HMGB1 (Cell Signaling Technology, #6893), and β-actin (Cell Signaling Technology, #8457). Non-specific binding was removed and target proteins were detected using corresponding secondary antibodies. Protein bands were then detected and developed using enhanced West Femto Maximum Sensitivity Substrate (ThermoFisher, 34096) and the Touch Imager (e-BLOT, Pudong, Shanghai, China).

4.9. Molecular Modeling of Crassolide and MAPK14 Interaction

To further investigate the binding interaction between crassolide and MAPK14 kinase, the crassolide was docked into the active site of MAPK14 using the GOLD docking tool in BIOVIA Discovery Studio 2021 (BIOVIA Corp., San Diego, CA, USA). The crystal structure of human MAPK14 (P38 kinase) was obtained from the RCSB Protein Data Bank (PDB ID: 1DI9) and the protein and crassolide compound atoms were assigned CHARMm force field.

4.10. Z′-LYTE Kinase Assay

An IC50 value of crassolide for inhibition of MAPK14 kinase activity was evaluated using a fluorescence resonance energy transfer-based Z′-LYTE kinase assay performed by Thermo Fisher Scientific's SelectScreen™ Profiling Service. Briefly, the 2X MAPK14 (p38 alpha) direct/Ser/Thr 15 mixture was prepared in 50 mM HEPES (pH 6.5), 0.01% BRIJ-35, 10 mM MgCl2, 1 mM EGTA, and 0.02% NaN3. The final 10 μL kinase reaction consisted of 7.14–103 ng MAPK14 (p38 alpha) direct and 2 μM Ser/Thr 15 in 50 mM HEPES (pH 7.0), 0.01% BRIJ-35, 10 mM MgCl2, 1 mM EGTA, and 0.01% NaN3. After a 1-h kinase reaction incubation, the reaction was developed and terminated, and the fluorescence ratio was calculated according to the manufacturer's protocol.

5. Conclusions

We have demonstrated that the marine natural product crassolide induces immunogenic cell death of tumor cells by blocking MPAK14 activation, thereby stimulating anti-tumor immunity. Our study not only highlights the immunotherapeutic effects of crassolide in activating antic ancer immune responses, but also provides a novel approach to developing marine natural products for clinical applications.

Author Contributions: Conceptualization, K.-C.T., C.-S.C., J.-H.S., Y.-C.L. and W.-C.W.; methodology, K.-C.T., C.-S.C., J.-H.S. and Y.-C.L.; formal analysis, K.-C.T., C.-S.C., Y.-H.T. and W.-C.W.; funding acquisition, W.-C.W. and J.-H.S.; investigation, K.-C.T. and C.-S.C.; project administration, K.-C.T. and W.-C.W.; resources, J.-H.S.; validation, K.-C.T. and W.-C.W.; writing—original draft, K.-C.T. and C.-S.C.; writing—review and editing, J.-H.S., Y.-H.T., Y.-C.L. and W.-C.W. All authors have read and agreed to the published version of the manuscript.

Funding: This research was funded by the National Science and Technology Council of Republic of China grant (108-2320-B-291-001-MY3) and Kaohsiung Armed Forces General Hospital grant (KAFGH_A_110018).

Institutional Review Board Statement: All animals were treated in accordance with the Institutional Animal Care and Use Committee (IACUC) of the National Research Institute of Chinese Medicine (NRICM), and the experiment was approved by the Committee on Animal Research and Care in NRICM (ref no: NRICM-IACUC-109-355-1).

Data Availability Statement: Data are available in the manuscript.

Acknowledgments: The authors would like to thank Pei-Wen Hsiao from Academia Sinica in Taipei, Taiwan for kindly providing the 4T1-luc2 cell line, as well as the members of the authors' laboratory at the NRICM for their assistance and support in this study.

Conflicts of Interest: The authors declare no conflict of interest.

References

1. Arnold, M.; Morgan, E.; Rumgay, H.; Mafra, A.; Singh, D.; Laversanne, M.; Vignat, J.; Gralow, J.R.; Cardoso, F.; Siesling, S.; et al. Current and future burden of breast cancer: Global statistics for 2020 and 2040. *Breast* **2022**, *66*, 15–23. [CrossRef] [PubMed]
2. Sung, H.; Ferlay, J.; Siegel, R.L.; Laversanne, M.; Soerjomataram, I.; Jemal, A.; Bray, F. Global Cancer Statistics 2020: GLOBOCAN Estimates of Incidence and Mortality Worldwide for 36 Cancers in 185 Countries. *CA Cancer J. Clin.* **2021**, *71*, 209–249. [CrossRef] [PubMed]
3. Pardoll, D.M. The blockade of immune checkpoints in cancer immunotherapy. *Nat. Rev. Cancer* **2012**, *12*, 252–264. [CrossRef] [PubMed]
4. Greenwald, R.J.; Freeman, G.J.; Sharpe, A.H. The B7 family revisited. *Annu. Rev. Immunol.* **2005**, *23*, 515–548. [CrossRef]
5. Ishida, Y.; Agata, Y.; Shibahara, K.; Honjo, T. Induced expression of PD-1, a novel member of the immunoglobulin gene superfamily, upon programmed cell death. *EMBO J.* **1992**, *11*, 3887–3895. [CrossRef]
6. Sharpe, A.H.; Pauken, K.E. The diverse functions of the PD1 inhibitory pathway. *Nat. Rev. Immunol.* **2018**, *18*, 153–167. [CrossRef]
7. Han, Y.; Liu, D.; Li, L. PD-1/PD-L1 pathway: Current researches in cancer. *Am. J. Cancer Res.* **2020**, *10*, 727–742.
8. Bradley, C.A. CD24—A novel 'don't eat me' signal. *Nat. Rev. Cancer* **2019**, *19*, 541. [CrossRef]
9. Takimoto, C.H.; Chao, M.P.; Gibbs, C.; McCamish, M.A.; Liu, J.; Chen, J.Y.; Majeti, R.; Weissman, I.L. The Macrophage 'Do not eat me' signal, CD47, is a clinically validated cancer immunotherapy target. *Ann. Oncol.* **2019**, *30*, 486–489. [CrossRef]
10. Fucikova, J.; Kepp, O.; Kasikova, L.; Petroni, G.; Yamazaki, T.; Liu, P.; Zhao, L.; Spisek, R.; Kroemer, G.; Galluzzi, L. Detection of immunogenic cell death and its relevance for cancer therapy. *Cell Death Dis.* **2020**, *11*, 1013. [CrossRef]
11. Zhou, J.; Wang, G.; Chen, Y.; Wang, H.; Hua, Y.; Cai, Z. Immunogenic cell death in cancer therapy: Present and emerging inducers. *J. Cell Mol. Med.* **2019**, *23*, 4854–4865. [CrossRef] [PubMed]
12. Jimenez, C. Marine Natural Products in Medicinal Chemistry. *ACS Med. Chem. Lett.* **2018**, *9*, 959–961. [CrossRef] [PubMed]
13. Ercolano, G.; De Cicco, P.; Ianaro, A. New Drugs from the Sea: Pro-Apoptotic Activity of Sponges and Algae Derived Compounds. *Mar. Drugs* **2019**, *17*, 31. [CrossRef]
14. Wang, L.T.; Wang, S.K.; Soong, K.; Duh, C.Y. New cytotoxic cembranolides from the soft coral Lobophytum michaelae. *Chem. Pharm. Bull.* **2007**, *55*, 766–770. [CrossRef] [PubMed]
15. Lai, K.M.; Wang, J.H.; Lin, S.C.; Wen, Y.; Wu, C.L.; Su, J.H.; Chen, C.C.; Lin, C.C. Crassolide Induces G2/M Cell Cycle Arrest, Apoptosis, and Autophagy in Human Lung Cancer Cells via ROS-Mediated ER Stress Pathways. *Int. J. Mol. Sci.* **2022**, *23*, 5624. [CrossRef] [PubMed]
16. Kroemer, G.; Galluzzi, L.; Kepp, O.; Zitvogel, L. Immunogenic cell death in cancer therapy. *Annu. Rev. Immunol.* **2013**, *31*, 51–72. [CrossRef] [PubMed]
17. Kuzmanic, A.; Sutto, L.; Saladino, G.; Nebreda, A.R.; Gervasio, F.L.; Orozco, M. Changes in the free-energy landscape of p38alpha MAP kinase through its canonical activation and binding events as studied by enhanced molecular dynamics simulations. *Elife* **2017**, *6*, e22175. [CrossRef] [PubMed]

18. Fabian, K.P.; Wolfson, B.; Hodge, J.W. From Immunogenic Cell Death to Immunogenic Modulation: Select Chemotherapy Regimens Induce a Spectrum of Immune-Enhancing Activities in the Tumor Microenvironment. *Front. Oncol.* **2021**, *11*, 728018. [CrossRef]
19. Zhao, Y.; Liu, X.; Liu, X.; Yu, J.; Bai, X.; Wu, X.; Guo, X.; Liu, Z.; Liu, X. Combination of phototherapy with immune checkpoint blockade: Theory and practice in cancer. *Front. Immunol.* **2022**, *13*, 955920. [CrossRef]
20. Lin, R.A.; Lin, J.K.; Lin, S.Y. Mechanisms of immunogenic cell death and immune checkpoint blockade therapy. *Kaohsiung J. Med. Sci.* **2021**, *37*, 448–458. [CrossRef]
21. Patel, S.A.; Minn, A.J. Combination Cancer Therapy with Immune Checkpoint Blockade: Mechanisms and Strategies. *Immunity* **2018**, *48*, 417–433. [CrossRef] [PubMed]
22. Chen, X.; Cubillos-Ruiz, J.R. Endoplasmic reticulum stress signals in the tumour and its microenvironment. *Nat. Rev. Cancer* **2021**, *21*, 71–88. [CrossRef] [PubMed]
23. Garg, A.D.; Maes, H.; van Vliet, A.R.; Agostinis, P. Targeting the hallmarks of cancer with therapy-induced endoplasmic reticulum (ER) stress. *Mol. Cell Oncol.* **2015**, *2*, e975089. [CrossRef]
24. Garg, A.D.; Dudek-Peric, A.M.; Romano, E.; Agostinis, P. Immunogenic cell death. *Int. J. Dev. Biol.* **2015**, *59*, 131–140. [CrossRef] [PubMed]
25. Zhang, W.; Liu, H.T. MAPK signal pathways in the regulation of cell proliferation in mammalian cells. *Cell Res.* **2002**, *12*, 9–18. [CrossRef]
26. Kim, E.K.; Choi, E.J. Pathological roles of MAPK signaling pathways in human diseases. *Biochim. Biophys. Acta* **2010**, *1802*, 396–405. [CrossRef]
27. Cargnello, M.; Roux, P.P. Activation and function of the MAPKs and their substrates, the MAPK-activated protein kinases. *Microbiol. Mol. Biol. Rev.* **2011**, *75*, 50–83. [CrossRef] [PubMed]
28. Darling, N.J.; Cook, S.J. The role of MAPK signalling pathways in the response to endoplasmic reticulum stress. *Biochim. Biophys. Acta* **2014**, *1843*, 2150–2163. [CrossRef]
29. Lin, C.C.; Chang, Y.K.; Lin, S.C.; Su, J.H.; Chao, Y.H.; Tang, K.T. Crassolide Suppresses Dendritic Cell Maturation and Attenuates Experimental Antiphospholipid Syndrome. *Molecules* **2021**, *26*, 2492. [CrossRef]

marine drugs

MDPI

Article

Sphaerococcenol A Derivatives: Design, Synthesis, and Cytotoxicity

Dídia Sousa [1,†], Milene A. G. Fortunato [2,†], Joana Silva [1], Mónica Pingo [1], Alice Martins [1], Carlos A. M. Afonso [2], Rui Pedrosa [1], Filipa Siopa [2,*] and Celso Alves [1,*]

1 MARE—Marine and Environmental Sciences Centre/ARNET—Aquatic Research Network, ESTM, Politécnico de Leiria, 2520-614 Peniche, Portugal

2 Research Institute for Medicines (iMed.ULisboa), Faculty of Pharmacy, Universidade de Lisboa, Av. Prof. Gama Pinto, 1649-003 Lisboa, Portugal

* Correspondence: filipasiopa@ff.ulisboa.pt (F.S.); celso.alves@ipleiria.pt (C.A.); Tel.: +351-217-946-400 (F.S.); +351-262-783-607 (C.A.)

† These authors contributed equally to this work.

Abstract: Sphaerococcenol A is a cytotoxic bromoditerpene biosynthesized by the red alga *Sphaerococcus coronopifolius*. A series of its analogues (**1–6**) was designed and semi-synthesized using thiol-Michael additions and enone reduction, and the structures of these analogues were characterized by spectroscopic methods. Cytotoxic analyses (1–100 μM; 24 h) were accomplished on A549, DU-145, and MCF-7 cells. The six novel sphaerococcenol A analogues displayed an IC_{50} range between 14.31 and 70.11 μM on A549, DU-145, and MCF-7 malignant cells. Compound **1**, resulting from the chemical addition of 4-methoxybenzenethiol, exhibited the smallest IC_{50} values on the A549 (18.70 μM) and DU-145 (15.82 μM) cell lines, and compound **3**, resulting from the chemical addition of propanethiol, exhibited the smallest IC_{50} value (14.31 μM) on MCF-7 cells. The highest IC_{50} values were exhibited by compound **4**, suggesting that the chemical addition of benzylthiol led to a loss of cytotoxic activity. The remaining chemical modifications were not able to potentiate the cytotoxicity of the original compounds. Regarding A549 cell viability, analogue **1** exhibited a marked effect on mitochondrial function, which was accompanied by an increase in ROS levels, Caspase-3 activation, and DNA fragmentation and condensation. This study opens new avenues for research by exploring sphaerococcenol A as a scaffold for the synthesis of novel bioactive molecules.

Keywords: marine natural products; anticancer; apoptosis; reactive oxygen species; algae; hemi-synthesis

1. Introduction

Cancer is one of the deadliest diseases in the world, having a huge impact on global health and representing a critical barrier to the life expectancy increase. The GLOBOCAN predicts the occurrence of 28.4 million new cases by 2040, corresponding to an increase of 47% compared to 2020 [1]. Assuming the current incidence trends, it is expected that this value will duplicate until 2070, tending to be one of the main causes of precocious death (>70 years old) [2]. Distinct therapeutic strategies such as classical therapies, e.g., surgery, radiotherapy, immunotherapy, targeted therapy, and chemotherapy, and more recently advanced approaches such as stem cell therapy, ablation therapy, and nanoparticles, among others, have been used [3,4]. Some of them are based on the induction of apoptosis through different stimuli, including radiation, hypoxia, toxins, hyperthermia, the production of reactive oxygen species, the activation of death receptors, etc., aiming at the effective elimination of malignant cells [5]. Despite the advances in the last decades, drug resistance to classical and/or new anticancer medicines and the side effects that result from non-specific treatments leading to healthy tissue damage continue to be one of the major cornerstones in cancer treatment [6]. Hence, in pursuing an increase in the quality and life expectancy of oncologic patients, it is imperative to persistently search and develop novel therapeutic tools with heightened efficacy and impact in cancer treatments, including new anticancer drugs.

Between 1981 and 2019, a total of 247 drugs with an indication for cancer treatment were approved, and their origins were traced back to compounds of natural provenance. Among these, 18 were developed directly from unaltered natural compounds' structures, while 29 were the result of a synthesis. Furthermore, 36 drugs were meticulously designed to mimic natural compounds, and an additional 43 were formulated using derivatives sourced from natural precursors [7]. These data attest the key role of nature as a source of chemical structures with anticancer potential, inspiring the development of innovative therapeutic agents. Opposite to the terrestrial environment, the marine environment remains poorly explored but exhibits a rich biological and chemical diversity, key factors in discovering bioactive compounds with pharmacological potential [8]. Due to their great diversity, marine natural products have shown an immense potential to inspire the development of innovative drugs with distinct mechanisms of action and great effectiveness in the treatment of many diseases [9]. However, their translation from basic scientific findings in the laboratory to clinical trials has been limited by several factors, such as low stability, bioavailability, water solubility, efficacy, pharmacokinetics, etc. [10]. To overcome these restrictions, the synthesis or hemi-synthesis of analogous molecules of resemblant nature with slight structural deviations can enhance the potency and efficacy of the inherent properties exhibited by a given compound, while concurrently mitigating its limitations.

In recent years, algae have been extensively studied as a source of bioactive compounds with health-beneficial properties such as antioxidant, antimicrobial, anti-inflammatory, immunomodulatory, and anticancer activities [11,12]. The red alga *Sphaerococcus coronopifolius*, Stackhouse 1797, has been revealed to be a great source of diterpenes, most of them brominated, with diverse molecular structures [13]. Sphaerococcenol A is one of the major compounds found in this algae, which is characterized to possess a sphaerane carbon skeleton and has revealed distinct biological activities, including anti-malarial [14] and antitumor [15–18] properties. Regarding cytotoxic activities, sphaerococcenol A has been displayed to affect the cell viability of different malignant cell lines in 2D, 3D, and co-culture models and stimulate the production of H_2O_2 and apoptosis [15–18]. It also exhibited a cytostatic effect on human apoptosis-resistant U373 cells, inhibiting the cell entry into the mitosis phase [18].

Despite the interesting activities evidenced by sphaerococcenol A, the hemi-synthesis of new analogues based on its structure was only approached by Cafieri and collaborators in 1978 (Scheme 1A) [19]. A base-catalyzed sphaerococcenol A rearrangement allowed the formation of the new hemi-synthetic compound A, which originated four derivatives (A1–A4) through its reduction, hydrogenation, and acetylation (Scheme 1A). Herein, we report for the first time the synthesis of four novel sulfur-containing sphaerococcenol A analogues (Scheme 1B). Sulfur-containing drugs present an important role in different medicinal areas (e.g., dexlansoprazole, a proton pump inhibitor; emtricitabine, an inhibitor of reverse transcriptase; ceritinib, an antineoplastic kinase inhibitor; and sugammadex, a selective relaxant binding agent) and constitute a large portion of newly approved drugs by the FDA [20]. In addition, sphaerococcenol A derivatives resulting from its reduction were also prepared (Scheme 1B). The cytotoxicity of the novel sphaerococcenol A analogues was further studied in malignant cell lines derived from lung (A549), breast (MCF-7), and prostate (DU-145) tissues as well as biomarkers related to oxidative stress and apoptosis.

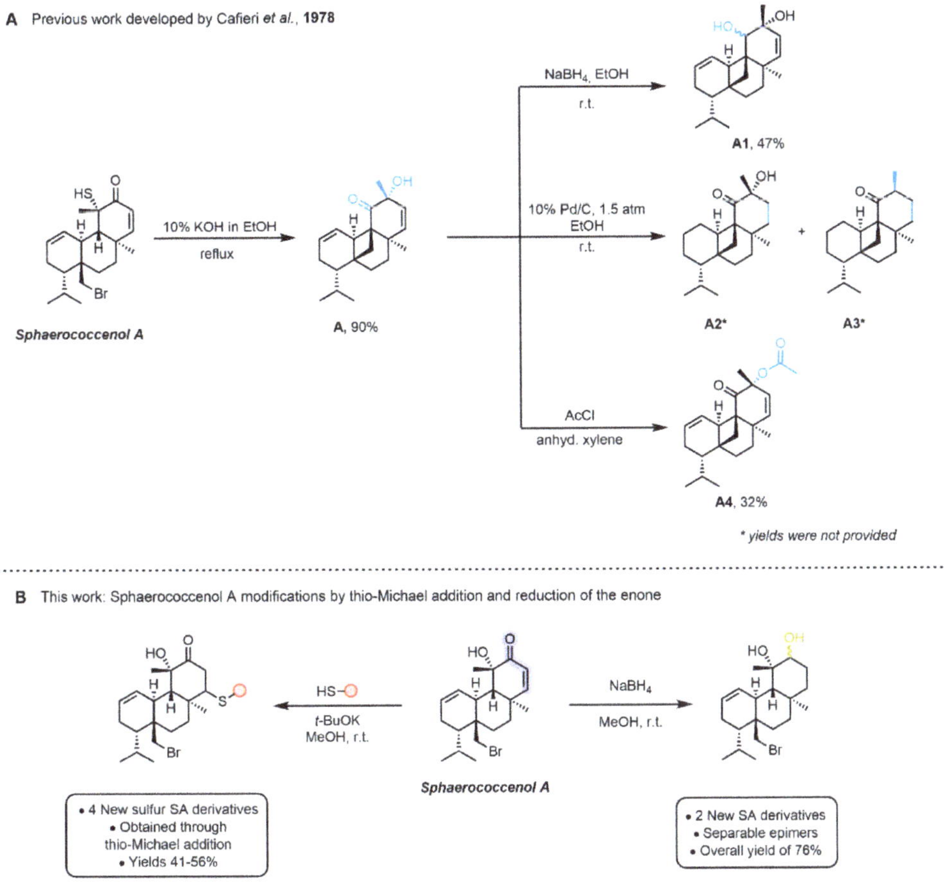

Scheme 1. Work on sphaerococcenol A reactions performed by Cafieri and collaborators [19] (**A**). Chemical modifications were performed in this study using sphaerococcenol A as scaffold (**B**).

2. Results

2.1. Hemi-Synthesis of New Sphaerococcenol A Analogues

The synthesis of novel sphaerococcenol A derivatives (**1–6**) was achieved by the reaction on the enone function via thiol-Michael addition and reduction (Scheme 2).

Thio-Michael addition allowed the preparation of four novel sulfur derivatives of sphaerococcenol A (**1–4**) (Scheme 2). The reactions were performed using the corresponding thiol nucleophile in methanol in the presence of potassium *tert*-butoxide (*t*-BuOK). In the case of using 4-methoxybenzenethiol and benzylthiol as the nucleophile, compounds **1** and **4** were obtained at yields of 56% and 41%, respectively. While using propanethiol, a mixture of diastereomers was delivered at a yield of 46% with a diastereomeric ratio of 1:1.55. The sphaerococcenol A reduction with sodium borohydride in methanol also resulted in a mixture of diastereomers with a 1:1 diastereomeric ratio. The new hydroxyl analogues (**5** and **6**) were obtained at a yield of 76% (Scheme 2). The proposed structure of the new hemi-synthetic analogues was assigned based on NMR and HRMS data, and the purity was checked by HPLC and/or ^{1}H-NMR and proved to be higher than 85%. The relevant protons for structural identification were H-14 and H-13 for compounds **1–4** and H-12 for compounds **5–6** (see Supporting Information, Table S1). For diastereoisomers **5** and **6**, a change in the corresponding chemical shifts for H-12 is visible (**5**: δH12 3.30 ppm;

6: δH12 3.61 ppm, Figure 1). Compound **5** corresponds to the diastereoisomer with the hydroxyl group behind the plane and **6** with the hydroxyl group to the front of the plane.

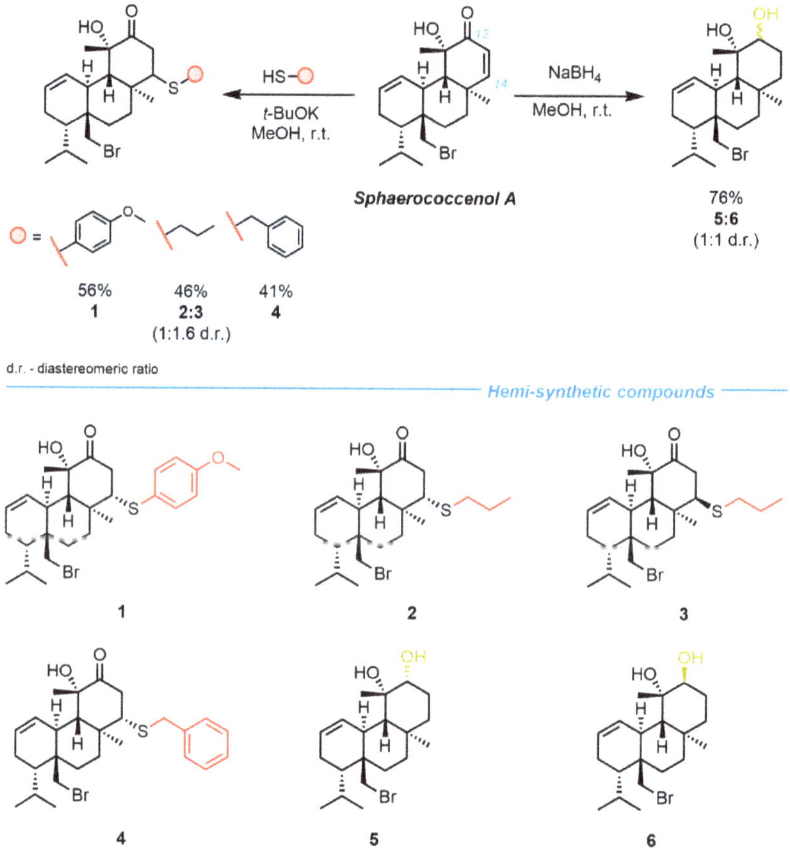

Scheme 2. Hemi-synthetic compounds of sphaerococcenol A obtained by thio-Michael addition and reduction.

2.2. Cytotoxicity on Malignant Cell Lines

The cytotoxicity of sphaerococcenol A and its derivatives (**1–6**) was evaluated in A549, DU-145, and MCF-7 cells. The results are presented in Table 1.

In the malignant cell lines DU-145, MCF-7, and A549, sphaerococcenol A displayed IC_{50} values of 3.75, 6.53, and 14.99 μM, respectively (Table 1). Between the synthesized derivatives (**1–6**), compounds **1**, **3**, and **5** exhibited the smallest IC_{50} values across the three cell lines. Amongst the compounds tested, compound **4** and compound **2** showed the highest IC_{50} values. Specifically, compound **4** displayed the highest IC_{50} values in the A549 (35.45 μM) and DU-145 (70.11 μM) cell lines, while compound **2** demonstrated the highest IC_{50} value among the MCF-7 cells (70.26 μM). Regarding the selectivity index, the original compound exhibited the highest value on DU-145 (10.0) and MCF-7 (5.7) malignant cells followed by compound **3** and compound **5** on MCF-7 (4.0) and DU-145 (4.4.) cells, respectively. On the other hand, compound **4** displayed the smallest selectivity index (0.6–1.3). Since analogue **1** demonstrated heightened potency in all three cell lines, with an IC_{50} value that closely paralleled the one obtained from the original compound in the A549 cell line and a selectivity index around 2, further studies were conducted in A549 cells to investigate the potential mechanisms of action underlying the cytotoxic activity previously observed with sphaerococcenol A.

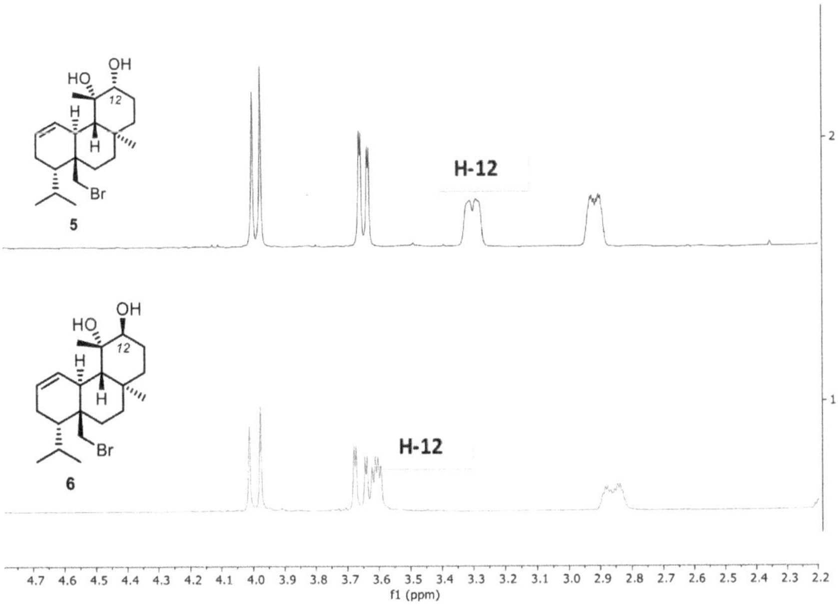

Figure 1. Partial stacking ^{1}H NMR spectra of diastereosiomers **5** and **6**.

Table 1. Determination of the IC_{50} value of sphaerococcenol A and its derivatives (**1–6**) in malignant (A549, DU-145, and MCF-7) and non-malignant (FL83B) cell lines after treatment for 24 h at different concentrations (1–100 μM). The effects were estimated by the MTT assay. The values in parentheses represent the confidence intervals for 95%. The selective index (SI) was also determined.

	IC_{50} (μM)						
	A549	**SI**	**DU-145**	**SI**	**MCF-7**	**SI**	**FL83B**
Sphaerococcenol A	14.99 * (12.30–18.19)	2.5	3.75 [c,e,*] (3.17–4.44)	10.0	6.53 [c,*] (4.43–9.57)	5.7	37.40 (31.49–44.92)
Compound **1**	18.70 (12.82–26.76)	1.8	15.82 [c,e] (13.33–18.92)	2.2	16.44 [c] (11.46–22.40)	2.1	34.56 (17.89–64.68)
Compound **2**	33.78 (27.63–41.19)	1.4	25.80 [e] (17.97–36.39)	1.9	70.26 * (49.57–101.7)	0.7	48.02 [a] (36.77–64.07)
Compound **3**	22.53 (18.36–27.56)	2.5	20.13 [e] (16.43–24.52)	2.8	14.31 [c,*] (10.01–21.61)	4.0	56.69 (35.40–98.96)
Compound **4**	35.45 [a] (29.72–42.43)	1.1	70.11 [a] (39.63–145.8)	0.6	30.40 [c] (23.46–39.22)	1.3	40.32 (32.10–50.92)
Compound **5**	22.68 * (18.17–27.88)	3.7	18.53 [e,*] (16.25–21.68)	4.4	31.95 [c,*] (23.36–45.45)	2.6	82.12 [a,b,c,d,e] (67.32–n.d.)
Compound **6**	33.54 * (29.48–38.55)	1.9	20.46 [e,*] (16.73–24.92)	3.1	22.19 [c,*] (14.49–31.98)	2.9	63.29 [b,*] (53.21–75.49)

Significant differences ($p < 0.05$) inside of the cell line group when compared with [a] sphaerococcenol A; [b] compound **1**; [c] compound **2**; [d] compound **3**; [e] compound **4**. Significant differences ($p < 0.05$) between different cells lines treated with the same compound when compared with * FL83B; SI = IC_{50} of FL83B/IC_{50} on the malignant cell lines. n.d., not defined.

2.3. Effects of Analogue 1 on Cell Viability and Mitochondrial Function

The effects of compound **1** on different cellular targets of A549 cells were estimated by the MTT, LDH, and calcein-AM assays (Figure 2).

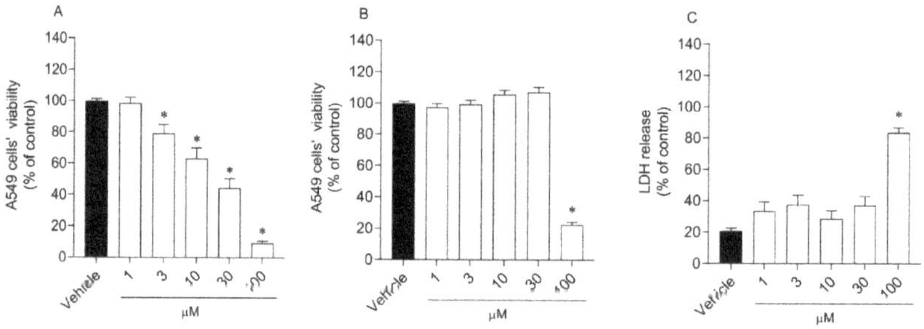

Figure 2. Effects of compound 1 (1–100 μM; 24 h) in A549 cell viability estimated by MTT (**A**), calcein-AM (**B**), and LDH (**C**) assays. Symbols represent significant differences (ANOVA, Dunnett's test, $p < 0.05$) when compared to vehicle. At least three independent experiments were carried out in triplicate.

The treatment with compound **1** for 24 h induced a significant progressive decline in the mitochondrial function of A549 cells starting at the concentration of 3 μM, with a more pronounced reduction at 100 μM (Figure 2A). On the other hand, the effects of compound **1** revealed by calcein-AM and LDH assays on A549 cell viability were only significant when tested at the maximum concentration (Figure 2B,C).

2.4. Reactive Oxygen Species Levels

Reactive oxygen species levels were estimated on A549 cells following treatment with compound **1** (10, 30, and 100 μM) for 3 and 6 h (Figure 3).

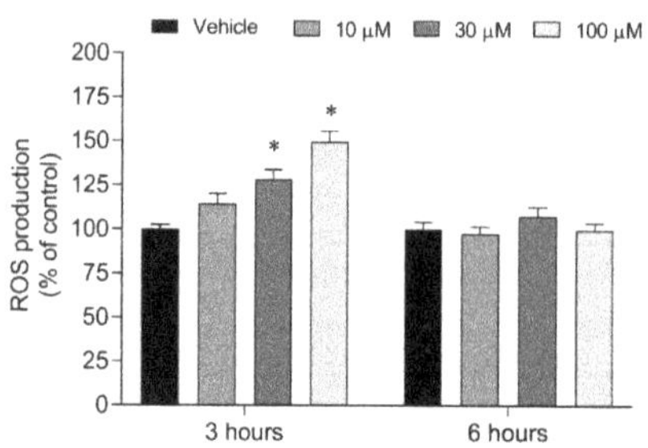

Figure 3. Reactive oxygen species levels produced by A549 cells following treatment with compound 1 (10, 30, and 100 μM) for 3 and 6 h. Symbols represent significant differences (two-way ANOVA, Bonferroni's test, $p < 0.05$) when compared to vehicle. At least three independent experiments were carried out in triplicate.

The A549 cells increased the production of reactive oxygen species after treatment with compound **1** for 3 h when tested at 30 and 100 μM (Figure 3). After a span of 6 h, no significant differences were observed in the levels of ROS when compared with the vehicle.

2.5. Mitochondrial Dysfunction and Apoptosis

Biomarkers related to mitochondrial dysfunction and apoptosis, including alterations in the mitochondrial membrane potential, Caspase-3 activity, and changes in nuclear morphology, were evaluated in A549 cells following the treatment with compound **1** at distinct times (Figure 4A–C).

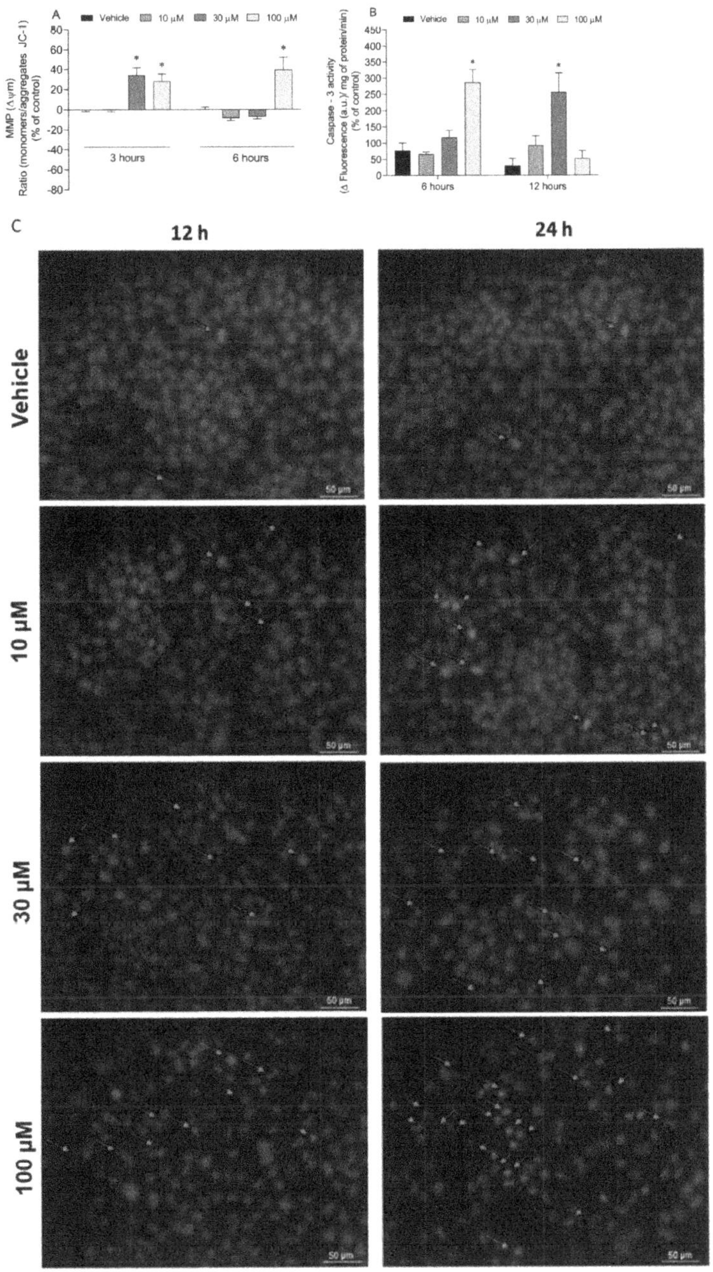

Figure 4. Effects of compound **1** treatment (10, 30, and 100 μM) on A549 cells regarding alterations in mitochondrial membrane potential after 3 and 6 h (**A**), Caspase-3 activity after 6 and 12 h (**B**), and alterations in DNA morphology after 12 and 24 h (**C**). Symbols represent significant differences (two-way ANOVA, Bonferroni's test, $p < 0.05$) when compared to vehicle. At least three independent experiments were carried out in triplicate. Images are representative of one well of each treatment condition and were obtained using an inverted fluorescence microscope at ×400. Red arrows indicate alterations in DNA compared to vehicle.

Analogue **1** induced a depolarization of the mitochondrial membrane potential of A549 malignant cells after treatment for 3 h at 30 and 100 μM. After 6 h of exposure, only the concentration of 100 μM maintained the effect (Figure 4A). Concerning the activity of Caspase-3, it is possible to observe a stimulation of its activity after 6 h of exposure for a concentration of 100 μM, and likewise after 12 h for a concentration of 30 μM (Figure 4B). All three concentrations induced DNA fragmentation and condensation after 12 and 24 h of treatment, which becomes evident in the regions demarcated by red arrows. The effects were more marked at the concentration of 100 μM (Figure 4C).

3. Discussion

Over the centuries, nature has been revealed to be an exceptional reservoir of new and uncommon chemical structures, on which the development of innovative drugs with distinct mechanisms of action was achieved, especially for the treatment of infectious diseases and cancer [21]. Despite the great pharmacological potential evidenced by natural products on laboratory assays, their translation to clinical applications is challenging due distinct factors [22]. However, these chemical structures represent a valuable source of scaffolds on which the development of new analogues can be inspired, improving their efficacy and mitigating limiting factors such as stability, bioavailability, solubility, pharmacokinetics, metabolism, toxicity, etc. [10]. The modification of natural products by semi-synthesis has been revealed to be a starting point for the generation of new analogue libraries with distinct properties from the original compounds, creating new lead structures for drug discovery [23]. Despite the red seaweed *Sphaerococcus coronopifolius* being revealed to be a prolific source of terpenes, most of them halogenated and with cytotoxic properties, there are only two studies that explore its chemical diversity as scaffolds for the synthesis of novel hemi-synthetic compounds [11,19,24]. As previously referenced, sphaerococcenol A was subjected to a base-catalyzed rearrangement, originating the new hemi-synthetic compound A, which by reduction, hydrogenation, and acetylation originated four new A analogues [19]. In addition to this, in 2022, Prousis et al. [24] reported the synthesis of hemi-synthetic analogues of bromosphaerol by reactions such as epoxidation and sequential hydroboration/oxidation. The newly synthesized bromosphaerol derivatives were evaluated regarding their antifouling activity [24]. Herein, we reported for the first time the synthesis of four novel sulfur-containing sphaerococcenol A analogues (**1–4**) and two derivatives (**5** and **6**) resulting from its enone reduction, aiming to improve the cytotoxic activity of the original compound. This library of new hemi-synthetic sphaerococcenol A derivatives allowed us to study key structure modifications, namely the effects of losing the enone function, the insertion of an alcohol function group at C-12 and its respective orientation (derivatives **5** and **6**), and the insertion of sulfur-containing moieties at C-14 (derivatives **1–4**). In the latter, the aliphatic and aromatic thiol substituent can also be compared.

The thio-Michael addition provided four novel sphaerococcenol A derivatives (**1–4**). Using 4-methoxybenzenethiol and benzylthiol as nucleophiles, only one epimer was obtained (**1** and **4**), while using propanethiol, two epimers were provided (**2** and **3**), resulting from the attack on both faces of the enone.

Sphaerococcenol A has a complex structure with distinct functional groups, such as alcohols, enones, olefins, and alkyl halides, which can undergo different chemical transformations. Thiols, in addition to engaging in the thio-Michael addition to enones, can also attack alkyl halides in a S_N2 fashion. Since sphaerococcenol A has an enone and an alkyl bromide function, the bromine substitution product could be expected. We proved the single formation of the thio-Michael product by subjecting the sphaerococcenol A to a large excess of thiol (20.0 equiv) and just observing the correspondent thio-Michael product. Additionally, when 1-bromo-2,2-dimethylpropane (a neopentyl bromide) was submitted to the standard reaction's conditions (2.0 equiv of thiol), it did not react. Concerning the enone reduction using sodium borohydride, two alcohol epimers (**5** and **6**) were originated in the same ratio derived from the 1,2- and 1,4-reduction.

The configuration of the newly formed stereocenters, C-14 for compounds **1–4** and C-12 for compounds **5** and **6**, was inferred by chemical shift values, an analysis of the coupling constants, and by a comparison with similar compounds isolated from the red alga *Sphaerococcus coronopifolius* [25] (Table S1). Compounds **1**, **2**, and **4** present high coupling constants of H-14 with the vicinal protons H-13α and H-13β. This is compatible with H-14 being in an axial configuration. On the opposite side, compound **3** presents a low coupling constant between H-14 and H-13β, indicative of an equatorial–equatorial configuration. This supported the equatorial configuration of H-14. Compounds **5** and **6** are epimers, and by comparing the coupling constants of H-12 with H-13, it is noticeable that **5** has a higher coupling constant than **6**, and this is consistent with H-12 being on an axial configuration on **5**. These findings are also supported by a comparison to similar compounds isolated from *Sphaerococcus coronopifolius* that have the same stereochemistry (Table S1).

Concerning the cytotoxic activities, the synthesized compounds displayed moderate effects ranging from 14.31 to 70.11 μM, never exceeding the IC_{50} values exhibited by the treatment with sphaerococcenol A. The only exceptions were observed with compounds **2** and **4**, which displayed significant differences when compared with the original compound. The extra methylene group in compound **4** seems to not be essential for sphaerococcenol A cytotoxicity, since compound **1** maintained similar activity to sphaerococcenol A and compound **4** lost the activity. Developing drugs with high selectivity for cancer cells is essential for creating more effective treatments for cancer patients. Achieving this selectivity not only enhances therapeutic efficacy but also minimizes damage to healthy tissues, thereby reducing side effects and improving patient outcomes. In this study, the original compound exhibited the highest selectivity index in DU-145 and MCF-7 cells, with only compound **5** surpassing it in the A549 cell line. The chemical modifications introduced did not appear to enhance the selectivity index. However, evaluating these compounds in additional cellular models could provide a more comprehensive understanding of their cytotoxic potential.

The effects of compounds on cell viability have been estimated through different assays, which have distinct cellular targets [26]. The MTT assay is widely used to estimate cellular metabolism through its reduction by mitochondrial dehydrogenases. On the other hand, the LDH assay allows us to understand if the cell membrane integrity was lost by measuring the levels of lactate dehydrogenase that leak from the cytoplasm into the culture medium [27]. In turn, calcein-AM is a lipid-soluble diester fluorogenic esterase substrate that can be converted by intracellular esterases in a hydrophilic, strongly fluorescent compound that is retained in the cytoplasm staining the viable cells [28]. Here, analogue **1** was able to induce a significant reduction in the cell metabolism at concentrations higher than 3 μM, while the significant effects estimated by the calcein-AM and LHD assays were only significant at the maximum concentration of 100 μM. These data suggest that compound **1** can target the cell metabolism instead to induce a disruption of the cell membrane.

The abnormal levels of ROS are often associated with changes in cellular metabolic activities and the occurrence of oxidative stress conditions, which affects both the development and maintenance of cancer [29]. The stimulation of ROS generation until achieving unsustainable cellular levels has been explored as a therapeutic strategy in cancer, leading to the activation of antitumorigenic signaling pathways and inducing cell senescence and cell death by apoptosis [30]. Usually, malignant cells display higher ROS levels due to their elevated metabolic rate becoming more vulnerable to further ROS damage than normal cells, which can regulate these levels through the antioxidant defense system [31–33]. Previous studies carried out with sphaerococcenol A in MCF-7 cells suggested that the decrease in cell viability was accompanied by the production of hydrogen peroxide, changes in mitochondrial membrane potential, the stimulation of Caspase-9 activity, and nuclear morphology alterations [15]. Although compound **1** did not potentiate the cytotoxic effects of the original compound in A549 cells, it seems that it induces cell viability reduction by similar mechanisms of the original compound. It was also able to increase the production of

ROS, decrease the mitochondrial membrane potential, stimulate the Caspase-3 activity, and induce DNA fragmentation and condensation. However, to establish a potential relation between the increase in ROS levels mediated by compound **1** and the activation of apoptosis, it will be essential to treat the cells with compound **1** in the presence of an antioxidant molecule such as N-acetylcysteine (NAC) to understand if the activation of apoptosis is directly activated by the ROS production or by other mechanisms. Furthermore, although the new derivatives do not enhance the cytotoxic effects of sphaerococcenol A, other factors such as solubility, stability, and additional biological activities, such as anti-inflammatory, immunomodulatory, and anti-angiogenic properties, should be explored in future studies to assess their potential contributions to cancer treatment.

4. Materials and Methods

4.1. Hemi-Synthesis of Analogues

4.1.1. Reagents

Reagents and solvents were purchased from commercial sources. All solvents were distilled before use. Methanol was distilled with calcium hydride under nitrogen and stored with 3 Å molecular sieves under inert gas. NMR spectra were recorded in a Bruker Fourier 300 (Bruker, Billerica, MA, USA) or a Bruker 400 (Bruker, Billerica, MA, USA) using $CDCl_3$ as a deuterated solvent. All coupling constants are expressed in Hz and chemical shifts (δ) in ppm. Multiplicities are given as s (singlet), d (doublet), dd (double doublet), dt (double triplet), t (triplet), td (triple triplet), tt (triple triplet), q (quartet), quint (quintuplet), and m (multiplet). High-Resolution Mass spectra were recorded in a Thermo Scientific Q Exactive hybrid quadrupole-Orbitrap mass spectrometer (Thermo Scientific Q Exactive Plus, Waltham, MA, USA). Reaction mixtures were analyzed by thin-layer chromatography using Merck silica gel 60F254 aluminum plates and visualized by UV light or stained with phosphomolybdic acid stain. Column chromatography was performed with silica gel Geduran® Si 60 (0.040–0.063 mm) purchased from Merck. Compounds **2** and **3** were purified using the HPLC equipment Thermo Scientific™ UltiMate™ 3000 UHPLC coupled with a semi-preparative column (Surf C18 100A 10 µM 250 × 10).

4.1.2. Extraction and Isolation of Sphaerococcenol A

Sphaerococcus coronopifolius specimens were collected from Berlenga Nature Reserve (39°24′47.9″ N 9°30′28.2″ W), Peniche, Portugal, with previous authorization of the Instituto da Conservação da Natureza e das Florestas (ICNF). Freeze-dried and powered biomass (60 g) was sequentially extracted with 1.2 L of a solution of 1:1 dichloromethane–methanol (72 h) and then with 1.2 L of methanol (48 h). The resulting extracts (1.43 g) were purified by silica gel chromatography (eluent: *n*-hexane/ethyl acetate (9:1)), yielding pure sphaerococcenol A (190 mg, 13% wt). The spectral data are in accordance with the literature [34]. ^{1}H NMR (300 MHz, $CDCl_3$) δ 6.81 (d, *J* = 9.9 Hz, 1H), 6.05 (dd, *J* = 10.0, 4.1 Hz, 2H), 5.76–5.69 (m, 1H), 3.88 (d, *J* = 10.7 Hz, 1H), 3.70 (dd, *J* = 10.7, 2.0 Hz, 1H), 2.99 (s, 1H), 2.88 (ddt, *J* = 12.2, 4.8, 2.4 Hz, 1H), 2.22–2.09 (m, 1H), 2.02–1.87 (m, 3H), 1.85–1.42 (m, 6H), 1.32 (s, 3H), 1.07 (s, 3H), 0.93 (dd, *J* = 14.3, 6.8 Hz, 6H). ^{13}C NMR (75 MHz, $CDCl_3$) δ 204.1, 162.9, 128.4, 127.0, 124.6, 75.5, 45.7, 42.2, 40.4, 40.0, 37.0, 35.6, 33.2, 31.5, 26.1, 26.0, 24.7, 22.5, 21.5, 19.6.

4.1.3. General Procedure for Thio-Michael Addition to Sphaerococcenol A (GP1)

In a Schlenk equipped with a stir bar, flame-dried and purged under an argon atmosphere, a solution of sphaerococcenol A (10.0 mg, 0.026 mmol) was prepared in distilled methanol (0.9 mL) with the respective thiol (2.0 equiv, 0.052 mmol) and potassium tert-butoxide (1.5 equiv, 0.039 mmol). The mixture was stirred at room temperature (25 °C). After consumption of sphaerococcenol A, a saturated solution of sodium bicarbonate (3 mL) was added to the mixture, and an extraction was performed using dichloromethane (4 × 3 mL). The organic phase was dried with anhydrous magnesium sulphate, filtered, and concentrated under reduced pressure. The crude product was purified by a chromatographic technique.

(4S,4aS,4bS,8S,8aS,10aS)-8a-(Bromomethyl)-4-hydroxy-8-isopropyl-4,10a-dimethyl-1-(phenylthio)-1,4,4a,4b,7,8,8a,9,10,10a-decahydrophenanthren-3(2H)-one (**1**)

The above was prepared according to general procedure GP1 from sphaerococcenol A (21.0 mg, 0.055 mmol), methanol (1.8 mL), 4-methoxybenzenethiol (13.6 μL, 2.0 equiv, 0.110 mmol), and potassium *tert*-butoxide (9.2 mg, 1.5 equiv, 0.082 mmol). The reaction was stirred for 40 min. The crude product was purified by silica gel chromatography (eluent: *n*-hexane/ethyl acetate (9:1)) to afford the product as a beige, amorphous solid (15.0 mg, 56%). ^{1}H NMR (400 MHz, $CDCl_3$) δ 7.39 (d, *J* = 8.7 Hz, 2H), 6.87 (d, *J* = 8.8 Hz, 1H), 5.99 (d, *J* = 10.4 Hz, 1H), 5.78–5.70 (m, 1H), 4.01 (d, *J* = 10.8 Hz, 1H), 3.81 (s, 3H), 3.78 (dd, *J* = 11.0, 1.8 Hz, 1H), 3.47 (s, 1H), 3.25 (dd, *J* = 7.3, 3.2 Hz, 1H), 2.93–2.91 (m, 2H), 2.80–2.72 (m, 1H), 2.50–2.41 (m, 2H), 2.19–2.14 (m, 1H), 2.03 (s, 1H), 2.00–1.92 (m, 1H), 1.77 (d, *J* = 6.0 Hz, 1H), 1.68 (s, 1H), 1.56 (dt, *J* = 13.9, 3.7 Hz, 1H), 1.44 (s, 3H), 1.15–1.08 (m, 1H), 0.95 (d, *J* = 6.0 Hz, 6H), 0.89 (d, *J* = 6.8 Hz, 3H). ^{13}C NMR (101 MHz, $CDCl_3$) δ 216.9, 159.9, 135.4, 128.7, 128.0, 125.3, 115.1, 76.5, 57.8, 55.5, 45.1, 42.0, 41.3, 40.3, 40.2, 40.0, 35.8, 31.9, 31.3, 26.0, 25.9, 25.3, 22.7, 19.9, 19.4. HRMS (ESI+): exact mass calculated for $[M + H]^+$ ($C_{27}H_{37}BrO_3S$) requires *m/z* 521.1720, found *m/z* 521.1718.

(4S,4aS,4bS,8S,8aS,10aS)-8a-(Bromomethyl)-4-hydroxy-8-isopropyl-4,10a-dimethyl-1-(propylthio)-1,4,4a,4b,7,8,8a,9,10,10a-decahydrophenanthren-3(2H)-one (**2** and **3**)

The above was prepared according to general procedure GP1 from sphaerococcenol A (20.7 mg, 0.054 mmol), methanol (1.4 mL), propanethiol (9.8 μL, 2.0 equiv, 0.108 mmol), and potassium tert-butoxide (9.1 mg, 1.5 equiv, 0.081 mmol). The reaction was stirred for 4 h. The crude product was purified by silica gel preparative thin-layer chromatography (eluent: 100% toluene). The mixture of the epimers was isolated as a translucid oil (11.3 mg, 46%, diastereomeric ratio 1.0:1.55) and was submitted to reverse-phase semi-preparative HPLC (water–acetonitrile 50–95%) obtaining 2.3 mg of compound **2** and 3.7 mg of compound **3**.

Compound **2**: ^{1}H NMR (400 MHz, $CDCl_3$) δ 5.98 (d, 1H), 5.75–5.70 (m, 1H), 3.83 (d, J = 10.7 Hz, 1H), 3.74 (dd, *J* = 10.7, 1.8 Hz, 1H), 3.28 (dd, *J* = 18.1, 10.4 Hz, 1H), 3.02 (dd, *J* = 10.4, 7.3 Hz, 1H), 2.83–2.69 (m, 2H), 2.56 (t, *J* = 7.3 Hz, 2H), 2.20–2.08 (m, 1H), 2.03 (d, *J* = 9.2 Hz, 1H), 1.98–1.91 (m, 2H), 1.86 (d, *J* = 12.2 Hz, 1H), 1.79–1.73 (m, 1H), 1.72–1.64 (m, 1H), 1.63 (dd, *J* = 7.3, 2.2 Hz, 1H), 1.58 (s, 10H), 1.53 (t, *J* = 3.4 Hz, 1H), 1.31 (s, 4H), 1.01 (t, *J* = 7.3 Hz, 3H), 0.95 (d, *J* = 6.8 Hz, 3H), 0.91–0.83 (m, 7H), 0.81 (s, 3H). ^{13}C NMR (101 MHz, $CDCl_3$) δ 215.7, 128.7, 128.2, 76.0, 53.3, 51.6, 42.3, 42.0, 40.3, 40.1, 40.0, 36.0, 34.8, 33.9, 31.7, 25.9, 25.8, 25.0, 23.2, 22.7, 19.3, 13.7, 13.2. HRMS (ESI+): exact mass calculated for $[M + H]^+$ ($C_{23}H_{37}BrO_2S$) requires *m/z* 457.1770, found *m/z* 457.1772.

Compound **3**: ^{1}H NMR (400 MHz, $CDCl_3$) δ 5.95 (d, *J* = 10.5 Hz, 1H), 5.74–5.69 (m, 1H), 3.97 (d, *J* = 10.7 Hz, 1H), 3.73 (dd, *J* = 10.7, 1.9 Hz, 1H), 3.16 (dd, *J* = 19.2, 9.0 Hz, 1H), 2.91 (dd, *J* = 19.2, 1.8 Hz, 1H), 2.79 (dd, *J* = 9.0, 1.9 Hz, 1H), 2.76–2.68 (m, 1H), 2.60 (t, *J* = 7.3 Hz, 2H), 2.41–2.33 (m, 2H), 2.18–2.10 (m, 1H), 2.03 (d, *J* = 14.6 Hz, 1H), 1.95 (qd, *J* = 6.9, 2.3 Hz, 1H), 1.76 (d, *J* = 6.0 Hz, 2H), 1.70–1.52 (m, 3H), 1.38 (s, 3H), 1.08 (d, *J* = 4.4 Hz, 1H), 1.02 (t, *J* = 7.3 Hz, 3H), 0.95 (d, *J* = 6.9 Hz, 3H), 0.93 (s, 3H), 0.89 (d, *J* = 6.8 Hz, 3H). ^{13}C NMR (101 MHz, $CDCl_3$) δ 217.1, 128.8, 128.0, 76.5, 53.3, 45.0, 42.8, 42.0, 40.5, 40.2, 39.8, 36.0, 35.8, 31.8, 31.4, 26.0, 25.9, 25.3, 23.2, 22.7, 19.8, 19.4, 13.7. HRMS (ESI+): exact mass calculated for $[M + H]^+$ ($C_{23}H_{37}BrO_2S$) requires *m/z* 457.1770, found *m/z* 457.1772.

(4S,4aS,4bS,8S,8aS,10aS)-1-(Benzylthio)-8a-(bromomethyl)-4-hydroxy-8-isopropyl-4,10a-dimethyl-1,4,4a,4b,7,8,8a,9,10,10a-decahydrophenanthren-3(2H)-one (**4**)

The above was prepared according to general procedure GP1 from sphaerococcenol A (21.0 mg, 0.055 mmol), methanol (1.4 mL), benzylthiol (12.9 μL, 2.0 equiv, 0.110 mmol), and potassium tert-butoxide (9.2 mg, 1.5 equiv, 0.082 mmol). The reaction was stirred for 22 h. The crude product was purified by two consecutive silica gel preparative thin-layer chromatography runs (eluent: *n*-hexane–ethyl acetate (9.5:0.5)) to afford the product as a translucid oil (11.0 mg, 41%). ^{1}H NMR (300 MHz, CDC_{13}) δ 7.37–7.27 (m, 5H), 5.95 (d, *J* = 10.4 Hz, 1H), 5.71 (ddt, *J* = 10.4, 5.3, 2.9 Hz, 1H), 3.79 (d, *J* = 3.2 Hz, 2H), 3.70 (d, *J* = 1.5 Hz, 2H), 3.49 (s, 1H), 3.09 (dd, *J* = 17.7, 10.2 Hz, 1H), 2.87 (dd, *J* = 10.2, 6.8 Hz, 1H), 2.81–2.63 (m, 1H), 2.20–2.05 (m, 1H), 2.04–1.89 (m, 1H), 1.80–1.72 (m, 2H), 1.67 (dd, *J* = 13.9, 4.0 Hz, 1H), 1.49 (t, *J* = 3.6 Hz, 1H), 1.26 (s, 3H), 1.24 (s, 3H), 0.94 (d, *J* = 6.8 Hz, 3H), 0.88 (d, *J* = 6.8 Hz, 3H), 0.81 (s, 3H). ^{13}C NMR (101 MHz, $CDCl_3$) δ 215.5, 137.8, 129.0, 128.8, 128.6, 128.2, 127.6, 76.0, 52.2, 51.5, 42.0, 41.9, 40.3, 40.0, 39.9, 36.9, 35.9, 33.8, 31.6, 29.8, 25.9, 25.8, 25.0, 22.7, 19.3, 13.5. HRMS (ESI+): exact mass calculated for $[M - H_2O]^+$ ($C_{27}H_{37}BrO_2S$) requires *m*/*z* 487.1665, found *m*/*z* 487.1668.

4.1.4. Reduction of Sphaerococcenol A

In a round-bottom flask equipped with a stir bar, flame-dried and purged under an argon atmosphere, a solution of sphaerococcenol A (16.0 mg, 0.041 mmol) was prepared in distilled methanol (1.4 mL). Then, sodium borohydride (2 equiv, 0.082 mmol) was added and the mixture was left reacting for 40 min. A saturated solution of ammonium chloride (6 mL) was added to the mixture and extracted with dichloromethane (4 × 4 mL). The organic phases were combined and dried with anhydrous magnesium sulphate, filtered, and concentrated under reduced pressure. The crude product was purified by silica gel column chromatography (eluent: *n*-hexane–ethyl acetate (7.5:2.5). The two epimers were isolated as pale oils (6.0 mg of each epimer, 76% overall yield).

Compound **5**: ^{1}H NMR (400 MHz, $CDCl_3$) δ 6.04 (d, *J* = 10.6 Hz, 1H), 5.69–5.63 (m, 1H), 3.99 (d, *J* = 10.5 Hz, 1H), 3.65 (dd, *J* = 10.5, 2.3 Hz, 1H), 3.30 (d, *J* = 11.4 Hz, 1H), 2.94–2.89 (m, 1H), 2.20–2.09 (m, 1H), 2.07 (s, 1H), 2.02–1.88 (m, 2H), 1.88–1.81 (m, 2H), 1.78–1.72 (m, 2H), 1.61 (qt, *J* = 5.6, 2.7 Hz, 3H), 1.47 (dd, *J* = 4.4, 2.5 Hz, 1H), 1.43 (s, 4H), 1.40 (t, *J* = 3.5 Hz, 1H), 1.32 (d, *J* = 3.5 Hz, 1H), 1.29 (d, *J* = 5.5 Hz, 1H), 1.23 (q, *J* = 2.3 Hz, 1H), 1.19 (q, *J* = 2.2 Hz, 1H), 1.13 (s, 3H), 0.96 (d, *J* = 6.8 Hz, 3H), 0.91 (d, *J* = 6.9 Hz, 3H). ^{13}C NMR (101 MHz, CDC_{13}) δ 129.6, 126.0, 78.3, 73.8, 49.0, 42.8, 41.2, 41.0, 40.1, 38.0, 37.1, 36.3, 31.0, 26.4, 26.0, 25.0, 22.1, 20.1, 19.3. HRMS (ESI+): exact mass calculated for $[M - H_2O]^+$ ($C_{20}H_{33}BrO_2$) requires *m*/*z* 367.1631, found *m*/*z* 367.1632.

Compound **6:** ^{1}H NMR (300 MHz, $CDCl_3$) δ 6.02 (d, *J* = 10.4 Hz, 1H), 5.72–5.65 (m, 1H), 3.99 (d, *J* = 10.6 Hz, 1H), 3.66 (dd, *J* = 10.6, 2.1 Hz, 1H), 3.61 (dd, *J* = 5.6, 3.0 Hz, 1H), 2.90–2.83 (m, 1H), 2.21–1.87 (m, 5H), 1.80 (ddd, *J* = 14.5, 5.1, 2.1 Hz, 1H), 1.74–1.70 (m, 1H), 1.65–1.57 (m, 1H), 1.56–1.46 (m, 1H), 1.43 (s, 3H), 1.37–1.18 (m, 4H), 1.16 (s, 3H), 0.96 (d, *J* = 6.8 Hz, 3H), 0.91 (d, *J* = 6.9 Hz, 3H). ^{13}C NMR (75 MHz, $CDCl_3$) δ 129.3, 127.3, 78.1, 77.4, 75.3, 45.6, 42.8, 41.4, 41.1, 38.9, 36.2, 36.1, 35.8, 30.7, 26.2, 26.1, 25.4, 25.0, 22.2, 21.0, 19.8. HRMS (ESI+): exact mass calculated for $[M - H_2O]^+$ ($C_{20}H_{33}BrO_2$) requires *m*/*z* 367.1631, found *m*/*z* 367.1631.

4.1.5. Studies on Thiol Attack: Thiol-Michael Addition versus SN2

Sphaerococcenol A with Nucleophile in Excess (20.0 equiv)

The above was prepared according to general procedure GP1 from sphaerococcenol A (50.0 mg, 0.131 mmol), methanol (5 mL), 4-methoxybenzenethiol (32.5 µL, 20.0 equiv, 0.262 mol), and potassium *tert*-butoxide (15.0 equiv, 0.197 mol). The reaction was stirred for 3 h. The crude product was purified by silica gel chromatography (eluent: *n*-hexane–ethyl acetate (9:1)) to afford the product as a beige, amorphous solid (37.5 mg, 55%).

1-Bromo-2,2-d′imethylpropane as Surrogate Molecule

The above was prepared according to general procedure GP1 from a solution of 1-bromo-2,2-dimethylpropane (17 µL, 0.132 mmol), methanol (4 mL), 4-methoxybenzenethiol (32.7 µL, 2.0 equiv, 0.265 mmol), and potassium *tert*-butoxide (22.3 mg, 1.5 equiv, 0.198 mmol). The reaction was stirred for 24 h. No reaction occurred.

4.2. Cell Culture Conditions

Three malignant cell lines (between passages 10 and 25) obtained from the DMSZ-German Collection of Microorganisms and Cell Cultures GmbH biobank were used: A549 (lung carcinoma), DU-145 (prostate carcinoma), and MCF-7 (breast adenocarcinoma). MCF-7 (ACC-115) and DU-145 (ACC-261) cells were maintained in RPMI 1640 medium (Merck, Darmstadt, Germany) supplemented with 10% FBS (fetal bovine serum, Biowest, Riverside, MO, USA) and 1% antimycotic and antibiotic solution (Biowest, Nuaillé, France). A549 (ACC-107) cells were maintained in DMEM:F12 medium (Merck, Darmstadt, Germany) and also supplemented with 10% FBS (Biowest, Riverside, MO, USA) and a 1% solution of antimycotic and antibiotic (Biowest, Nuaillé, France). FL83B hepatocytes (FL83B; ATCC: CLR-2390) were used as the non-malignant cell line. The cells were cultured in F-12K medium supplemented with FBS 10% (Biowest, Riverside, MO, USA) and 1% solution of antimycotic and antibiotic (Biowest, Nuaillé, France).

Upon reaching a confluency of about 80%, subculturing was initiated. The cells were lifted from the plate with a 1% trypsin solution (Sigma-Aldrich, St. Louis, MO, USA), and the neutralization was accomplished by adding culture medium. The cells were then subjected to centrifugation at 290× g for 5 min at room temperature. The supernatant was removed and cells were resuspended in fresh medium with a 1:8 split. Subsequently, they were planted in 25 cm^2 T-flasks and placed in the incubator at a temperature of 37 °C and 5% CO_2.

4.2.1. Cytotoxicity of Compounds

The effects of sphaerococcenol A and its analogues (**1–6**) on the viability of malignant cell lines were studied through three distinct assays, 3-(4,5-dimethylthiazol-2-yl)-2,5-diphenyltetrazolium bromide (MTT), lactate dehydrogenase (LDH) activity, and calcein-AM, targeting different cellular biomarkers. Untreated cells with DMSO (<0.2%) were used as control, and saponin (0.4 mg/mL) (Sigma, Darmstadt, Germany) was used as the positive control for cell death.

4.2.2. 3-(4,5-Dimethylthiazol-2-yl)-2,5-diphenyltetrazolium Bromide (MTT)

The cells were incubated with compounds at different concentrations (1–100 μM) for 24 h. After the 24 h was over, cells were washed with PBS buffer (pH = 7.4) and incubated for 60 min with the MTT solution (1.2 mM) previously prepared in a fresh medium. The MTT solution was then removed, and 100 μL of dimethyl sulfoxide (DMSO) was added to dissolve the formazan crystals. The results were expressed as the half-maximal inhibitory concentration (IC_{50}) after reading the absorbance at 570 nm using a microplate reader (Synergy H1, BioTek Instruments, USA). The selectivity index (SI) was calculated as the ratio of the IC_{50} value for a normal cell line to the IC_{50} value for the corresponding tumor cell line (SI = IC_{50} of non-malignant cell line/IC_{50} of malignant cell line), where an SI ≥ 2 of a compound represents a selective toxicity towards malignant cells, while an SI value < 2 is considered generally toxic [35].

4.2.3. Lactate Dehydrogenase (LDH) Activity

The cytotoxicity was measured by the LDH cytotoxicity assay kit (Pierce™ LDH Cytotoxicity Assay Kit; ThermoScientifc, Rockford, IL, USA) according to the manufacturer's instructions. Cell death was quantified and expressed as the percentage of control untreated cells.

4.2.4. Calcein-AM Assay

The cell viability was evaluated through the activity of esterases that interact with the calcein-AM probe by transforming it into calcein, a molecule that emits fluorescence and is trapped in the cytoplasm of living cells. After exposure to compounds (1–100 μM; 24 h), the cells were washed with PBS buffer and loaded with 2 μM of a calcein-AM (Invitrogen, Carlsbad, CA, USA) solution, which was previously dissolved in a PBS buffer and incubated for 30 min at room temperature protected from the light. The fluorescence emitted was measured using a microplate reader (Synergy H1, BioTek Instruments, Winooski, VT, USA) at wavelengths of 485 nm (excitation) and 530 nm (emission). The cell viability was expressed in percentage of control untreated cells.

4.3. Levels of Reactive Oxygen Species

This assay is based on the degree of fluorescence that is generated by the reaction of carboxy-H2DCFDA, which is a non-fluorescent probe that when in contact with reactive oxygen species (ROS) becomes oxidized, emitting fluorescence. Cells were seeded in 96-well plates and further incubated with compounds (10, 30, and 100 µM) for 3 and 6 h. After that, cells were washed with PBS and incubated with 100 µL of 20 µM carboxy-H2DCFDA solution (Invitrogen, C400) for 60 min. The fluorescence was read at wavelengths of 527 nm (emission) and 495 nm (excitation) using a microplate reader (Synergy H1, BioTek Instruments, Winooski, VT, USA). The results were expressed in the percentage of control untreated cells.

4.4. Mitochondrial Membrane Potential

To evaluate changes in the mitochondrial membrane potential, assays were carried out with a JC-1 fluorescent probe (Molecular Probes, Eugene, OR, USA), which evaluates the membrane potential through a ratio between the number of monomers and existing aggregates. Cells were incubated with compounds (10, 30, and 100 µM) for 3 and 6 h. The measurement of JC-1 aggregates (λ excitation: 490 nm; λ emission: 590 nm) and monomers (λ excitation: 490 nm; λ emission: 530 nm) was performed using a microplate reader (Synergy H1, BioTek Instruments, Winooski, VT, USA). The results were expressed in percentage of control untreated cells.

4.5. Biomarkers Related to Apoptosis

4.5.1. Caspase-3 Activity

The activity of Caspase-3 was determined using a commercial kit (Sigma, Casp3f, St. Louis, MO, USA) according to the manufacturer's instructions. To carry out this assay, cells were seeded in 6-well plates and subsequently incubated with compounds (10, 30, and 100 µM) for 6 and 12 h. Cells were then washed with PBS, transferred to a microtube, and centrifuged at 3200× *g* for 5 min at 4 °C. The resulting pellet was resuspended in 50 µL of lyse buffer and then kept on ice for 20 min. After that, cells were centrifugated at 15,300× *g* for 20 min at 4 °C. The supernatant was used to quantify Caspase-3 activity and the pellet for protein quantification. The fluorescence read was performed in a microplate reader (Synergy H1, BioTek Instruments, Winooski, VT, USA) during 60 min at wavelengths of 360 nm (excitation) and 460 nm (emission). The results were expressed in percentage of control untreated cells (Δfluorescence (u.a)/mg of protein/min).

4.5.2. DAPI Staining

The purpose of employing the 4′,6-Diamidino-2-Phenylindole, Dihydrochloride (DAPI) method is to investigate alterations occurring at the DNA level. DAPI serves as a fluorescent stain, exhibiting an affinity for binding to regions abundant in A and T content, which enables the visualization of genetic material condensation or fragmentation occurrences. For this assay, 6-well plates were seeded and subsequently exposed to compounds (10, 30, and 100 µM) for 12 and 24 h. After this, cells were stained with DAPI, as previously described by Silva et al. [36]. A representative image of each treatment condition was taken with a camera (AxioCam MRC-ZEISS, Jena, Germany) coupled to a fluorescence inverted microscope (ZEISS Axio, VERT. A1, Jena, Germany).

4.6. Data and Statistical Analysis

The data were obtained from at least three independent experiments (n = 3) carried out in triplicate and presented as mean ± standard error of the mean (SEM). The data were checked for normality and homoscedasticity. Data that did not meet normal distribution were analyzed by the Kruskal–Wallis non-parametric test. A one-way analysis of variance (ANOVA) with Dunnett's multiple comparison of group means was employed to determine significant differences to the control treatment and/or a two-way ANOVA with Bonferroni's test. All other post hoc analyses were conducted using Tukey's test. The differences were considered significant at a level of 0.05 ($p < 0.05$). The inhibitory concentrations (IC_{50}) were determined by means of the equation $y = 100/(1 + 10(x - \log IC_{50}))$. All data were analyzed using the software SPSS v28.0.0.0 (SPSS Inc., Chicago, IL, USA) and GraphPad v8.0.2 (GraphPad Software, Inc., La Jolla, CA, USA).

5. Conclusions

In conclusion, the data here reported correspond to the first study regarding the semi-synthesis of sphaerococcenol A analogues prepared through thiol-Michael additions and enone reduction, resulting in six new derivatives. The chemical alterations did not enhance the cytotoxic activity of the original compound, and the extra methylene group in compound **4** seems to contribute to the loss of activity. The semi-synthetic compound **1**, synthesized using 4-methoxybenzenethiol, exhibited similar cytotoxic activity of sphaerococcenol A in A549 malignant cells, which was accompanied by an increase in ROS generation and by the alterations of different biomarkers related to apoptosis cell death. This study opens new research opportunities to fully explore the potential use of this bromoditerpene as a scaffold for the synthesis of new molecules.

Supplementary Materials: The following supporting information can be downloaded at: https://www.mdpi.com/article/10.3390/md22090408/s1, Table S1: Relevant ^{1}H NMR spectral data of compounds **1–6**, and similar structures isolated from *Sphaerococcus coronopifolius*.

Author Contributions: D.S.: investigation, formal analysis, methodology, writing—original draft; M.A.G.F.: investigation, formal analysis, methodology, writing—original draft; J.S.: investigation, formal analysis, methodology, writing—review and editing; M.P.: investigation, formal analysis, methodology; A.M.: investigation, formal analysis, writing—review and editing; C.A.M.A.: funding acquisition, validation, writing—review and editing; R.P.: funding acquisition, validation, writing—review and editing; F.S.: funding acquisition, supervision, validation, writing—original draft, writing—review and editing; C.A.: funding acquisition, supervision, validation, writing—original draft, writing—review and editing. All authors have read and agreed to the published version of the manuscript.

Funding: The authors acknowledge Fundação para a Ciência e Tecnologia (FCT) for financial support (UIDP/04292/2020, LA/P/0069/2020, 2022.09196.PTDC (doi.org/10.54499/2022.09196.PTDC), UIDB/04138/2020, UIDP/04138/2020 and 2021.06598.BD). The project leading to this application has received funding from the European Union's Horizon 2020 research and innovation programme under grant agreement no. 951996. The NMR spectrometer part of the National NMR Network (PTNMR) is partially supported by Infrastructure Project no. 022161 (co-financed by FEDER through COMPETE 2020, POCI, and PORL and FCT through PIDDAC). This work was also supported by the BEAP-MAR (EAPA_0032/2022) project through the Interreg Atlantic Area Co-funded by the European Union.

Institutional Review Board Statement: Not applicable.

Data Availability Statement: The data presented in this study are available on request from the corresponding author.

Conflicts of Interest: The authors declare no conflicts of interest.

References

1. Sung, H.; Ferlay, J.; Siegel, R.L.; Laversanne, M.; Soerjomataram, I.; Jemal, A.; Bray, F. Global Cancer Statistics 2020: Globocan Estimates of Incidence and Mortality Worldwide for 36 Cancers in 185 Countries. *CA A Cancer J. Clin.* **2021**, *71*, 209–249. [CrossRef]
2. Soerjomataram, I.; Bray, F. Planning for tomorrow: Global cancer incidence and the role of prevention 2020–2070. *Nat. Rev. Clin. Oncol.* **2021**, *18*, 663–672. [CrossRef]

3. Tripathi, D.; Hajra, K.; Maity, D. Recent Advancement of Bio-Inspired Nanoparticles in Cancer Theragnostic. *J. Nanotheranostics* **2023**, *4*, 299–322. [CrossRef]
4. Debela, D.T.; Muzazu, S.G.; Heraro, K.D.; Ndalama, M.T.; Mesele, B.W.; Haile, D.C.; Kitui, S.K.; Manyazewal, T. New approaches and procedures for cancer treatment: Current perspectives. *SAGE Open Med.* **2021**, *9*, 20503121211034366. [CrossRef]
5. Singh, V.; Khurana, A.; Navik, U.; Allawadhi, P.; Bharani, K.K.; Weiskirchen, R. Apoptosis and Pharmacological Therapies for Targeting Thereof for Cancer Therapeutics. *Sci* **2022**, *4*, 15. [CrossRef]
6. Wang, X.; Zhang, H.; Chen, X. Drug resistance and combating drug resistance in cancer. *Cancer Drug Resist.* **2019**, *2*, 141–160. [CrossRef] [PubMed]
7. Newman, D.J.; Cragg, G.M. Natural Products as Sources of New Drugs over the Nearly Four Decades from 01/1981 to 09/2019. *J. Nat. Prod.* **2020**, *83*, 770–803. [CrossRef] [PubMed]
8. Karthikeyan, A.; Joseph, A.; Nair, B.G. Promising bioactive compounds from the marine environment and their potential effects on various diseases. *J. Genet. Eng. Biotechnol.* **2022**, *20*, 14. [CrossRef]
9. Ghareeb, M.A.; Tammam, M.A.; El-Demerdash, A.; Atanasov, A.G. Insights about clinically approved and Preclinically investigated marine natural products. *Curr. Res. Biotechnol.* **2020**, *2*, 88–102. [CrossRef]
10. Seyhan, A.A. Lost in translation: The valley of death across preclinical and clinical divide—*Identification* of problems and overcoming obstacles. *Transl. Med. Commun.* **2019**, *4*, 18. [CrossRef]
11. Alves, C.; Silva, J.; Pinteus, S.; Gaspar, H.; Alpoim, M.C.; Botana, L.M.; Pedrosa, R. From marine origin to therapeutics: The antitumor potential of marine algae-derived compounds. *Front. Pharmacol.* **2018**, *9*, 777. [CrossRef]
12. Lomartire, S.; Gonçalves, A.M.M. An overview of potential seaweed-derived bioactive compounds for pharmaceutical applications. *Mar. Drugs* **2022**, *20*, 141. [CrossRef] [PubMed]
13. Smyrniotopoulos, V.; Vagias, C.; Roussis, V. Sphaeroane and neodolabellane diterpenes from the red alga *Sphaerococcus coronopifolius*. *Mar. Drugs* **2009**, *7*, 184–195. [CrossRef] [PubMed]
14. Etahiri, S.; Bultel-Poncé, V.; Caux, C.; Guyot, M. New Bromoditerpenes from the Red Alga *Sphaerococcus coronopifolius*. *J. Nat. Prod.* **2001**, *64*, 1024–1027. [CrossRef]
15. Alves, C.; Silva, J.; Afonso, M.B.; Guedes, R.A.; Guedes, R.C.; Alvariño, R.; Pinteus, S.; Gaspar, H.; Goettert Márcia, I.; Alfonso, A.; et al. Disclosing the antitumour potential of the marine bromo diterpene sphaerococcenol A on distinct cancer cellular models. *Biomed. Pharmacother.* **2022**, *149*, 112886. [CrossRef]
16. Alves, C.; Serrano, E.; Silva, J.; Rodrigues, C.; Pinteus, S.; Gaspar, H.; Botana, L.M.; Alpoim, M.C.; Pedrosa, R. *Sphaerococcus coronopifolius* bromoterpenes as potential cancer stem cell-targeting agents. *Biomed. Pharmacother.* **2020**, *128*, 110275. [CrossRef]
17. Rodrigues, D.; Alves, C.; Horta, A.; Pinteus, S.; Silva, J.; Culioli, G.; Thomas, O.P.; Pedrosa, R. Antitumor and Antimicrobial Potential of Bromoditerpenes Isolated from the Red Alga, *Sphaerococcus coronopifolius*. *Mar. Drugs* **2015**, *13*, 713–726. [CrossRef] [PubMed]
18. Smyrniotopoulos, V.; Vagias, C.; Bruyère, C.; Lamoral-Theys, D.; Kiss, R.; Roussis, V. Structure and in vitro antitumor activity evaluation of brominated diterpenes from the red alga *Sphaerococcus coronopifolius*. *Bioorganic Med. Chem.* **2010**, *18*, 1321–1330. [CrossRef] [PubMed]
19. Cafieri, F.; Napoli, L.D.; Fattorusso, E. Base-induced rearrangement of Sphaerococcenol A. *Tetrahedron* **1978**, *34*, 1225–1226. [CrossRef]
20. Scott, K.A.; Njardarson, J.T. Analysis of US FDA-Approved Drugs Containing Sulfur Atoms. *Top. Curr. Chem.* **2018**, *376*, 5. [CrossRef]
21. Atanasov, A.G.; Zotchev, S.B.; Dirsch, V.M.; Orhan, I.E.; Banach, M.; Rollinger, J.M.; Barreca, D.; Weckwerth, W.; Bauer, R.; Bayer, E.A.; et al. Natural products in drug discovery: Advances and opportunities. *Nat. Rev. Drug Discov.* **2021**, *20*, 200–216. [CrossRef]
22. Sorkin, B.C.; Kuszak, A.J.; Bloss, G.; Fukagawa, N.K.; Hoffman, F.A.; Jafari, M.; Barrett, B.; Brown, P.N.; Bushman, F.D.; Casper, S.J.; et al. Improving natural product research translation: From source to clinical trial. *FASEB J. Off. Publ. Fed. Am. Soc. Exp. Biol.* **2020**, *34*, 41–65. [CrossRef]
23. Majhi, S.; Das, D. Chemical derivatization of natural products: Semisynthesis and pharmacological aspects—A decade update. *Tetrahedron* **2021**, *78*, 131801. [CrossRef]
24. Prousis, K.C.; Kikionis, S.; Ioannou, E.; Morgana, S.; Faimali, M.; Piazza, V.; Calogeropoulou, T.; Roussis, V. Synthesis and Antifouling Activity Evaluation of Analogs of Bromosphaerol, a Brominated Diterpene Isolated from the Red Alga *Sphaerococcus coronopifolius*. *Mar. Drugs* **2022**, *20*, 7. [CrossRef] [PubMed]
25. Smyrniotopoulos, V.; Quesada, A.; Vagias, C.; Moreau, D.; Roussakis, C.; Roussis, V. Cytotoxic bromoditerpenes from the red alga *Sphaerococcus coronopifolius*. *Tetrahedron* **2008**, *64*, 5184–5190. [CrossRef]
26. Riss, T.; Moravec, R.A.; Niles, A.L.; Duellman, S.; Benink, H.A.; Worzella, T.J.; Minor, L. *Cell Viability Assays*; Eli Lilly & Company and the National Center for Advancing Translational Sciences: Bethesda, MD, USA, 2016.
27. Riss, T.; Niles, A.; Moravec, R.; Karassina, N.; Vidugiriene, J. *Cytotoxicity Assays: In Vitro Methods to Measure Dead Cells*; Eli Lilly & Company and the National Center for Advancing Translational Sciences: Bethesda, MD, USA, 2019.
28. Neri, S.; Mariani, E.; Meneghetti, A.; Cattini, L.; Facchini, A. Calcein-acetyoxymethyl cytotoxicity assay: Standardization of a method allowing additional analyses on recovered effector cells and supernatants. *Clin. Diagn. Lab. Immunol.* **2001**, *8*, 1131–1135. [CrossRef] [PubMed]

29. Zhao, Y.; Ye, X.; Xiong, Z.; Ihsan, A.; Ares, I.; Martínez, M.; Lopez-Torres, B.; Martínez-Larrañaga, M.R.; Anadón, A.; Wang, X.; et al. Cancer Metabolism: The Role of ROS in DNA Damage and Induction of Apoptosis in Cancer Cells. *Metabolites* **2023**, *13*, 796. [CrossRef]
30. Pelicano, H.; Feng, L.; Zhou, Y.; Carew, J.S.; Hileman, E.O.; Plunkett, W.; Keating, M.J.; Huang, P. Inhibition of Mitochondrial Respiration: A Novel Strategy to Enhance Drug-Induced Apoptosis in Human Leukemia Cells by a Reactive Oxygen Species-Mediated Mechanism. *J. Biol. Chem.* **2003**, *278*, 37832–37839. [CrossRef] [PubMed]
31. Zhang, Y.-L.; Chen, G.-L.; Liu, Y.; Zhuang, X.-C.; Guo, M.-Q. Stimulation of ROS Generation by Extract of *Warburgia ugandensis* Leading to G0/G1 Cell Cycle Arrest and Antiproliferation in A549 Cells. *Antioxidants* **2021**, *10*, 1559. [CrossRef]
32. Hasanzadeh, D.; Mahdavi, M.; Dehghan, G.; Charoudeh, H.N. Farnesiferol C induces cell cycle arrest and apoptosis mediated by oxidative stress in MCF-7 cell line. *Toxicol. Rep.* **2017**, *4*, 420–426. [CrossRef]
33. Perillo, B.; Di Donato, M.; Pezone, A.; Di Zazzo, E.; Giovannelli, P.; Galasso, G.; Castoria, G.; Migliaccio, A. ROS in cancer therapy: The bright side of the moon. *Exp. Mol. Med.* **2020**, *52*, 192–203. [CrossRef]
34. Rosa, S.D.; Stefano, S.D.; Scarpelli, P.; Zavodnik, N. Terpenes from the Red Alga *Spaherococcus coronopifolius* of the North Adriatic Sea. *Phytochemistry* **1988**, *27*, 1875–1878. [CrossRef]
35. Chipoline, C.; Fonseca, A.C.C.d.; Costa, G.R.M.; de Souza, M.P.; Rabelo, V.W.-H.; de Queiroz, L.N.; de Souza, T.L.F.; de Almeida, E.C.P.; Abreu, P.A.; Pontes, B.; et al. Molecular mechanism of action of new 1,4-naphthoquinones tethered to 1,2,3-1H-triazoles with cytotoxic and selective effect against oral squamous cell carcinoma. *Bioorg. Chem.* **2020**, *101*, 103984.
36. Silva, J.; Alves, C.; Freitas, R.; Martins, A.; Pinteus, S.; Ribeiro, J.; Gaspar, H.; Alfonso, A.; Pedrosa, R. Antioxidant and Neuroprotective Potential of the Brown Seaweed *Bifurcaria bifurcata* in an in vitro Parkinson's Disease Model. *Mar. Drugs* **2019**, *17*, 85. [CrossRef] [PubMed]

marine drugs

Article

An Investigation of Structure–Activity Relationships and Cell Death Mechanisms of the Marine Alkaloids Discorhabdins in Merkel Cell Carcinoma Cells

Maria Orfanoudaki [1,†], Emily A. Smith [1,2,†], Natasha T. Hill [3], Khalid A. Garman [3], Isaac Brownell [3], Brent R. Copp [4], Tanja Grkovic [1,5,*] and Curtis J. Henrich [1,2,*]

1 Molecular Targets Program, Center for Cancer Research, National Cancer Institute, Frederick, MD 21702, USA; maria.orfanoudaki@nih.gov (M.O.); emily.smith2@nih.gov (E.A.S.)
2 Basic Science Program, Frederick National Laboratory for Cancer Research, Frederick, MD 21702, USA
3 Dermatology Branch, National Institute of Arthritis and Musculoskeletal and Skin Diseases, Bethesda, MD 20891, USA; natasha.hill@nih.gov (N.T.H.); khalid.garman@nih.gov (K.A.G.); isaac.brownell@nih.gov (I.B.)
4 School of Chemical Sciences, University of Auckland, Auckland 1142, New Zealand; b.copp@auckland.ac.nz
5 Natural Products Branch, Developmental Therapeutics Program, Division of Cancer Treatment and Diagnosis, National Cancer Institute, Frederick, MD 21702, USA
* Correspondence: tanja.grkovic@nih.gov (T.G.); curtis.henrich2@nih.gov (C.J.H.); Tel.: +1-301-846-5688 (T.G.); +1-301-846-6054 (C.H.)
† These authors contributed equally to this work.

Abstract: A library of naturally occurring and semi-synthetic discorhabdins was assessed for their effects on Merkel cell carcinoma (MCC) cell viability. The set included five new natural products and semi-synthetic compounds whose structures were elucidated with NMR, HRMS, and ECD techniques. Several discorhabdins averaged sub-micromolar potency against the MCC cell lines tested and most of the active compounds showed selectivity towards virus-positive MCC cell lines. An investigation of structure–activity relationships resulted in an expanded understanding of the crucial structural features of the discorhabdin scaffold. Mechanistic cell death assays suggested that discorhabdins, unlike many other MCC-active small molecules, do not induce apoptosis, as shown by the lack of caspase activation, annexin V staining, and response to caspase inhibition. Similarly, discorhabdin treatment failed to increase MCC intracellular calcium and ROS levels. In contrast, the rapid loss of cellular reducing potential and mitochondrial membrane potential suggested that discorhabdins induce mitochondrial dysfunction leading to non-apoptotic cell death.

Keywords: Merkel cell carcinoma; discorhabdin; structure–activity relationship; mechanism of action

1. Introduction

Merkel cell carcinoma (MCC) is a rare, aggressive, and rapidly metastatic neuroendocrine skin cancer [1–4]. Although rare, the incidence of MCC is increasing [5] due to the aging population, UV exposure [1–4], and immune suppression [6]. The majority of MCC cases result from chromosomal integration of Merkel cell polyomavirus (MCPyV) and expression of large T antigen and small T antigen [1]. These MCC virus-positive cases (VP-MCC) have disruptions in a variety of cell signaling pathways [1]. The other 20% of MCC cases have mutagenesis induced by UV light damage [1]. These virus-negative cases (VN-MCC) have a higher mutational burden with frequent mutations in oncogenes and tumor suppressor genes [1], and generally have poorer prognosis than VP-MCC patients [7]. The primary treatment of MCC is surgery and radiation for local disease and immune checkpoint inhibitors for metastasis [1–4,8]. Despite high response rates to immunotherapy, fewer than half of patients have a durable response, and thus, novel effective treatments are needed [9]. Genomic and expression analysis of MCC tumors has suggested a variety of potential therapeutic targets [10,11].

The ongoing opportunity for development of new MCC-active therapeutics has driven a number of drug discovery efforts over the years, typically based on in vitro MCC cell viability applied to chemical libraries or to small numbers of known compounds and leading to the identification of a range of potential drugs and probes [12–21]. In particular, a recent high-throughput screening campaign resulted in the identification of a substantial number of synthetic and naturally occurring small molecules as differential modulators of MCC cell viability compared to immortalized skin cells [22]. Among these were natural products not previously demonstrated to be MCC-selective agents, including the terpenes glaucarubin, englerin A, and thapsigargin; the lignan etoposide; naphtoquinone plumbagin, macrolide borrelidin; and the alkaloids discorhabdin D, petrosamine A, mitomycin C, and pluripotin. Discorhabdin D, a natural product isolated from marine sponges [23,24], was one of the most potent and selective of the active compounds identified in the screen. The discorhabdins are a group of marine alkaloids containing a core pyrido [2,3-*h*]pyrrolo [4,3,2-*de*]quinoline tetracyclic skeleton bound to various *spiro*-substituents at the C-6 position (Figure 1). The compounds have been associated with potent cytotoxic, antimicrobial, antiviral, antimalarial, and immunomodulatory activities [23,25]; however, their general toxicity towards mammalian cell lines and lack of selectivity have hampered their progress towards drug development. Recently, several trends on the structure/activity of the discorhabdins have been established—analogues containing the redox-active iminoquinone moiety and the electrophilic spirodienone ring are cytotoxic in the sub micromolar ranges, but these two reactive structural features were hypothesized to be involved in the generation of an oxygen radical and nucleophilic substitution, respectively, which is likely responsible for the broad cytotoxic activity observed for the group [23,26,27]. Compounds which possess an additional ring between C-2 and *N*-18 atoms and substitution at the C-1 position have neither of these reactive structural features and tend to be less cytotoxic to mammalian and cancer cell lines [27].

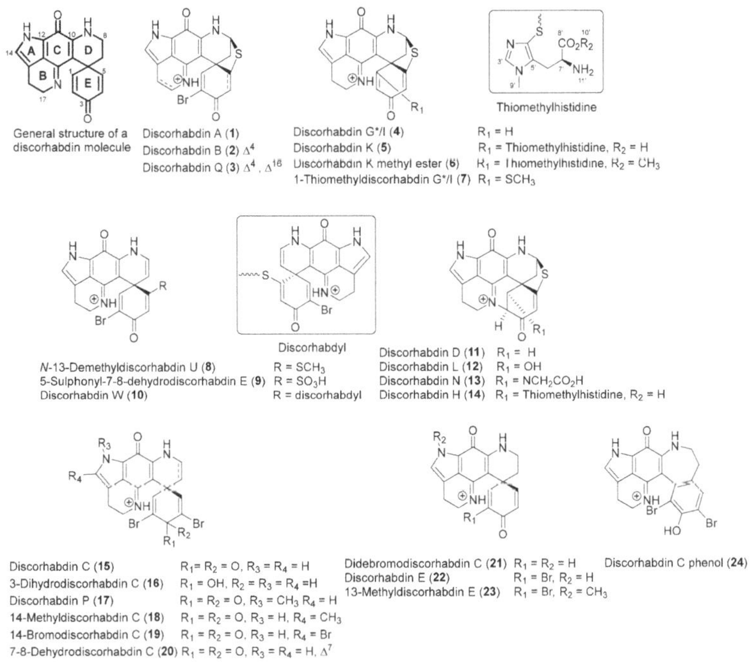

Figure 1. Structures of the naturally occurring and semi-synthetic molecules used in this study.

Investigation of cell death mechanisms of action for cytotoxic compounds is an increasingly important activity in drug discovery and development [28], and cell death mechanisms have been probed for a number of MCC-active compounds. In most cases, induction of apoptosis in the MCC cells was observed [29–36]. Ferroptosis [37,38] and autophagy/necroptosis/autophagic cell death [39] have also been reported as potential mechanisms of action in targeted MCC cell death. On the other hand, relatively little has been reported in the literature regarding molecular targets and mechanisms of action of discorhabdins beyond general toxicity in a variety of cell types. There are a few reports of effects of various discorhabdins on specific molecular targets, including acetylcholinesterases [40], calcineurin [41], caspase-3 [41], heat shock proteins [42], and HIF1α-P300 binding interaction [43] in tumor and angiogenesis models [44]. However, cell death mechanisms have not been extensively investigated for cytotoxic activities of discorhabdins.

In the current study, a large library of discorhabdins was assessed for effects on MCC cell viability. The discorhabdins were sourced from in house pure compound libraries as well as new natural products isolated and described herein. Investigation of structure–activity relationships (SAR) resulted in the identification of crucial structural features driving the activity and has allowed for an expanded understanding of discorhabdin SAR. Analysis of cell death mechanisms induced in MCC cells by discorhabdins suggested induction of non-apoptotic cell death involving mitochondrial dysfunction in all tested MCC cells. Active discorhabdins induced cell death at higher potency in VP-MCC cell lines compared to VN-MCC lines, but without apparent mechanistic differences.

2. Results

The library of twenty-four molecules shown in Figure 1 represents the majority of structural diversity reported for the monomeric discorhabdins. In addition to eighteen known natural products (**1–5**, **7**, **10–16**, **19**, **21**, **22**,) sourced from pure compound libraries and three previously reported semi-synthetic derivatives (**8**, **17**, and **24**), the set was expanded to include the structures of three new structures, namely, discorhabdin K methyl ester (**6**), 5-sulphonyl-7,8-discorhabdin E (**9**), and 7–8-dehydrodiscorhabdin C (**20**), as well as two new alkylated semi-synthetic discorhabdins, namely, 14-methyl discorhabdin C (**18**) and 13-methyl discorhabdin E (**23**) (Figure 1). A summary of the physicochemical properties of compounds **1–24** is presented in Supporting Information (Figure S2) and shows molecular weights ranging from 400 to 700 (with the exception of the dimer discorhabdin W at Mw = 1055), clogP ranging from −4 to 3, polar surface area ranging from 60 to 180, hydrogen bond acceptors ranging from 3 to 9, and hydrogen bond donor ranging from 1 to 7, all showing favorable physicochemical properties for drug-like small molecules. The twenty-four structures can be classified into three distinct groups represented by discorhabdins B, C, and D as prototypical compounds. The discorhabdin B series is characterized by the core pentacyclic pyrridopyroloiminoquinone structures **1–10** containing a *spiro* ring at C-6 and either a thioether bridge between C-5 and C-8 (**1–7**) or a thiol substitution at C-5 (**8–10**). The discorhabdin D series (**11–14**) is characterized by an additional ring between *N*-18 and C-2 positions and various -*O*, -*N*, and -*S* atom substitutions at C-1. The discorhabdin C series is characterized by pentacyclic pyrridopyroloiminoquinone structures **15–24** containing a *spiro* ring at C-6, thioether or sulfur substitution at C-5, and bromine or alkyl substitutions at C-2, C-4, *N*-13, and C-14.

2.1. Structure Elucidation

Compound **6** was assigned the molecular formula $C_{26}H_{25}N_6O_4S_2$ as established by the quasi-molecular ion at m/z 549.1374 (calculated for $C_{26}H_{25}N_6O_4S_2$ 549.1379) observed in HRESIMS. ^{1}H and ^{13}C NMR data indicated high similarity with the known compound discorhabdin K (**5**) [26]. Additionally, an extra methyl group (δ_H 3.61, δ_C 53.0) at the carboxylic acid on the thiohistidine residue of the molecule was observed, supported by lower chemical shifts of the carbonyl group at position C-8′ (δ_C 168.7) and the methine group at position C-7′ (δ_C 50.9), as well as a higher chemical shift of proton H-7′ (δ_H 4.20).

Key ^1H–^{13}C HMBC correlations from H-10′ (δ_H 3.61) to C-8′ (δ_C 168.7) (Figure 2) confirmed the location of the methyl group. In order to annotate the stereochemical assignment of compound **6**, its experimental ECD spectrum was compared to that of a structurally related discorhabdin with a previously defined configuration, namely (+)-(6*S*,8*S*,7′S*)-discorhabdin K (**5**). The two structures showed high similarity of the ECD spectra (Figure S3) and the same sign of optical rotary dispersion values at three different wavelengths, thereby establishing that the two molecules have the same configuration and identifying compound **6** as (+)-(6*S*,8*S*,7′S*)-discorhabin K methyl ester. In an effort to determine if compound **6** was an isolation procedure artefact of the co-occurring metabolite discorhabdin K (**5**), we heated **6** in methanol [0.1% TFA] as well as methanol-water (1:1) [0.1% TFA] at 40 °C and monitored the stability of the compound over 72 h. These conditions represented an extreme version of the steps involved in the isolation procedure where the fractions were subjected to semi-preparative HPLC using acidified water and methanol and then dried overnight in a centrifugal evaporator at 40 °C. The results showed a small but detectable appearance of an ion at *m*/*z* 549.1374 corresponding to discorhabdin K methyl ester, and the authors conclude that **6** may be an isolation procedure artefact of the natural product **5**.

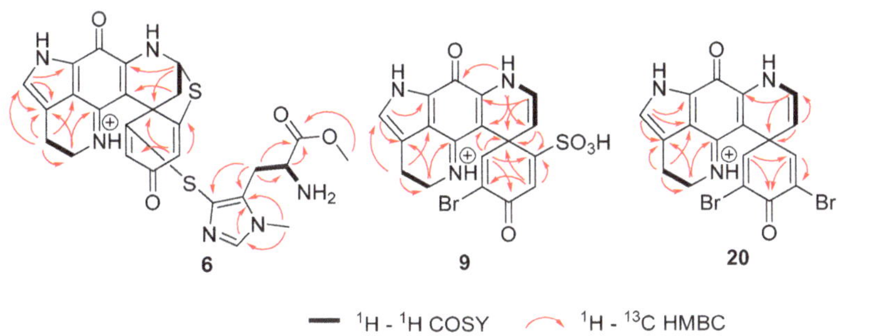

Figure 2. Crucial 2D NMR correlations used to establish the structures of **6**, **9**, and **20**.

Compound **9** was assigned the molecular formula $C_{18}H_{13}BrN_3O_5S$ as established from the quasi-molecular ions at *m*/*z* 461.9751 (calculated for $C_{18}H_{13}{}^{79}BrN_3O_5S$, 461.9754) and 463.9730 (calculated for $C_{18}H_{13}{}^{81}BrN_3O_5S$, 463.9734) observed in HRESIMS spectra. ^1H and ^{13}C NMR data indicated high similarity with the known semisynthetic compound *N*-13-demethyldiscorhabdin U (**8**) [45], with one major difference at the substitution of C-5. The existence of the sulfonyl group at C-5 was indicated by two IR characteristic bands at 1210 and 1137 cm^{-1} [46,47] and a loss of *m*/*z* 79.9567 (negative mode) in the high-resolution product ion spectra (Figure S4). The sulphonyl group while relatively rare in nature, has been reported in metabolites from both marine and terrestrial organisms, for example in nakijiquinone R isolated from marine sponges of the family Spongiidae [48], in the triterpene glycoside koreoside A isolated from the sea cucumber *Cucumaria koraiensis* [49], and in diterpenoid alkaloids from *Aconitum carmichaelii* [50]. In order to complete the stereochemical assignment of compound **9**, the experimental ECD spectrum of the natural product was compared to the calculated ECD spectrum of the 6*S* enantiomer of **9** using TDDFT calculations. A good agreement between the measured and calculated ECD spectra of **9** (Table S1, Figure 3) was supportive of the *S* configuration at C-6 to complete the structure of (+)-(6*S*)-5-sulphonyl-7,8-dehydro-discorhabdin E. Additionally, here for the first time, the absolute configuration of discorhabdin E (**22**) has been established to be 6*S* by comparison of the experimental and calculated ECD spectra (Table S2, Figure S1).

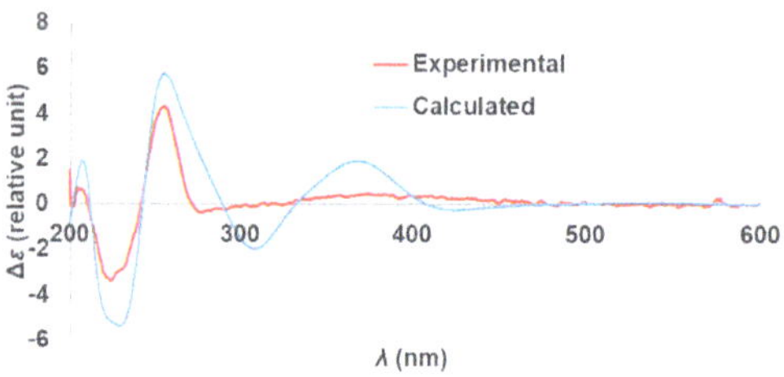

Figure 3. Calculated ECD spectrum (blue line) for compound **9** compared to the experimental spectrum observed for compound **9** (red line).

Compound **20** was assigned the molecular formula $C_{18}H_{12}Br_2N_3O_2$ as established from the quasi-molecular ions at *m*/*z* 459.930 (calculated for $C_{18}H_{12}{}^{79}Br_2N_3O_2$, 459.930), 461.9276 (calculated for $C_{18}H_{12}{}^{79}Br^{81}BrN_3O_2$, 461.9271), and 463.9260 (calculated for $C_{18}H_{12}{}^{81}Br_2N_3O_2$, 463.9250) observed in HRESIMS spectra. ^1H and ^{13}C NMR data had high similarity with the known compound discorhabdin C (**15**) [51]. However, one difference could be observed, the presence of an additional olefin at dihydropyridine ring between C-7 and C-8 which was indicated by higher chemical shifts of position C-7 (δ_H 4.71, δ_C 109.8) and position C-8 (δ_H 6.53, δ_C 125.6) and were consistent with literature values [52–54]. ^1H–^1H COSY correlations of the protons H-7/H-8/H-9 and ^1H–^{13}C HMBC correlations from H-7 (δ_H 4.71) to C-20 at δ_C 95.4 and H-8 (δ_H 6.53) to C-6, C-7, and C-10, (δ_C 47.1, 109.8 and 145.2) (Figure 2) confirmed the placement of the double bond and completed the structure of compound **20** which was assigned the trivial name 7,8-dehydro-discorhabdin C.

Additionally, two semisynthetic compounds were made: 14-methyldiscorhabdin C (**18**) and (+)-(6*S*)-*N*-13-methyldiscorhabdin E (**23**). 14-Methyldiscorhabdin C (**18**) was prepared with the addition of $FeCl_2$ and H_2O_2 in a DMSO solution of discorhabdin C based on the protocol described in Zhang et al., [55] which resulted in the addition of a methyl group at C-14 of discorhabdin C. The position of the extra methyl group was indicated by specific chemical shifts of the methyl group (δ_H 2.25, δ_C 11.1) and ^1H–^{13}C HMBC correlations from H-22 (δ_H 2.25) to C-15 at δ_C 118.1 and C-14 at δ_C 139.3. (+)-(6*S*)-*N*-13-Methyldiscorhabdin E (**23**) was prepared using a previously established semi-synthetic route [45] which included the addition of CH_3I and K_2CO_3 to an acetone solution of discorhabdin E and resulted in the addition of a methyl group at position C-13 of discorhabdin E. The placement of the extra methyl group was indicated by specific chemical shifts at δ_H 3.92, δ_C 36.5 and ^1H–^{13}C HMBC correlations from H-22 (δ_H 3.92) to C-12 at δ_C 124.8 and C-14 at δ_C 132.0 for compound **23**.

2.2. *Assay Activity*

The discorhabdins were assessed for activity against seven cell lines: three virus-negative (VN-MCC) cell lines (MCC13, MCC26, and UISO), three virus-positive (VP-MCC) cell lines (MKL-1, MKL-2, and Waga), and one non-cancerous skin cell line used as a control (HaCaT). Dose–response curves, discorhabdin structures, and IC_{50} values for each cell line/discorhabdin pair are shown in Figure S39. Activity of the discorhabdins against the MCC cell lines ranged from low nano molar values to greater than 10 μM (highest concentration tested). Eight discorhabdins averaged sub-micromolar potency (IC_{50}) across all MCC cell lines tested. These were (in decreasing order of potency) discorhabdin A (**1**), discorhabdin B (**2**), N-13-demethyldiscorhabdin U (**8**), discorhabdin P (**17**), 14-bromodiscorhabdin discorhabdin C (**19**), discorhabdin L (**12**), discorhabdin E (**22**), and discorhabdin G*/I (**4**). Discorhabdins A (**1**), B (**2**), and N-13-demethyl U (**8**) also had IC_{50} values at or below 1 μM for control cells. Five compounds were essentially inactive (>5 μM average IC_{50}) against all the cell lines: discorhabdin K (**5**), didebromodiscorhabdin C (**21**), 7-8-dehydrodiscorhabdin C (**20**), discorhabdin H (**14**), and 5-sulphonyl-7,8 dehydrodiscorhabdin E (**9**).

In order to compare and visualize differences in the activity of the compounds, all of the dose–response curves used identical dilution series, and area under the curve (AUC) was determined for each cell line/discorhabdin pair (Table S3). AUC is a parameter that incorporates potency and efficacy and is useful for comparing activity across multiple cell lines and drugs [56]. The data showed a very high linear correlation between IC_{50} and AUC (R^2 = 0.98, Figure S40). Subsequent analyses generally utilized AUC, since comparisons could also then include compounds with minimal effect on specific cell lines at the concentrations tested. Figure 4 shows the effects of the discorhabdin alkaloids on Merkel cell viability using AUC and sorted into discorhabdin structural classes. As expected, the AUC data led to similar general conclusions as noted above from IC_{50} data. Figure S41 details selectivity among VN-MCC and VP-MCC cells compared to the control. Interestingly, only 14-bromo discorhabdin C (**19**) and 14-methyl discorhabdin C (**18**) showed substantially increased activity against VN-MCC compared to control cells (>3-fold difference). In contrast, seven discorhabdins had >10-fold increased activity against VP-MCC compared to the control—in order of decreasing relative activity: 14-methyldiscorhabdin C (**18**), 14-bromodiscorhabdin C (**19**), discorhabdin B (**2**), discorhabdin W (**10**), discorhabdin E (**22**), N-13-demethyldiscorhabdin U (**8**), and discorhabdin P (**17**).

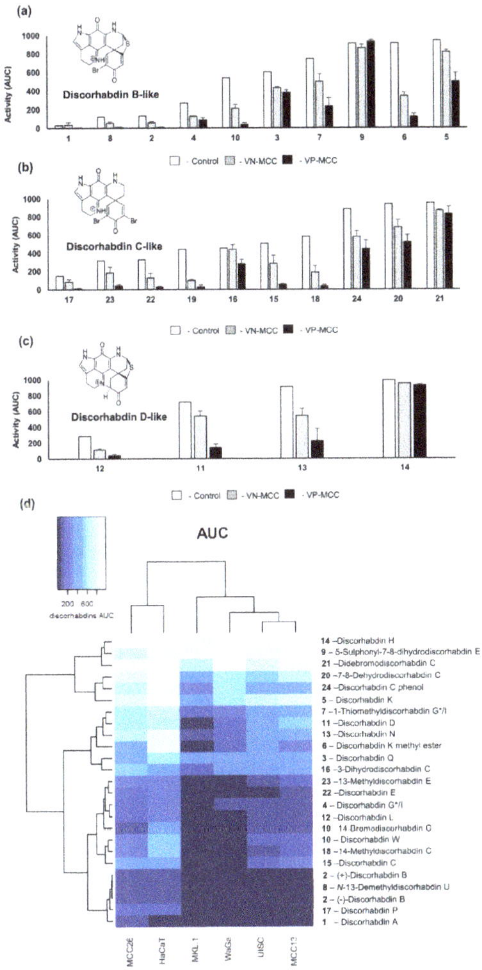

Figure 4. (**a**–**c**) Effects of the discorhabdins on MCC cell viability. Cytotoxicity data are presented from most active (lowest AUC) to least active (highest AUC) based on activity against control cells.

VN-MCC and VP-MCC data are averages across each class of cell lines. (AUC, arbitrary units—see Table S3). For VN-MCC and VP-MCC cells, error bars represent se (n = 3) or range. Data for discorhabdin B-like structures **1–10** is shown in panel (**a**); data for discorhabdin D-like structures. **12–14** is shown in panel (**b**); and data for discorhabdin C-like structures **17–21** is shown in panel (**c**). (**d**) Heat map of the discorhabdin cytotoxicity data organized by inhibitory effect by AUC where darker regions indicate higher activity of each discorhabdin on VN-MCC (MCC13, MCC26, and UISO), VP-MCC (MKL-1, WaGa), and HaCaT control cells. The heatmap was generated in R version 1.3.1073 (R Core Team (2013). R: A language and environment for statistical computing, Vienna, Austria, http://www.R-project.org/ (accessed on 12 January 2023). Dendrograms indicate cell line and compound similarities based on unsupervised hierarchical clustering. Darker shades indicate higher activity.

Among the discorhabdin B-like structures **1–10** (Figure 4a), the most potent compounds were discorhabdins A (**1**), *N*-13 demethyl U (**8**), and B (**2**), which all had the α-bromo enone moiety, suggesting, as others have found [57], that increased cytotoxicity is potentiated by electrophilic reactivity. However, the C-5 sulphonyl-substituted α-bromo enone **9** was practically inactive, while the C-5 thiomethyl-substituted compound **8** was one of the most active compounds tested, suggesting the size and polarity of the C-5 substituent on the discorhabdin B-like scaffold is also crucial for the activity. Discorhabdin B (**2**) was >10-fold more active than discorhabdin Q (**3**) against MCC cells. Discorhabdin Q (**3**) has additional oxidation between C-16 and C-17 as compared to **2**, suggesting that unsaturation on ring B has a deleterious effect on cytotoxicity possibly because of the unstable nature of this metabolite, which may degrade to complex mixtures [57]. Discorhabdin C*/I (**4**) lacking the bromine substitution at C-2 showed a loss of activity compared to compound **2** (compound **2** was 3-fold more active against MCC cells compared to **3**), and substitution at C-1 further decreased activity of the scaffold, in particular the addition of a large thiohistidine group. Interestingly, the presence of the methoxy group in **6** drastically improved the selectivity compared to the free acid group on the thiohistidine in compound **5**. As the discorhabdins are known to occur in enantiomeric configurations, both forms of discorhabdin B were tested. It was found that (+)-**2** and (−)-**2** had comparable activity against MCC and control cell lines.

In the discorhabdin D-like series **11–14** (Figure 4b), the presence of an additional ring between C-2 and *N*-18 positions generally reduced potency compared to the discorhabdin B and C analogues. The size of the C-1 substituents had a drastic effect on the potency, with the hydroxy substituted discorhabdin L (**12**) being most active while the glycine and thiohistidine analogues showed a loss of activity. Among the discorhabdin C-like structures **15–24** (Figure 4c), the crucial features that enhanced the activity of discorhabdin C were *N*-13 methylation, as seen in compounds **17** and **23**, and the presence of an α-bromo enone moiety. The mono-brominated discorhabdin E (**22**) had comparable activity to the 14-bromodiscorhabdin C (**15**) as well as discorhabdin C (**15**), suggesting that a bromine substitution at positions C-4 and C-14 is not essential for the activity. Additionally, changes in the conjugation of the spirodienone ring E and addition of a C-7 and C-8 olefin had detrimental effects for all cell lines tested, as shown by the results for discorhabdin C phenol (**24**), 3-dihydrodiscorhabdin C (**16**), and 7,8 dehydrodiscorhabdin C (**20**).

2.3. Cell Death Mechanisms

Apoptotic cell death was first investigated in MCC cells in response to discorhabdins. Three methods were utilized: activation of effector caspases 3 and/or 7, annexin V binding, and effects of caspase inhibitors. The data in Figure 5a demonstrates lack of caspase-3/7 activation by discorhabdins B (**2**), C (**15**), and L (**12**) against UISO (representative VN-MCC) and MKL-1 (representative of VP-MCC) cells. By comparison, bortezomib treatment robustly activates caspase in these cells (Figure S42). As reported in the literature [39], appreciable caspase activation in MCC cells by bortezomib took up to 24 h. Similarly, discorhabdin treatment did not significantly increase binding of labeled annexin V (Figure 5b, open symbols). Figures S42 and S43 include caspase activation and annexin V-binding/cell permeability results for other discorhabdins and additional MCC cell lines. Pretreatment of cells with the pan-caspase inhibitor Z-VAD-FMK reduced bortezomib-induced, but not discorhabdin-induced MCC cell death (Figure S44). By contrast, rapid increases in cell permeability were observed for discorhabdin-treated MCC cells as measured by accessibility of a cell-impermeant fluorescent DNA-binding compound (closed symbols, Figure 5b). The magnitude of the increase in the fluorescence (i.e., necrotic) signal roughly correlates with the potency of individual discorhabdins against each cell line (Figure S43). Together, these results suggest that discorhabdins induce necrotic rather than apoptotic cell death in MCC cells.

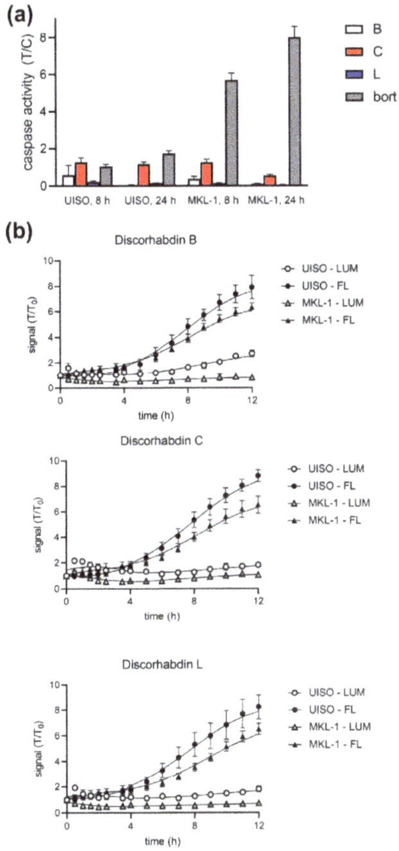

Figure 5. Representative data for effects of pentacyclic (C), hexacyclic (B), and heptacyclic (L) discorhabdins on UISO (VN) and MKL-1 (VP) MCC cells, bort: bortezomib. (**a**) Caspase activation. Cells were treated for 8 or 24 h with indicated discorhabdins or bortezomib. Caspase-3/7 activity was determined (Promega CaspaseGLO-3/7) and normalized to untreated (DMSO) control cells. Error bars represent sd (n = 4). (**b**). Apoptosis/necrosis. Cells were treated for up to 24 h with the indicated discorhabdins and assessed for Annexin binding and cell permeability using the Promega RealTime-Glo™ Annexin V Apoptosis and Necrosis Assay kit. Luminescence indicates Annexin binding, fluorescence indicates membrane permeability. Values were normalized to 0 time control. Error bars represent sd (n = 4). $p < 0.01$ (vs. DMSO control) for all fluor points at $\geq$ 6 h, insignificant for luminescence.

2.4. Mitochondrial Dysfunction

Three aspects of mitochondrial function, mitochondrial membrane potential (MMP), cell reducing potential, and cellular ATP content were investigated (Figure 6). MMP was significantly reduced in UISO and MKL-1 cells after treatment with discorhabdins B (**2**), C (**15**), and L (**12**). Cellular reducing potential also dropped significantly. Similarly, loss of cellular ATP content was dramatic and rapid. The drop in cellular reducing potential was faster and more dramatic than the increase in cell permeability (compare Figure S45 and Figure 5b). The effects of discorhabdins on all three measures of mitochondrial function generally correlated with discorhabdin potency (Figures S45 and S46). As with caspase, the effects of discorhabdins on mitochondrial function were dramatically different to the effects of the apoptotic drug bortezomib (Figures S45 and S46). Induction of mitochondrial dysfunction is often caused by, accompanied by, or followed by generation of reactive oxygen species (ROS) and/or increasing intracellular Ca^{2+}. ROS generation and calcium mobilization in MCC cells in response to discorhabdins were assessed using DCFDA and Fluo-4, respectively. None of the discorhabdins tested induced ROS generation or Ca^{2+} mobilization in any of the five MCC cell lines tested although appropriate controls were active in all five cell lines (see Figures S47 and S48, respectively).

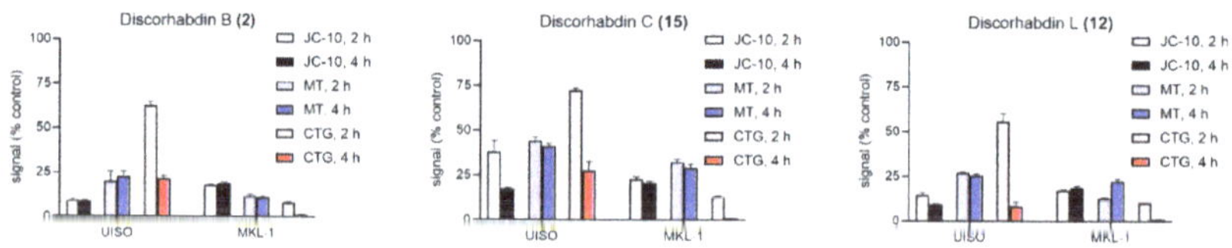

Figure 6. Mitochondrial effects of discorhabdins.

Cells were treated with the indicated discorhabdins (10 μM) and assessed for mitochondrial membrane potential (MMP) using JC-10 ratiometric dye. JC-10 was added for the last hour of incubation. Cellular reducing potential was assessed using a RealTimeGlo MT Cell Viability kit, and cellular ATP levels using CellTiterGlo. All values were normalized to DMSO control. Error bars (n = 3–4) represent sd. See Figures S45 and S46 for additional cell line/discorhabdin combinations, concentrations, and time points for reducing potential and MMP, respectively.

3. Discussion

The discorhabdin SAR confirmed many of the previously established trends for this group of natural products [27,57,58]. Compounds containing an α-bromo enone moiety were the most potent, while analogues with an additional bridge between C-2 and *N*-14 were less active. Large, bulky substituents such as thiohistidine on position C-1 in both discorhabdin B-type or D-type structures had a detrimental effect on the activity. Changes in the *spiro*-dienone ring E, such as reduction at C-3 or rearrangement to a phenol, had detrimental effects on the activity. Here, we have expanded the discorhabdin SAR (Figure 7) to show that, in MCC cells, methylation of the pyrrole ring A enhances the activity, as does the presence of a thioether ring between C-5 and C-8 positions. Addition of an olefin between C-7 and C-8 was found to have a detrimental effect on the activity of the group, as does the addition of large polar substituents on C-5.

Several pairs of the discorhabdins used in this study may also give some insights into features relevant to effects on cell viability and/or selectivity for MCC-VP cells. Discorhabdin A (**1**) differs from the rest of the discorhabdin B series in that it lacks the C-4–C-5 olefin. It was the most generally toxic compound tested and considerably less selective. Discorhabdin P (**17**) was previously reported to be considerably less cytotoxic than discorhabdin C (**15**) [45,58], whereas, in the present work, it was more potent than discorhabdin C in all seven cell lines, albeit with very similar VP-MCC selectivity. With regard to bromination of the spirodienone ring, discorhabdin G*/I (**4**) had similar potency, but lost selectivity by comparison to discorhabdin B (**2**).

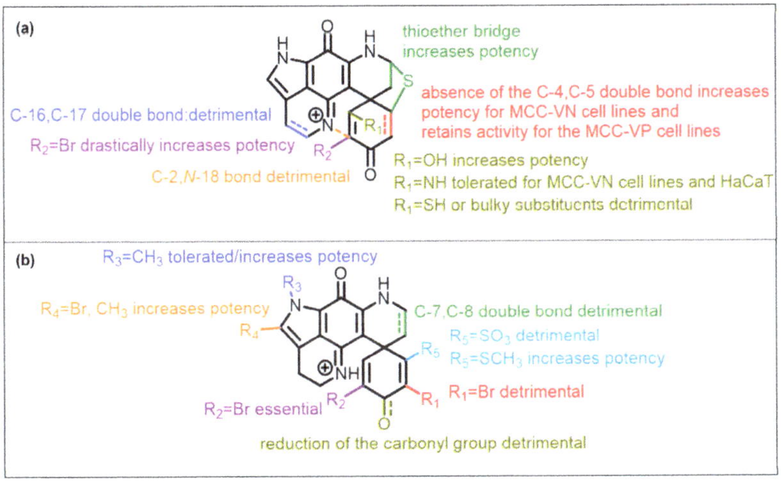

Figure 7. Discorhabdin SAR summary: (**a**) discorhabdin B and L series, (**b**) discorhabdin C series.

There is very little in the literature regarding cell death mechanisms in response to discorhabdins in susceptible cells. One of the more extensive mechanistic studies involved analysis of discorhabdin A and semi-synthetic discorhabdin analogs. No effects on kinases, HDACs, telomerase, or proteasome were found. NCI-60 cell analysis provided no significant insights [59]. Discorhabdin P has been reported to inhibit caspase-3 [41]. Given this paucity of information related to discorhabdins cell death mechanisms were investigated for discorhabdins and MCC cells.

A range of regulated cell death mechanisms have been described and extensively reviewed in the literature [28,60]. Several of these have been implicated in drug-induced MCC cell death. As noted, many drugs have been reported to induce apoptotic cell death in MCC. Based on multiple assessments of apoptotic cell death (caspase 3/7 activation, annexin V binding, caspase inhibitor effects, and cell permeability), it seems clear that discorhabdin-induced loss of cell viability is not due to the induction of apoptosis. Comparisons to effects of bortezomib, known to induce apoptosis in MCC cells [39], further corroborate this conclusion. Mitochondria are critical regulators of a number of cell death modalities, including apoptosis [2,61]. It has also long been known that oxidative stress and increased intracellular calcium can induce apoptotic cell death [3,62]. However, neither ROS generation nor increased intracellular [Ca^{2+}] were observed in discorhabdin-treated MCC cells.

The characteristics of discorhabdin-induced MCC cell death are somewhat consistent with caspase-independent necroptotic cell death [63]. However, pre-treatment of MCC cells with necrostatin-1 did not block discorhabdin effects suggesting a non-necroptotic mechanism [64]. Furthermore, necroptosis and ROS generation typically correlate [65], but ROS was not detected in response to discorhabdins. Examples of necroptosis-inducing drugs described in the literature include aurora kinase inhibitors [63]. Interestingly, aurora kinase inhibition has recently been reported to affect MCC, albeit by induction of apoptosis rather than necroptosis [32].

Ferroptosis is another caspase-independent cell death mechanism observed in drug-treated MCC [37], but is also generally ROS-dependent [66]. Autophagy/autophagic cell death has been observed in drug-treated MCC cells [38,39]. Pretreatment of cells with autophagy inhibitors [67] MRT68921, bafilomycin, or chloroquine did not block discorhabdin-induced MCC cell death. LC3-II, a common marker of autophagy, was not detected by Western blot analysis of discorhabdin-treated cells. Similarly, pretreatment with the commonly used parthanatos inhibitor DPQ [68] did not block the effects of discorhabdins on MCC cells.

Discorhabdin-induced cell death appeared to be equivalent for all of the discorhabdins tested and for both VN-MCC and VP-MCC cell lines. No significant differential other than potency was observed with regard to discorhabdin type, target cells, or cell death mechanistic assays. These results suggest that the effects of discorhabdins on MCC cells are due to the induction of mitochondrial dysfunction. However, the lack of differential activities or mechanisms between classes of discorhabdins suggests that discorhabdin electrophilic reactivity with mitochondrial or other cellular targets may not be the driving factor in their effects on Merkel cell carcinoma cells. The difference in susceptibility between VN-MCC and VP-MCC cells also appears to be subtle. On the other hand, the marked increased activity of discorhabdins against VP-MCC cells may be important. Although VP-MCC disease tends to have a better prognosis, MCPyV, in particular small T antigen, has been reported to enhance metastatic potential [69].

Discorhabdins B, C, and L are highlighted as representative of the three main structural classes of discorhabdins. Discorhabdin L has also been highlighted in this work in part because it is one of the few (if not the only) discorhabdins that has been shown to have minimal in vivo toxicity in animals, in this case in a prostate cancer xenograft model [44]. Further development of this discorhabdin for application in prostate cancer may allow for parallel development for targeting MCC.

4. Materials and Methods

4.1. General Experimental Procedures

Optical rotations were measured on a Rudolph research analytical AUTOPOL IV automatic polarimeter (Rudolph Research Analytical, Hackettstown, NJ, USA) using a cell of 0.25 dm pathlength and MeOH as the solvent at 20 °C, ECD experiments were recorded on a J-1500 CD spectrophotometer (JASCO Inc., Easton, MD, USA). IR spectra were recorded with a Bruker ALPHA II FT-IR spectrometer (Bruker, Billerica, MA, USA), and UV spectra were measured with an HP 8453 UV-VIS spectrophotometer (Agilent Technologies, Palo Alto, CA, USA) and a Varian Cary 50 Bio spectrophotometer (Agilent, Santa Clara, CA, USA). HPLC separations were performed on a Gilson HPLC system (Middleton, WI, USA) equipped with a 322 pump, a 172-diode array detector, and a GX-281 liquid handler. Samples were dried on a Thermo Savant Explorer-220 speed vacuum system and a SP Genevac vacuum system (SP, Warminster, PA, USA). NMR spectra were obtained with either a 600 MHz Bruker Avance III NMR spectrometer (Bruker, Billerica, MA, USA) equipped with a 3 mm cryogenic probe or a 600 MHz Bruker Avance III HD spectrometer (Bruker, Billerica, MA, USA), equipped with a triple resonance 5 mm CPP TCI cryo-probe, both operating at a frequency of 600.0 MHz for the ^{1}H nucleus and 150.9 MHz for the ^{13}C nucleus. Spectra were calibrated to residual solvent signals at δ_H 2.50 and δ_C 39.5 (DMSO-d_6). All 2D NMR experiments were acquired with non-uniform sampling (NUS) set to 50% or 25%. HMBC experiments were run with $^{n}J_{CH}$ = 8.0 Hz. HRESIMS data were acquired on a 6230 Accurate-Mass TOF LC/MS system (1260 Infinity II) equipped with a dual AJS ESI source and a 6545 Accurate-mass Q-TOF LC/MS (1260 Infinity II) (Agilent Technologies, Santa Clara, CA, USA), whereas low-resolution mass spectra were measured with an Agilent InfinityLab LC/MSD System comprising an Agilent HPLC 1260 HPLC, equipped with a binary pump, autosampler, column oven, and photodiode array detector Agilent 1260 HPLC (Santa Clara, CA, USA).

4.2. Chemicals and Reagents

All chemicals were purchased from Sigma Aldrich (St. Louis, MO, USA) and Merck KGaA (Darmstadt, Germany). All solvents required for isolation and analytical experiments were purchased from Sigma Aldrich (St. Louis, MO, USA). The isolated compounds were dissolved in deuterated DMSO-d_6 and methanol-d_4 from Cambridge Isotope Laboratories (Tewksbury, MA, USA). Ultrapure water was produced with a Hydro® (Hydro, NC, USA) purification system. HP-20 SS, Sephadex LH-20, and C18 silica (55–105 μm, 125 Å) material were purchased from Sigma-Aldrich (St. Louis, MO, USA), GE Healthcare (Chicago, IL, USA), and Waters (Milford, MA, USA), respectively.

4.3. Natural Product Isolation

Compound **1**: (+)-(5*R*,6*S*,8*S*) discorhabdin A was isolated from *Latrunculia brevis*, collection and isolation details of which have previously been reported [43].

Compound **2**: (+)-(6*S*,8*S*) and (−)-(6*R*,8*R*) discorhabdins B were isolated from *Latrunculia* sp., collection and isolation details of which have previously been reported [70].

Compound **3**: (+)-(6*S*,8*S*) discorhabdin Q was isolated from *Latrunculia purpurea*, collection and isolation details of which have previously been reported [71].

Compound **4**: (+)-(6*S*,8*S*) discorhabdin G*/I was isolated from *Latrunculia brevis*, collection and isolation details of which have previously been reported [43].

Compound **5**: (+)-(6*S*,8*S*,7′S*) discorhabdin K was isolated from *Latrunculia kaakaariki*, collection and isolation details of which are reported in the SI.

Compound **6**: (+)-(6*S*,8*S*,7′S*) discorhabdin K methyl ester was isolated from *Latrunculia kaakaariki*, collection and isolation details of which are reported in the SI.

Compound **7**: (+)-(6*R*,8*S*) thiomethyldiscorhabdin G*/I was isolated from *Latrunculia purpurea*, collection and isolation details of which are reported in the SI.

Compound **8**: (+)-(6*S*) *N*-13-demethyldiscorhabdin U was semi-synthesized from (+)-(6*S*,8*S*) discorhabdin B details of which are reported below.

Compound **9**: (+)-(6*S*) sulphonyl-7,8-dehydrodiscorhabdin E was isolated from *Latrunculia brevis*, collection and isolation details of which are reported in the SI.

Compound **10**: (−)-(6*S*,6′*S*) discorhabdin W from *Latrunculia* sp., collection and isolation details of which have previously been reported [70].

Compound **11**: (+)-(2*S*,6*R*,8*S*) discorhabdin D was isolated from *Latrunculia brevis*, collection and isolation details of which have previously been reported [43].

Compound **12**: (−)-(1*R*,2*S*,6*R*,8*S*) discorhabdin L was isolated from *Latrunculia brevis*, collection and isolation details of which have previously been reported [43].

Compound **13**: (−)-(1*R*,2*S*,6*R*,8*S*) discorhabdin N was isolated from *Latrunculia brevis*, collection and isolation details of which have previously been reported [43].

Compound **14**: (−)-(1*R*,2*R*,6*R*,8*S*,7′S*) discorhabdin H was isolated from *Latrunculia brevis*, collection and isolation details of which have previously been reported [43].

Compound **15**: discorhabdin C was isolated from *Latrunculia* sp., collection and isolation details of which have previously been reported [45].

Compound **16**: 3-dihydrodiscorhabdin C was isolated from *Latrunculia brevis*, collection and isolation details of which have previously been reported [43].

Compound **17**: discorhabdin P was semi-synthesized from discorhabdin C details of which have previously been reported [45].

Compound **18**: 14-methyldiscorhabdin C was semi-synthesized from discorhabdin C details of which are reported below.

Compound **19**: 14-bromodiscorhabdin C was isolated from *Tsitsikamma pedunculata* collection and isolation details of which are reported in the SI.

Compound **20**: 7,8-dehydrodiscorhabdin C was isolated from *Latrunculia brevis* collection and isolation details of which are reported in the SI.

Compound **21**: didebromodiscorhabdin C was isolated from *Latrunculia brevis* collection and isolation details of which are reported in the SI.

Compound **22**: (+)-(6*S*)-discorhabdin E was isolated from *Latrunculia brevis* collection and isolation details of which are reported in the SI.

Compound **23**: (+)-(6*S*)-*N*-13-methyldiscorhabdin E was semi-synthesized from discorhabdin E details of which are reported below.

Compound **24**: discorhabdin C phenol was semi-synthesized from discorhabdin C details of which are reported below.

4.4. Preparation of Semi-Synthetic Derivatives

Compound **8** was prepared using a previously established semi-synthetic route [45]. Discorhabdin B trifluoroacetate salt (**2**) (3.0 mg, 7.2 µmol) was dissolved in dry acetone (3 mL) to which CH_3I (1 µL, 16.2 µmol) and K_2CO_3 (8 mg) were added. The reaction mixture was kept under N_2 at reflux at 80 °C for 2 h. After the end of the reaction, which was indicated by LC-MS analysis, the products were loaded onto a pre-column cartridge filled with dental cotton, dried overnight, and purified by C_{18} chromatography with a Luna C_{18} (10 µm, 150 × 21.2 mm) column (water acidified with 0.1% TFA/methanol from 98:2 to 6:4 over 70 min) yielding *N*-13-demethyldiscorhabdin U **8** (1.4 mg, 46% yield).

Compound **18**: Discorhabdin C trifluoroacetate salt (**15**) (5.9 mg, 12.8 µmol) was dissolved in DMSO (200 µL) to which $FeCl_2$ (0.36 mg, 2.8 µmol) and H_2O_2 (2 µL, 85.2 µmol) were added. The reaction mixture was kept under N_2 at reflux at 25 °C for five hours. After the end of the reaction which was indicated by LC-MS analysis, the products were loaded onto a pre-column cartridge filled with dental cotton, dried overnight, and purified with C_8 chromatography with a Phenomenex Kinetex C_8 (5 µm, 150 × 21.2 mm) column (water acidified with 0.1% TFA/methanol from 98:2 to 6:4 over 50 min) yielding 14-methyldiscorhabdin C **18** (1.5 mg, 25% yield).

Compound **23**: Discorhabdin E trifluoroacetate salt (**22**) (2.4 mg, 8.9 µmol) was dissolved in dry acetone (2 mL), to which CH_3I (8.3 µL, 133.0 µmol) and K_2CO_3 (10.4 mg) were added. The reaction mixture was kept under N_2 at reflux at 80 °C for three hours. After the end of the reaction which was indicated by LC-MS analysis, the products were loaded onto a pre-column cartridge filled with dental cotton, dried overnight and purified using C_{18} chromatography with a Luna C_{18} (10 µm, 150 × 21.2 mm) column (water acidified with 0.1% TFA/methanol from 98:2 to 75:25 over 50 min) yielding 13-methyl-discorhabdin E **23** (0.3 mg, 12.5% yield).

Compound **24** was prepared using a previously established semi-synthetic route [72]. Discorhabdin C trifluoroacetate salt (**15**) (4.5 mg, 9.7 µmol) was dissolved in concentrated H_2SO_4 (3 mL) and left at room temperature for 5 min. The reaction mixture was neutralized by the addition of solid $NaHCO_3$. The products were loaded onto a pre-column cartridge filled with dental cotton and purified by C_4 chromatography with a Luna C_4 (10 µm, 250 × 10 mm) column (water acidified with 0.1% TFA/methanol from 98:2 to 7:3 over 70 min) yielding discorhabdin C phenol **24** (0.9 mg, 25% yield).

4.5. Compound Characterization

Compound **5**: (+)-(6*S*,8*S*,7′*S**) discorhabdin K TFA salt, brown amorphous powder; $[\alpha]_D$ = +177.8, $[\alpha]_{546}$ = −50.8, $[\alpha]_{633}$ = +311.1 (*c* 0.06, MeOH); NMR spectroscopic and chiroptical data in agreement with those previously reported [26]; (+)-HRESIMS *m*/*z* $[M + H - CF_3COO^-]^+$ 535.1219 (calculated for $C_{25}H_{23}N_6O_4S_2^+$, 535.1217).

Compound **6**: (+)-(6*S*,8*S*,7′*S**) discorhabdin K methyl ester TFA salt, brown amorphous powder; $[\alpha]_D$ = +407.2, $[\alpha]_{546}$ = −142.0, $[\alpha]_{633}$ = +688.0 (*c* 0.1, MeOH); UV (MeOH) λ_{max} (log ε) 242 (3.76), 279 (3.97), 332 (3.87), 409 (3.65) nm; ECD (MeOH) λ (Δε) 212 (−13.2), 240 (−4.4), 262 (−15.8), 306 (−7.6), 332 (0), 363 (+14.2), 433 (0) nm; IR (film) 3006, 1677, 1634, 1529, 1436, 1418, 1364, 1331, 1308, 1203, 1132, 1030, 1004, 832, 801, 728 cm^{-1}; ^1H NMR (DMSO-d_6, 600 MHz) and ^{13}C NMR (DMSO-d_6, 151 MHz) data, see Table 1; (+)-HRESIMS *m*/*z* $[M + H - CF_3COO^-]^+$ 549.1374 (calculated for $C_{26}H_{25}N_6O_4S_2^+$, 549.1374).

Compound **7**: (+)-(6*R*,8*S*) thiomethyldiscorhabdin G*/I TFA salt, green-brown amorphous powder; $[\alpha]_D$ = +53.6, $[\alpha]_{546}$ = −31.6, $[\alpha]_{633}$ = +110.0 (*c* 0.1, MeOH); NMR spectroscopic and chiroptical data in agreement with those previously reported [73]; (+)-HRESIMS *m*/*z* $[M + H - CF_3COO^-]^+$ 382.0681 (calculated for $C_{19}H_{16}N_3O_2S_2^+$, 382.0679).

Compound **8**: (+)-(6*S*) *N*-13-demethyldiscorhabdin U TFA salt, green amorphous powder; $[\alpha]_D$ = +177.8, $[\alpha]_{546}$ = −50.8, $[\alpha]_{633}$ = +311.1 (*c* 0.06, MeOH); NMR spectroscopic and chiroptical data in agreement with those previously reported [45]; (+)-HRESIMS *m*/*z* $[M + H - CF_3COO^-]^+$ 428.0066 (calculated for $C_{19}H_{15}{}^{79}BrN_3O_2S^+$, 428.0063).

Table 1. ^{1}H and ^{13}C NMR (600/151 MHz, DMSO-d_6) spectroscopic data of compounds **6**, **9**, and **20**.

No.	Compound 6		Compound 9		Compound 20	
	δ_H Mult. (J Hz)	δ_C Mult.	δ_H Mult. (J Hz)	δ_C Mult.	δ_H Mult. (J Hz)	δ_C Mult.
1	-	160.1, C	7.77 s	150.1, CH	7.86 s	150.0, CH
2	5.75 s	125.3, CH	-	122.0, C	-	121.1, C
3	-	179.3, C	-	178.6, C	-	170.9, C
4	6.14 s	118.5, CH	6.61 s	124.2, CH	-	121.1, C
5	-	167.8, C	-	163.9, C	7.86 s	150.0, CH
6	-	50.7, C	-	46.3, C	-	47.1 *, C
7	2.59 dd (3.6,12.0) 2.93 m	42.1, CH_2	4.51 d (7.4)	113.5, CH	4.71 d (7.4)	109.8, CH
8	5.69 d (3.6)	59.2, CH	6.33 dd (5.0,7.4)	124.6, CH	6.53 dd (5.0,7.4)	125.6, CH
9	10.85 s	-	10.38 d (5.0)	-	10.71 d (5.0)	-
10	-	151.5, C	-	143.8, C	-	145.7 *, C
11	-	164.9, C	-	166.7, C	-	167.0, C
12	-	123.7, C	-	123.6, C	-	123.7, C
13	13.36 br d (2.0)	-	13.22 br d (2.2)	-	13.33 br d (2.0)	-
14	7.42 d (2.0)	127.6, CH	7.37 d (2.8)	126.9, CH	7.41 d (2.8)	127.2, CH
15	-	120.5, C	-	119.3, C	-	119.6, C
16	2.86 m	17.7, CH_2	2.82, m	18.0, CH_2	2.87, t (8.0)	17.8, CH_2
17	3.87 m 3.95 m	44.9, CH_2	3.61 m 3.75 m	44.4, CH_2	3.78 t (8.0)	44.5, CH_2
19	-	153.6, C	-	158.0, C	-	157.7, C
20	-	97.6, C	-	97.2, C	-	95.4 *, C
21	-	122.8, C	-	122.7, C	-	122.2, C
1′	-	123.1, C	-	-	-	-
3′	8.01 s	141.2, CH	-	-	-	-
5′	-	132.6, C	-	-	-	-
6′	3.19 dd (9.6,15.2) 3.26 dd (6.0,15.2)	24.2, CH_2	-	-	-	-
7′	4.20 m	50.9, CH	-	-	-	-
8′	-	168.7, C	-	-	-	-
9′	3.69 s	32.3, CH_3	-	-	-	-
10′	3.61 s	53.0, CH_3	-	-	-	-
11′	8.74 br s	-	-	-	-	-

[*] Chemical shift determined from the ^{1}H–^{13}C HMBC spectrum.

Compound **9**: (+)-(6*S*) 5-sulphonyl-7,8-dehydro-discorhabdin E TFA salt, green amorphous powder; $[\alpha]_D$ +29.9, $[\alpha]_{546}$ = +41.8, $[\alpha]_{633}$ = +23.9 (*c* 0.066, MeOH); UV (MeOH) λ_{max} (log ε) 246 (3.45), 307 (3.25), 433 (3.13) nm; ECD (MeOH) λ (Δε) 208 (+0.6), 227 (−3.7), 243

(0), 258 (+4.2), 274 (0), 372 (+0.4) nm; IR (film) 1683, 1442, 1202, 1143, 846, 803, 725 cm^{-1}; ^{1}H NMR (DMSO-d_6, 600 MHz) and ^{13}C NMR (DMSO- d_6, 151 MHz) data, see Table 1; (+)-HRESIMS m/z [M + H − CF_3COO^-]$^+$ 461.9751 (calculated for $C_{18}H_{13}{}^{79}BrN_3O_5S^+$, 461.9754), 463.9730 (calculated for $C_{18}H_{13}{}^{81}BrN_3O_5S^+$, 463.9734).

Compound **18**: 14-methyl-discorhabdin C TFA salt, brown amorphous powder; IR (film) 3119, 1674, 1589, 1551, 1518, 1324, 1202, 1137, 1024, 833, 799, 724, 700 cm^{-1}; ^{1}H NMR (DMSO-d_6, 600 MHz) 13.05 (s, H-13), 10.17 (s, H-9), 7.71 (s, H-1/H-5), 3.67 (m, H-17), 3.61 (m, H-8), 2.73, (t, J = 7.4 Hz, H-16), 2.25 (s, H-22), 2.00 (t, J = 5.6 Hz, H-7), ^{13}C NMR (DMSO-d_6, 151 MHz) 171.5 (C, C-3), 163.7 (C, C-11), 153.0 (C, C-19), 152.3 (C, C-10), 151.2 (CH, C-1, C-5), 139.3 (C, C-14), 124.5 (C, C-21), 122.6 (C, C-2, C-4), 121.1 (C, C-12), 118.1 (C, C-15), 91.4 (C, C-20), 44.7 (C, C-6), 43.7 (CH_2, C-17), 38.3 (CH_2, C-8), 33.6 (CH_2, C-7), 17.3 (CH_2, C-16), 11.1 (CH_3, C-22); (+)-HRESIMS m/z [M + H − CF_3COO^-]$^+$ 475.9600 (calculated for $C_{19}H_{16}{}^{79}Br_2N_3O_2{}^+$, 475.9604).

Compound **19**: 14 bromodiscorhabdin C TFA salt, dark purple oil; NMR spectroscopic data in agreement with those previously reported [54]; HRESIMS m/z [M + H − CF_3COO^-]$^+$ 539.85562 (calculated for $C_{18}H_{13}Br_3N_3O_2{}^+$, 539.85524).

Compound **20**: 7,8-dehydro-discorhabdin C TFA salt, green amorphous powder; UV (MeOH) λ_{max} 220, 262, 310, 440, 595 nm; IR (film) 3423, 1679, 1211, 1136, 1024, 1006, 843, 802, 727 cm^{-1}; ^{1}H NMR (DMSO-d_6, 600 MHz) and ^{13}C NMR (DMSO-d_6, 151 MHz) data, see Table 1; (+)-HRESIMS m/z [M + H − CF_3COO^-]$^+$ 459.93296 (calculated for $C_{18}H_{12}{}^{79}Br_2N_3O_2{}^+$, 459.9291), 461.9276 (calculated for $C_{18}H_{12}{}^{79}Br^{81}BrN_3O_2{}^+$, 461.9271), 463.9260 (calculated for $C_{18}H_{12}{}^{81}Br_2N_3O_2{}^+$, 463.9250).

Compound **21**: didebromodiscorhabdin C TFA salt, light pink amorphous powder; NMR spectroscopic data in agreement with those previously reported [74]; (+)-HRESIMS m/z [M + H − CF_3COO^-]$^+$ 306.1236 (calculated for $C_{18}H_{16}N_3O_2{}^+$, 306.1237).

Compound **22**: (+)-(6S) discorhabdin E TFA salt, purple amorphous powder; $[\alpha]_D$ = +17.2, $[\alpha]_{546}$ = +6.8, $[\alpha]_{633}$ = +28.0 (c 0.1, MeOH); ECD (MeOH) λ ($\Delta\varepsilon$) 207 (−5.9), 218 (−0.6), 230 (−1.4), 240 (0), 248 (+2.1), 261 (0), 274 (−0.7), 337 (0), 368 (+0.6), 445 (0), nm; NMR spectroscopic and chiroptical data in agreement with those previously reported [72]; (+)-HRESIMS m/z [M + H − CF_3COO^-]$^+$ 384.0341 (calculated for $C_{18}H_{15}{}^{79}BrN_3O_2{}^+$, 384.0343).

Compound **23**: (+)-(6S) N-13-methyldiscorhabdin E TFA salt, pink amorphous powder; $[\alpha]_D$ = +177.8, $[\alpha]_{546}$ = −50.8, $[\alpha]_{633}$ = +311.1 (c 0.06, MeOH); IR (film) 3255, 1681, 1447, 1207, 1135, 839, 804, 723; ^{1}H NMR (DMSO-d_6, 600 MHz) 10.08 (br s, H-9), 7.70 (d, J = 2.8, H-1), 7.39 (s, H-14), 7.12 (dd, J = 2.8, 9.8 Hz, H-5), 6.47 (d, J = 9.8 Hz, H-4), 3.92 (s, H-22), 3.66 (m, H-17), 3.62 (m, H-8), 2.78 (m, H-16), 1.90 (m, H-7), 1.96 (m, H-7); ^{13}C NMR (DMSO-d_6, 151 MHz) 178.1 (C, C-3), 154.2 (C, C-19), 152.0 (C, C-10), 151.8 (CH, C-5), 151.6 (CH, C-1), 132.0 (C, C-14), 129.6 (C, C-4), 125.5 (C, C-2), 124.8 (C, C-12), 123.1 (C, C-21), 119.4 (C, C-15), 92.6 (C, C-20), 44.1 (CH_2, C-17), 43.0 (C, C-6), 39.8 (CH_2, C-8), 36.5 (CH_3, C-22), 34.8 (CH_2, C-7), 18.9 (CH_2, C-16); (+)-HRESIMS m/z [M + H − CF_3COO^-]$^+$ 398.0499 (calculated for $C_{19}H_{17}{}^{79}BrN_3O_2{}^+$, 398.0499).

Compound **24**: discorhabdin C phenol TFA salt, purple amorphous powder; NMR spectroscopic data in agreement with those previously reported [72]; (+)-HRESIMS m/z [M + H − CF_3COO^-]$^+$ 461.9450 (calculated for $C_{18}H_{14}{}^{79}Br_2N_3O_2{}^+$, 461.9448).

4.6. Computational Methods

Three-dimensional structures of the molecules were drawn and subjected to conformational analysis in ComputeVOA (BioTools Inc., Jupiter, FL, USA) using MMFF94 as a force field and the GMMX methodology on a Windows operating system machine. Geometrical optimization and energy calculation of conformers occurring in an energy window (ΔE) of 0–3 Kcal/mol were done by implementation of B3LYP/DGDZVP using the COSMO solvation algorithm in Gaussian 16 software. The optimized structures (Tables S1 and S2) were used to calculate the thermochemical parameters estimated at 298 K and 1 atm. Calculations taking into account the solvent (MeOH) were carried out starting from DFT-optimized structures. Optimized conformers were then subjected to TDDFT calculations in MeOH on Gaussian 16 using B3LYP/DGDZVP to obtain the ECD spectra. All quantum mechanical calculations were carried out using the Gaussian 16 software on a Linux operating system in the Biowulf cluster. Obtained ECD spectra with half-band of 0.25 eV and UV shift of 0 nm were Boltzmann-averaged and scaled using the SpecDis program spectra and compared with experimental spectra obtained in MeOH.

4.7. Cell lines Used

Three VN-MCC cell lines (MCC13 and MCC26 [75], and UISO [76]), along with three VP-MCC cell lines (MKL-1 [77], MKL-2 [78], and Waga [79]) and HaCaT immortalized keratinocytes [80] (ThermoFisher, Waltham, MA, USA) were used. Cell identity was confirmed, and cells were maintained and utilized as previously described [22].

4.8. Cell Viability and Analysis of Cell Death Mechanisms

Three methods were employed for assessment of MCC and control cell survival/viability after discorhabdin treatment, two metabolic assays and a cell permeability assay. For all three methods, cells were plated in 384-well plates at 2500 cells/well and treated with various concentrations of discorhabdins for various time periods. CellTiterGlo™ (Promega, Madison, WI, USA) measures cellular ATP content and was used to estimate potency of discorhabdins in cell viability assays as previously described [22]. Continuous monitoring of metabolic activity was accomplished using a cellular reducing potential luminescence assay [81], the RealTime-Glo™ MT Cell Viability Assay (Promega, Madison, WI, USA) according to manufacturer's instructions. Loss of cell plasma membrane integrity was assessed using a cell-impermeant molecule that becomes fluorescent upon binding DNA [82] in parallel with apoptosis detection [83] per manufacturer's instructions (RealTimeGlo™ Annexin V Apoptosis and Necrosis Assay-Promega). Two additional assays of apoptotic cell death were also used. Caspase activation in response to treatment of MCC cells by discorhabdins or bortezomib (as a positive control) was measured using the CaspaseGlo® 3/7 Assay (Promega, Madison, WI, USA) according to the manufacturer's instructions at multiple time points. Inhibition of apoptotic cell death was investigated using pre-treatment of cells with for 1 h with the pan-caspase inhibitor Z-VAD-FMK (Enzo Life Sciences, Farmingdale, NY, USA) followed by treatment with discorhabdins or bortezomib and estimation of cell viability as outlined above.

Mitochondrial membrane potential (MMP) was assessed using the JC-10 ratiometric dye (Sigma, St. Louis, MO, USA). UISO or MKL-1 cells were treated in black-walled, clear-bottom 384-well plates (Corning Life Sciences, Durham, NC, USA) with discorhabdins or doxorubicin (Sigma, St. Louis, MO, USA) as a positive control for up to 24 h with JC-10 for the last 1 h of incubation. Red/green fluorescence signals were measured, the red/green ratio for each well was calculated and normalized to untreated (DMSO) control wells for the same cell line and incubation time to determine relative MMP.

For the detection of reactive oxygen species (ROS), cells in black-walled clear-bottom 384-well plates were preloaded with DCFDA per manufacturer's protocol (ThermoFisher, Waltham, MA, USA), washed, then treated with discorhabdins or TBHP (Sigma, St. Louis, MO, USA) as a positive control. Fluorescence intensity (485 nm excitation, 535 nm emission) was measured at multiple time intervals up to 4 h and normalized to untreated (DMSO) controls for each cell line at the same time point.

Calcium mobilization was assessed with Fluo-4 (Fluo-4 NW Calcium Assay Kit—ThermoFisher) per manufacturer's protocols. Cells in black-wall, clear-bottom 384-well plates were pre-loaded with Fluo-4 followed by treatment with 10 μM discorhabdins or 20 μM thapsigargin (Sigma, St. Louis, MO, USA) as a positive control to monitor fluorescence. Fluorescence signals were normalized to DMSO controls at the same time/cell line.

4.9. Data Analysis

In order to compare responses among all of the discorhabdins and cell lines (98 combinations), dose–response curves were generated using identical discorhabdin dilution series.

GraphPad Prism 8 (San Diego, CA, USA) software was utilized to graph dose–response data and to calculate IC_{50} values and area under the dose–response curves (AUC) along with 95% confidence interval estimates using four-parameter logistic nonlinear regression analysis. For further analysis and comparisons, AUC for each cell line/discorhabdin pair was visualized in a heatmap generated in R version 1.3.1073 (R Core Team (2013). R: A language and environment for statistical computing. R Foundation for Statistical Computing, Vienna, Austria, http://www.R-project.org/ (accessed on 12 January 2023).

Supplementary Materials: The following supporting information can be downloaded at: https://www.mdpi.com/article/10.3390/md21090474/s1, collection, extraction, and isolation procedures, HRMS, 1D and 2D NMR, IR spectra of compounds **6**, **9**, **18**, **20**, **23**, population of Boltzmann averaged conformers of compounds **9** and **22**, calculated and experimental ECD spectra for compound **6** and **22**, physicochemical properties of discorhabdins and effects of discorhabdins on MCC cells.

Author Contributions: Conceptualization, T.G. and C.J.H., Methodology, M.O., C.J.H., T.G., I.B., N.T.H. and K.A.G.; Investigation, M.O. and E.A.S.; Formal analysis, M.O., C.J.H., T.G., N.T.H., K.A.G. and I.B.; Resources, B.R.C.; Writing—original draft preparation, M.O., C.J.H. and E.A.S.; all co-authors contributed to writing/review/editing the manuscript; Visualization/data presentation, C.J.H., N.T.H., K.A.G., T.G. and M.O. All authors have read and agreed to the published version of the manuscript.

Funding: This project has been funded in whole or in part with federal funds from the National Cancer Institute, National Institutes of Health, under contract 75N91019D00024. The content of this publication does not necessarily reflect the views or policies of the Department of Health and Human Services, nor does mention of trade names, commercial products, or organizations imply endorsement by the U.S. Government. This research was supported (in part) by the Intramural Research Program of the NIH.

Institutional Review Board Statement: Not applicable.

Informed Consent Statement: Not applicable.

Data Availability Statement: All data are contained in this article and associated Supplementary Materials.

Acknowledgments: This research utilized the computational resources of the NIH HPC Biowulf cluster and was funded in part by the Intramural Research Program of the NIH, National Cancer Institute, Center for Cancer Research. Authors also thank Sergey G. Tarasov and Marzena Dyba of the Biophysics Resource in the Center for Structural Biology, NCI-Frederick for technical support and help with the ECD measurement and Lin Du of the Molecular Targets Program, NCI-Frederick and Lucero Martínez Fructuoso of the Natural Products Branch, NCI-Frederick for their help with the ECD calculations. Additionally, authors thank Tapas K. Das Gupta for providing early passage UISO cells, Patrick Moore and Jürgen Becker for providing WaGa, Mkl-1, and late-passage UISO cells and Patrick Moore for providing MCC13 and MCC26 cells.

Conflicts of Interest: The authors declare no conflict of interest.

References

1. Harms, P.W.; Harms, K.L.; Moore, P.S.; DeCaprio, J.A.; Nghiem, P.; Wong, M.K.K.; Brownell, I. The biology and treatment of Merkel cell carcinoma: Current understanding and research priorities. *Nat. Rev. Clin. Oncol.* **2018**, *15*, 763–776. [CrossRef]
2. Patel, P.; Hussain, K. Merkel cell carcinoma. *Clin. Exp. Dermatol.* **2021**, *46*, 814–819. [CrossRef]
3. Zwijnenburg, E.M.; Lubeek, S.F.K.; Werner, J.E.M.; Amir, A.L.; Weijs, W.L.J.; Takes, R.P.; Pegge, S.A.H.; van Herpen, C.M.L.; Adema, G.J.; Kaanders, J. Merkel Cell Carcinoma: New Trends. *Cancers* **2021**, *13*, 1614. [CrossRef] [PubMed]
4. Walsh, N.M.; Cerroni, L. Merkel cell carcinoma: A review. *J. Cutan. Pathol.* **2021**, *48*, 411–421. [CrossRef] [PubMed]
5. Banks, P.D.; Sandhu, S.; Gyorki, D.E.; Johnston, M.L.; Rischin, D. Recent Insights and Advances in the Management of Merkel Cell Carcinoma. *J. Oncol. Pract.* **2016**, *12*, 637–646. [CrossRef]
6. Angeles, C.V.; Sabel, M.S. Immunotherapy for Merkel cell carcinoma. *J. Surg. Oncol.* **2021**, *123*, 775–781. [CrossRef]
7. Harms, K.L.; Zhao, L.; Johnson, B.; Wang, X.; Carskadon, S.; Palanisamy, N.; Rhodes, D.R.; Mannan, R.; Vo, J.N.; Choi, J.E.; et al. Virus-positive Merkel Cell Carcinoma Is an Independent Prognostic Group with Distinct Predictive Biomarkers. *Clin. Cancer Res.* **2021**, *27*, 2494–2504. [CrossRef] [PubMed]

8. Samimi, M. Immune Checkpoint Inhibitors and Beyond: An Overview of Immune-Based Therapies in Merkel Cell Carcinoma. *Am. J. Clin. Dermatol.* **2019**, *20*, 391–407. [CrossRef]
9. Iyer, J.G.; Blom, A.; Doumani, R.; Lewis, C.; Tarabadkar, E.S.; Anderson, A.; Ma, C.; Bestick, A.; Parvathaneni, U.; Bhatia, S.; et al. Response rates and durability of chemotherapy among 62 patients with metastatic Merkel cell carcinoma. *Cancer Med.* **2016**, *5*, 2294–2301. [CrossRef]
10. Hill, N.T.; Kim, D.; Busam, K.J.; Chu, E.Y.; Green, C.; Brownell, I. Distinct Signatures of Genomic Copy Number Variants Define Subgroups of Merkel Cell Carcinoma Tumors. *Cancers* **2021**, *13*, 1134. [CrossRef]
11. Shao, Q.; Byrum, S.D.; Moreland, L.E.; Mackintosh, S.G.; Kannan, A.; Lin, Z.; Morgan, M.; Stack, B.C., Jr.; Cornelius, L.A.; Tackett, A.J.; et al. A Proteomic Study of Human Merkel Cell Carcinoma. *J. Proteom. Bioinform.* **2013**, *6*, 275–282. [CrossRef]
12. Liu, G.Y.; Frank, N.; Bartsch, H.; Lin, J.K. Induction of apoptosis by thiuramdisulfides, the reactive metabolites of dithiocarbamates, through coordinative modulation of NFκB, c-fos/c-jun, and p53 proteins. *Mol. Carcinog.* **1998**, *22*, 235–246. [CrossRef]
13. Schreck, R.; Meier, B.; Männel, D.N.; Dröge, W.; Baeuerle, P.A. Dithiocarbamates as potent inhibitors of nuclear factor kappa B activation in intact cells. *J. Exp. Med.* **1992**, *175*, 1181–1194. [CrossRef] [PubMed]
14. Singh, A.K.; Bishayee, A.; Pandey, A.K. Targeting Histone Deacetylases with Natural and Synthetic Agents: An Emerging Anticancer Strategy. *Nutrients* **2018**, *10*, 731. [CrossRef]
15. Tripathi, S.K.; Panda, M.; Biswal, B.K. Emerging role of plumbagin: Cytotoxic potential and pharmaceutical relevance towards cancer therapy. *Food Chem. Toxicol.* **2019**, *125*, 566–582. [CrossRef] [PubMed]
16. Binoy, A.; Nedungadi, D.; Katiyar, N.; Bose, C.; Shankarappa, S.A.; Nair, B.G.; Mishra, N. Plumbagin induces paraptosis in cancer cells by disrupting the sulfhydryl homeostasis and proteasomal function. *Chem. Biol. Interact.* **2019**, *310*, 108733. [CrossRef]
17. Blasiak, J. DNA-Damaging Anticancer Drugs—A Perspective for DNA Repair-Oriented Therapy. *Curr. Med. Chem.* **2017**, *24*, 1488–1503. [CrossRef]
18. Baldwin, E.L.; Osheroff, N. Etoposide, topoisomerase II and cancer. *Curr. Med. Chem. Anticancer Agents* **2005**, *5*, 363–372. [CrossRef] [PubMed]
19. Fukamiya, N.; Lee, K.H.; Muhammad, I.; Murakami, C.; Okano, M.; Harvey, I.; Pelletier, J. Structure-activity relationships of quassinoids for eukaryotic protein synthesis. *Cancer Lett.* **2005**, *220*, 37–48. [CrossRef] [PubMed]
20. Wu, Z.; Zhao, S.; Fash, D.M.; Li, Z.; Chain, W.J.; Beutler, J.A. Englerins: A Comprehensive Review. *J. Nat. Prod.* **2017**, *80*, 771–781. [CrossRef]
21. Martirosyan, A.; Leonard, S.; Shi, X.; Griffith, B.; Gannett, P.; Strobl, J. Actions of a histone deacetylase inhibitor NSC3852 (5-nitroso-8-quinolinol) link reactive oxygen species to cell differentiation and apoptosis in MCF-7 human mammary tumor cells. *J. Pharmacol. Exp. Ther.* **2006**, *317*, 546–552. [CrossRef]
22. Smith, E.A.; Hill, N.T.; Gelb, T.; Garman, K.A.; Goncharova, E.I.; Bokesch, H.R.; Kim, C.K.; Wendt, K.L.; Cichewicz, R.H.; Gustafson, K.R.; et al. Identification of natural product modulators of Merkel cell carcinoma cell growth and survival. *Sci. Rep.* **2021**, *11*, 13597. [CrossRef] [PubMed]
23. Hu, J.F.; Fan, H.; Xiong, J.; Wu, S.B. Discorhabdins and pyrroloiminoquinone-related alkaloids. *Chem. Rev.* **2011**, *111*, 5465–5491. [CrossRef] [PubMed]
24. Li, F.; Kelly, M.; Tasdemir, D. Chemistry, Chemotaxonomy and Biological Activity of the Latrunculid Sponges (Order Poecilosclerida, Family Latrunculiidae). *Mar. Drugs* **2021**, *19*, 27. [CrossRef] [PubMed]
25. Antunes, E.M.; Copp, B.R.; Davies-Coleman, M.T.; Samaai, T. Pyrroloiminoquinone and related metabolites from marine sponges. *Nat. Prod. Rep.* **2005**, *22*, 62–72. [CrossRef]
26. Grkovic, T.; Pearce, A.N.; Munro, M.H.G.; Blunt, J.W.; Davies-Coleman, M.T.; Copp, B.R. Isolation and Characterization of Diastereomers of Discorhabdins H and K and Assignment of Absolute Configuration to Discorhabdins D, N, Q, S, T, and U. *J. Nat. Prod.* **2010**, *73*, 1686–1693. [CrossRef]
27. Lam, C.F.C.; Cadelis, M.M.; Copp, B.R. Exploration of the Electrophilic Reactivity of the Cytotoxic Marine Alkaloid Discorhabdin C and Subsequent Discovery of a New Dimeric C-1/N-13-Linked Discorhabdin Natural Product. *Mar. Drugs* **2020**, *18*, 404. [CrossRef]
28. Peng, F.; Liao, M.; Qin, R.; Zhu, S.; Peng, C.; Fu, L.; Chen, Y.; Han, B. Regulated cell death (RCD) in cancer: Key pathways and targeted therapies. *Signal Transduct. Target. Ther.* **2022**, *7*, 286. [CrossRef]
29. Song, L.; Bretz, A.C.; Gravemeyer, J.; Spassova, I.; Muminova, S.; Gambichler, T.; Sriram, A.; Ferrone, S.; Becker, J.C. The HDAC Inhibitor Domatinostat Promotes Cell-Cycle Arrest, Induces Apoptosis, and Increases Immunogenicity of Merkel Cell Carcinoma Cells. *J. Investig. Dermatol.* **2021**, *141*, 903–912.e4. [CrossRef]
30. Fang, B.; Kannan, A.; Zhao, S.; Nguyen, Q.H.; Ejadi, S.; Yamamoto, M.; Camilo Barreto, J.; Zhao, H.; Gao, L. Inhibition of PI3K by copanlisib exerts potent antitumor effects on Merkel cell carcinoma cell lines and mouse xenografts. *Sci. Rep.* **2020**, *10*, 8867. [CrossRef]
31. Adam, C.; Baeurle, A.; Brodsky, J.L.; Wipf, P.; Schrama, D.; Becker, J.C.; Houben, R. The HSP70 modulator MAL3-101 inhibits Merkel cell carcinoma. *PLoS ONE* **2014**, *9*, e92041. [CrossRef] [PubMed]
32. Das, B.K.; Kannan, A.; Nguyen, Q.; Gogoi, J.; Zhao, H.; Gao, L. Selective Inhibition of Aurora Kinase A by AK-01/LY3295668 Attenuates MCC Tumor Growth by Inducing MCC Cell Cycle Arrest and Apoptosis. *Cancers* **2021**, *13*, 3708. [CrossRef] [PubMed]

33. Kadletz, L.; Bigenzahn, J.; Thurnher, D.; Stanisz, I.; Erovic, B.M.; Schneider, S.; Schmid, R.; Seemann, R.; Birner, P.; Helduschka, G. Evaluation of Polo-like kinase 1 as a potential therapeutic target in Merkel cell carcinoma. *Head Neck* **2016**, *38* (Suppl. S1), E1918–E1925. [CrossRef] [PubMed]
34. Verhaegen, M.E.; Mangelberger, D.; Weick, J.W.; Vozheiko, T.D.; Harms, P.W.; Nash, K.T.; Quintana, E.; Baciu, P.; Johnson, T.M.; Bichakjian, C.K.; et al. Merkel cell carcinoma dependence on bcl-2 family members for survival. *J. Investig. Dermatol.* **2014**, *134*, 2241–2250. [CrossRef]
35. Kannan, A.; Lin, Z.; Shao, Q.; Zhao, S.; Fang, B.; Moreno, M.A.; Vural, E.; Stack, B.C., Jr.; Suen, J.Y.; Kannan, K.; et al. Dual mTOR inhibitor MLN0128 suppresses Merkel cell carcinoma (MCC) xenograft tumor growth. *Oncotarget* **2016**, *7*, 6576–6592. [CrossRef]
36. Leiendecker, L.; Jung, P.S.; Krecioch, I.; Neumann, T.; Schleiffer, A.; Mechtler, K.; Wiesner, T.; Obenauf, A.C. LSD1 inhibition induces differentiation and cell death in Merkel cell carcinoma. *EMBO Mol. Med.* **2020**, *12*, e12525. [CrossRef]
37. Sarma, B.; Willmes, C.; Angerer, L.; Adam, C.; Becker, J.C.; Kervarrec, T.; Schrama, D.; Houben, R. Artesunate Affects T Antigen Expression and Survival of Virus-Positive Merkel Cell Carcinoma. *Cancers* **2020**, *12*, 919. [CrossRef] [PubMed]
38. Lin, Z.; McDermott, A.; Shao, L.; Kannan, A.; Morgan, M.; Stack, B.C., Jr.; Moreno, M.; Davis, D.A.; Cornelius, L.A.; Gao, L. Chronic mTOR activation promotes cell survival in Merkel cell carcinoma. *Cancer Lett.* **2014**, *344*, 272–281. [CrossRef]
39. Arora, R.; Shuda, M.; Guastafierro, A.; Feng, H.; Toptan, T.; Tolstov, Y.; Normolle, D.; Vollmer, L.L.; Vogt, A.; Dömling, A.; et al. Survivin is a therapeutic target in Merkel cell carcinoma. *Sci. Transl. Med.* **2012**, *4*, 133ra56. [CrossRef]
40. Botić, T.; Defant, A.; Zanini, P.; Žužek, M.C.; Frangež, R.; Janussen, D.; Kersken, D.; Knez, Ž.; Mancini, I.; Sepčić, K. Discorhabdin alkaloids from Antarctic *Latrunculia* spp. sponges as a new class of cholinesterase inhibitors. *Eur. J. Med. Chem.* **2017**, *136*, 294–304. [CrossRef]
41. Gunasekera, S.P.; McCarthy, P.J.; Longley, R.E.; Pomponi, S.A.; Wright, A.E.; Lobkovsky, E.; Clardy, J. Discorhabdin P, a new enzyme inhibitor from a deep-water Caribbean sponge of the genus *Batzella*. *J. Nat. Prod.* **1999**, *62*, 173–175. [CrossRef] [PubMed]
42. Amusengeri, A.; Tastan Bishop, Ö. Discorhabdin N, a South African Natural Compound, for Hsp72 and Hsc70 Allosteric Modulation: Combined Study of Molecular Modeling and Dynamic Residue Network Analysis. *Molecules* **2019**, *24*, 188. [CrossRef] [PubMed]
43. Goey, A.K.; Chau, C.H.; Sissung, T.M.; Cook, K.M.; Venzon, D.J.; Castro, A.; Ransom, T.R.; Henrich, C.J.; McKee, T.C.; McMahon, J.B.; et al. Screening and Biological Effects of Marine Pyrroloiminoquinone Alkaloids: Potential Inhibitors of the HIF-1α/p300 Interaction. *J. Nat. Prod.* **2016**, *79*, 1267–1275. [CrossRef] [PubMed]
44. Harris, E.M.; Strope, J.D.; Beedie, S.L.; Huang, P.A.; Goey, A.K.L.; Cook, K.M.; Schofield, C.J.; Chau, C.H.; Cadelis, M.M.; Copp, B.R.; et al. Preclinical Evaluation of Discorhabdins in Antiangiogenic and Antitumor Models. *Mar. Drugs* **2018**, *16*, 241. [CrossRef]
45. Grkovic, T.; Kaur, B.; Webb, V.L.; Copp, B.R. Semi-synthetic preparation of the rare, cytotoxic, deep-sea sourced sponge metabolites discorhabdins P and U. *Bioorgan. Med. Chem. Lett.* **2006**, *16*, 1944–1946. [CrossRef]
46. Nyquist, R.A. (Ed.) Chapter 5—Sulfoxides, Sulfones, Sulfates, Monothiosulfates, Sulfonyl Halides, Sulfites, Sulfonamides, Sulfonates, and N-Sulfinyl Anilines. In *Interpreting Infrared, Raman, and Nuclear Magnetic Resonance Spectra*; Academic Press: San Diego, CA, USA, 2001; pp. 85–117.
47. Schreiber, K.C. Infrared Spectra of Sulfones and Related Compounds. *Anal. Chem.* **1949**, *21*, 1168–1172. [CrossRef]
48. Takahashi, Y.; Ushio, M.; Kubota, T.; Yamamoto, S.; Fromont, J.; Kobayashi, J.I. Nakijiquinones J−R, Sesquiterpenoid Quinones with an Amine Residue from Okinawan Marine Sponges. *J. Nat. Prod.* **2010**, *73*, 467–471. [CrossRef]
49. Avilov, S.A.; Kalinovsky, A.I.; Kalinin, V.I.; Stonik, V.A.; Riguera, R.; Jiménez, C. Koreoside A, a New Nonholostane Triterpene Glycoside from the Sea Cucumber *Cucumaria koraiensis*. *J. Nat. Prod.* **1997**, *60*, 808–810. [CrossRef]
50. Guo, Q.; Xia, H.; Wu, Y.; Shao, S.; Xu, C.; Zhang, T.; Shi, J. Structure, property, biogenesis, and activity of diterpenoid alkaloids containing a sulfonic acid group from *Aconitum carmichaelii*. *Acta Pharm. Sin. B* **2020**, *10*, 1954–1965. [CrossRef]
51. Perry, N.B.; Blunt, J.W.; McCombs, J.D.; Munro, M.H.G. Discorhabdin C, a highly cytotoxic pigment from a sponge of the genus *Latrunculia*. *J. Org. Chem.* **1986**, *51*, 5476–5478. [CrossRef]
52. Yang, A.; Baker, B.J.; Grimwade, J.; Leonard, A.; McClintock, J.B. Discorhabdin Alkaloids from the Antarctic Sponge *Latrunculia apicalis*. *J. Nat. Prod.* **1995**, *58*, 1596–1599. [CrossRef]
53. Gunasekera, S.P.; Zuleta, I.A.; Longley, R.E.; Wright, A.E.; Pomponi, S.A. Discorhabdins S, T, and U, New Cytotoxic Pyrroloiminoquinones from a Deep-Water Caribbean Sponge of the Genus *Batzella*. *J. Nat. Prod.* **2003**, *66*, 1615–1617. [CrossRef] [PubMed]
54. Antunes, E.M.; Beukes, D.R.; Kelly, M.; Samaai, T.; Barrows, L.R.; Marshall, K.M.; Sincich, C.; Davies-Coleman, M.T. Cytotoxic Pyrroloiminoquinones from Four New Species of South African Latrunculid Sponges. *J. Nat. Prod.* **2004**, *67*, 1268–1276. [CrossRef] [PubMed]
55. Zhang, R.; Shi, X.; Yan, Q.; Li, Z.; Wang, Z.; Yu, H.; Wang, X.; Qi, J.; Jiang, M. Free-radical initiated cascade methylation or trideuteromethylation of isocyanides with dimethyl sulfoxides. *RSC Adv.* **2017**, *7*, 38830–38833. [CrossRef]
56. Fallahi-Sichani, M.; Honarnejad, S.; Heiser, L.M.; Gray, J.W.; Sorger, P.K. Metrics other than potency reveal systematic variation in responses to cancer drugs. *Nat. Chem. Biol.* **2013**, *9*, 708–714. [CrossRef]
57. Lam, C.F.; Grkovic, T.; Pearce, A.N.; Copp, B.R. Investigation of the electrophilic reactivity of the cytotoxic marine alkaloid discorhabdin B. *Org. Biomol. Chem.* **2012**, *10*, 3092–3097. [CrossRef]
58. Lam, C.F.; Cadelis, M.M.; Copp, B.R. Exploration of the influence of spiro-dienone moiety on biological activity of the cytotoxic marine alkaloid discorhabdin P. *Tetrahedron* **2017**, *73*, 4779–4785. [CrossRef]

59. Wada, Y.; Harayama, Y.; Kamimura, D.; Yoshida, M.; Shibata, T.; Fujiwara, K.; Morimoto, K.; Fujioka, H.; Kita, Y. The synthetic and biological studies of discorhabdins and related compounds. *Org. Biomol. Chem.* **2011**, *9*, 4959–4976. [CrossRef]
60. Tang, D.; Kang, R.; Berghe, T.V.; Vandenabeele, P.; Kroemer, G. The molecular machinery of regulated cell death. *Cell Res.* **2019**, *29*, 347–364. [CrossRef]
61. Bock, F.J.; Tait, S.W.G. Mitochondria as multifaceted regulators of cell death. *Nat. Rev. Mol. Cell Biol.* **2020**, *21*, 85–100. [CrossRef]
62. Ermak, G.; Davies, K.J. Calcium and oxidative stress: From cell signaling to cell death. *Mol. Immunol.* **2002**, *38*, 713–721. [CrossRef] [PubMed]
63. Molnár, T.; Mázló, A.; Tslaf, V.; Szöllősi, A.G.; Emri, G.; Koncz, G. Current translational potential and underlying molecular mechanisms of necroptosis. *Cell Death Dis.* **2019**, *10*, 860. [CrossRef] [PubMed]
64. Cao, L.; Mu, W. Necrostatin-1 and necroptosis inhibition: Pathophysiology and therapeutic implications. *Pharmacol. Res.* **2021**, *163*, 105297. [CrossRef] [PubMed]
65. Hsu, S.K.; Chang, W.T.; Lin, I.L.; Chen, Y.F.; Padalwar, N.B.; Cheng, K.C.; Teng, Y.N.; Wang, C.H.; Chiu, C.C. The Role of Necroptosis in ROS-Mediated Cancer Therapies and Its Promising Applications. *Cancers* **2020**, *12*, 2185. [CrossRef]
66. Kuang, F.; Liu, J.; Tang, D.; Kang, R. Oxidative Damage and Antioxidant Defense in Ferroptosis. *Front. Cell Dev. Biol.* **2020**, *8*, 586578. [CrossRef]
67. Pasquier, B. Autophagy inhibitors. *Cell Mol. Life Sci.* **2016**, *73*, 985–1001. [CrossRef]
68. Fatokun, A.A.; Dawson, V.L.; Dawson, T.M. Parthanatos: Mitochondrial-linked mechanisms and therapeutic opportunities. *Br. J. Pharmacol.* **2014**, *171*, 2000–2016. [CrossRef]
69. Krump, N.A.; You, J. From Merkel Cell Polyomavirus Infection to Merkel Cell Carcinoma Oncogenesis. *Front. Microbiol.* **2021**, *12*, 739695. [CrossRef] [PubMed]
70. Grkovic, T.; Ding, Y.; Li, X.-C.; Webb, V.L.; Ferreira, D.; Copp, B.R. Enantiomeric Discorhabdin Alkaloids and Establishment of Their Absolute Configurations Using Theoretical Calculations of Electronic Circular Dichroism Spectra. *J. Org. Chem.* **2008**, *73*, 9133–9136. [CrossRef]
71. Dijoux, M.-G.; Gamble, W.R.; Hallock, Y.F.; Cardellina, J.H.; van Soest, R.; Boyd, M.R. A New Discorhabdin from Two Sponge Genera. *J. Nat. Prod.* **1999**, *62*, 636–637. [CrossRef]
72. Copp, B.R.; Fulton, K.F.; Perry, N.B.; Blunt, J.W.; Munro, M.H.G. Natural and Synthetic Derivatives of Discorhabdin C, a Cytotoxic Pigment from the New Zealand Sponge *Latrunculia* cf. *bocagei*. *J. Org. Chem.* **1994**, *59*, 8233–8238. [CrossRef]
73. Grkovic, T.; Copp, B.R. New natural products in the discorhabdin A- and B-series from New Zealand-sourced *Latrunculia* spp. sponges. *Tetrahedron* **2009**, *65*, 6335–6340. [CrossRef]
74. Jeon, J.-e.; Na, Z.; Jung, M.; Lee, H.-S.; Sim, C.J.; Nahm, K.; Oh, K.-B.; Shin, J. Discorhabdins from the Korean Marine Sponge *Sceptrella* sp. *J. Nat. Prod.* **2010**, *73*, 258–262. [CrossRef] [PubMed]
75. Leonard, J.H.; Dash, P.; Holland, P.; Kearsley, J.H.; Bell, J.R. Characterisation of four Merkel cell carcinoma adherent cell lines. *Int. J. Cancer* **1995**, *60*, 100–107. [CrossRef]
76. Ronan, S.G.; Green, A.D.; Shilkaitis, A.; Huang, T.S.; Das Gupta, T.K. Merkel cell carcinoma: In vitro and in vivo characteristics of a new cell line. *J. Am. Acad. Dermatol.* **1993**, *29 Pt 1*, 715–722. [CrossRef] [PubMed]
77. Rosen, S.T.; Gould, V.E.; Salwen, H.R.; Herst, C.V.; Le Beau, M.M.; Lee, I.; Bauer, K.; Marder, R.J.; Andersen, R.; Kies, M.S.; et al. Establishment and characterization of a neuroendocrine skin carcinoma cell line. *Lab. Investig.* **1987**, *56*, 302–312. [PubMed]
78. Martin, E.M.; Gould, V.E.; Hoog, A.; Rosen, S.T.; Radosevich, J.A.; Deftos, L.J. Parathyroid hormone-related protein, chromogranin A, and calcitonin gene products in the neuroendocrine skin carcinoma cell lines MKL1 and MKL2. *Bone Miner.* **1991**, *14*, 113–120. [CrossRef]
79. Houben, R.; Shuda, M.; Weinkam, R.; Schrama, D.; Feng, H.; Chang, Y.; Moore, P.S.; Becker, J.C. Merkel cell polyomavirus-infected Merkel cell carcinoma cells require expression of viral T antigens. *J. Virol.* **2010**, *84*, 7064–7072. [CrossRef]
80. Boukamp, P.; Petrussevska, R.T.; Breitkreutz, D.; Hornung, J.; Markham, A.; Fusenig, N.E. Normal keratinization in a spontaneously immortalized aneuploid human keratinocyte cell line. *J. Cell Biol.* **1988**, *106*, 761–771. [CrossRef]
81. Duellman, S.J.; Zhou, W.; Meisenheimer, P.; Vidugiris, G.; Cali, J.J.; Gautam, P.; Wennerberg, K.; Vidugiriene, J. Bioluminescent, Nonlytic, Real-Time Cell Viability Assay and Use in Inhibitor Screening. *Assay Drug Dev. Technol.* **2015**, *13*, 456–465. [CrossRef]
82. Niles, A.L.; Riss, T.L. Multiplexed viability, cytotoxicity, and caspase activity assays. *Methods Mol. Biol.* **2015**, *1219*, 21–33. [PubMed]
83. Kupcho, K.; Shultz, J.; Hurst, R.; Hartnett, J.; Zhou, W.; Machleidt, T.; Grailer, J.; Worzella, T.; Riss, T.; Lazar, D.; et al. A real-time, bioluminescent annexin V assay for the assessment of apoptosis. *Apoptosis* **2019**, *24*, 184–197. [CrossRef] [PubMed]

marine drugs

MDPI

Article

The Salmon Oil OmeGo Reduces Viability of Colorectal Cancer Cells and Potentiates the Anti-Cancer Effect of 5-FU

Caroline H. H. Pettersen [1,2,3,*], Helle Samdal [1,2], Pål Sætrom [1,4,5,6], Arne Wibe [1,2], Erland Hermansen [3] and Svanhild A. Schønberg [1]

1 Department of Clinical and Molecular Medicine, Faculty of Medicine and Health Sciences, Norwegian University of Science and Technology (NTNU), 7491 Trondheim, Norway; helle.samdal@ntnu.no (H.S.); pal.satrom@ntnu.no (P.S.); arne.wibe@ntnu.no (A.W.); svanhild.schonberg@ntnu.no (S.A.S.)
2 Department of Surgery, St. Olav's University Hospital, 7006 Trondheim, Norway
3 Hofseth BioCare, Kipervikgata 13, 6003 Ålesund, Norway; ehe@hofsethbiocare.no
4 Department of Computer Science, Faculty of Information Technology and Electrical Engineering, Norwegian University of Science and Technology (NTNU), 7491 Trondheim, Norway
5 Bioinformatics Core Facility—BioCore, Norwegian University of Science and Technology (NTNU), 7006 Trondheim, Norway
6 K.G. Jebsen Center for Genetic Epidemiology, Norwegian University of Science and Technology (NTNU), 7006 Trondheim, Norway
* Correspondence: caroline.h.pettersen@ntnu.no; Tel.: +47-73598577

Abstract: Colorectal cancer (CRC) is one of the most common cancer types worldwide. Chemotherapy is toxic to normal cells, and combinatory treatment with natural well-tolerated products is being explored. Some omega-3 polyunsaturated fatty acids (n-3 PUFAs) and marine fish oils have anti-cancer effects on CRC cells. The salmon oil OmeGo (Hofseth BioCare) contains a spectrum of fatty acids, including the n-3 PUFAs docosahexaenoic acid (DHA) and eicosahexaenoic acid (EPA). We explored a potential anti-cancer effect of OmeGo on the four CRC cell lines DLD-1, HCT-8, LS411N, and LS513, alone and in combination with the chemotherapeutic agent 5-Fluorouracil (5-FU). Screening indicated a time- and dose-dependent effect of OmeGo on the viability of the DLD-1 and LS513 CRC cell lines. Treatment with 5-FU and OmeGo (IC20–IC30) alone indicated a significant reduction in viability. A combinatory treatment with OmeGo and 5-FU resulted in a further reduction in viability in DLD-1 and LS513 cells. Treatment of CRC cells with DHA + EPA in a concentration corresponding to the content in OmeGo alone or combined with 5-FU significantly reduced viability of all four CRC cell lines tested. The lowest concentration of OmeGo reduced viability to a higher degree both alone and in combination with 5-FU compared to the corresponding concentrations of DHA + EPA in three of the cell lines. Results suggest that a combination of OmeGo and 5-FU could have a potential as an alternative anti-cancer therapy for patients with CRC.

Keywords: colorectal cancer; CRC; fish oil; omega-3 fatty acids; salmon oil; OmeGo

1. Introduction

The outcome of colorectal cancer (CRC) has improved over the past decades; however, it is still the second and third most common cancer type worldwide among women and men, respectively. In Norway, CRC is the second most common cancer type for men and women together, with approximately 4500 new cases every year [1]. The incidence rate is high in Norway compared to other Nordic countries and has increased by 300% in the last 60 years [2]. In 2014, CRC was the costliest cancer in Norway, constituting a significant economic burden on Norwegian society [3].

For treatment of CRC, surgery is still the cornerstone of curative intent [4]. However, adjuvant cancer chemotherapy is commonly used after resection of advanced tumors [5]. One of the first-line chemotherapy drugs for CRC treatment is 5-fluorouracil (5-FU), which is commonly used alone or in combination with other anti-cancer drugs. Although 5-FU is considered one of the safest chemotherapy agents, chemotherapy may lead to development of drug resistance and toxicity towards normal cells [6]. This has led to an increased interest in exploring the potential anti-cancer effects of different natural dietary ingredients such as fish and fish oil in combination with chemotherapy to improve CRC treatment and patient quality of life.

Marine fish oil is a good dietary source of the omega-3 (n-3) polyunsaturated fatty acids (PUFAs) docosahexaenoic acid (DHA) and eicosapentaenoic acid (EPA), which have been shown to have anti-cancer properties (reviewed in [7,8]). The human body has limited capacity to synthesize these PUFAs; hence, they are considered essential and must be acquired through the diet. The Norwegian authorities recommend a daily intake of at least 1–2 g n-3 PUFAs or two to three fatty fish meals weekly [9], while the European Food Safety Authority (EFSA) recommends an intake of $\geq$2 fish meals weekly or an intake of 250–500 mg DHA and EPA daily [10]. However, both the Norwegian and American intake of DHA and EPA is below the recommended levels, and intake of fatty fish or fish oils should be increased to improve health [11,12].

Some epidemiological studies suggest that the intake of n-3 PUFAs reduces the risk of developing CRC [13] and that intake of fish and n-3 PUFAs may have the potential to affect the outcome of CRC treatment [14]. Observational data indicate reduced mortality after CRC diagnosis, and longer disease-free survival, in patients with high intake of n-3 PUFAs [15,16]. Some interventional studies demonstrate beneficial anti-cancer effects of n-3 PUFAs in CRC patients [17,18] and EPA supplementation was shown to reduce crypt cell hyperproliferation and increase mucosal apoptosis in patients with colorectal adenomas [18,19]. EPA supplementation given pre-surgically to patients with CRC metastases improved overall and disease-free survival compared to placebo [20]. Also, intake of n-3 PUFA-containing perioperative nutrition may reduce postoperative complications, pro-inflammatory cytokine levels and hospital stay for CRC patients [21]. Animal studies indicate that n-3 PUFAs and fish oil may decrease the formation and growth of CRC tumors in vivo [7,22,23] and improve the efficacy of chemotherapeutic drugs like 5-FU [7,14,22], and that fish oil may increase cellular uptake of 5-FU in the colon of mice, thereby reversing multi-drug resistance and restore 5-FU-mediated chemosensitivity [24]. In vitro studies confirm the anti-cancer potential of n-3 PUFAs alone and in combination with chemotherapeutic drugs like 5-FU and suggest a range of different molecular pathways involved [7,14,22,25]. Commercially, n-3 PUFAs are available in different formulations: as free fatty acids (FAs), phospholipids, triglycerides, and conjugated to ethyl esters. The effect of different formulations alone and in combination with chemotherapeutic drugs on cancer cells may vary [14]. DHA and EPA enhance the anti-cancer effect of chemotherapies on human cancer cells both in their pure forms [25–30] and when delivered as part of liposomes [31]. Fish oils may also enhance the effect of cytostatic treatment on cancer cells [32–35].

In this study, we tested a potential anti-cancer effect of the salmon oil OmeGo on CRC cells alone and in combination with the chemotherapeutic drug 5-FU. We also compared the effect to corresponding concentrations of the n-3 PUFAs DHA and EPA. We selected two DHA-sensitive cell lines, DLD-1 and HCT-8, and two less sensitive cell lines, LS411N and LS513. The choice of cell lines was based on a previous publication from our group where we tested the DHA sensitivity and basal level of autophagy on 10 CRC cell lines that represented different clinically relevant subtypes [36]. OmeGo is a natural fish oil liberated from Atlantic salmon using a patented enzymatic process (Hofseth BioCare). OmeGo contains ~99% fat, of which less than 1% is free FAs (21 different identified) and about 1% lipopeptides, and meets the FDA standards for New Dietary Ingredients (NDI) status [37]. Taken as Cardio capsules, it contains about 140 mg n-3 PUFAs per gram of salmon oil [38]. It also contains the natural carotenoid astaxanthin, an antioxidant, which originates from algal production and gives the red color of the salmon oil [39]. OmeGo has in previous studies demonstrated an anti-eosinophilic effect and may have beneficial effects on eosinophil-driven diseases such as asthma and Chronic obstructive pulmonary disease (COPD) [40,41], as well as cardio-vascular events through reduction of serum concentrations of Oxidized low-density lipoprotein-2-glycoprotein I complex x (oxLDL-GP) [42].

2. Results

2.1. 5-FU and OmeGo Treatment Reduce Viability of CRC Cell Lines

Four CRC cell lines were selected for testing the potential anti-cancer effect of OmeGo alone and in combination with 5-FU using the Resazurin viability assay. 5-FU was tested in the range of 0.5–64 µM based on previously reported blood [5-FU] in cancer patients undergoing 5-FU treatment (2.54–17.4 µM) [43,44] and previously reported [5-FU] tested on CRC cells in vitro [27,34,45,46]. 5-FU treatment reduced the viability of all four cell lines in a time- and dose-dependent manner ($p < 2.4 \times 10^{-56}$, Wald tests) (1–3 days, Figure 1, Supplementary Table S1). The reduction in cell viability did not exceed 70% for the highest [5-FU] tested (3 days) for all cell lines. LS513 cells were highly sensitive to 5-FU treatment; hence, the [5-FU] used for screening was reduced as indicated in Table S1 and Figure 1 to find the linear area of the dose–response curve for this cell line.

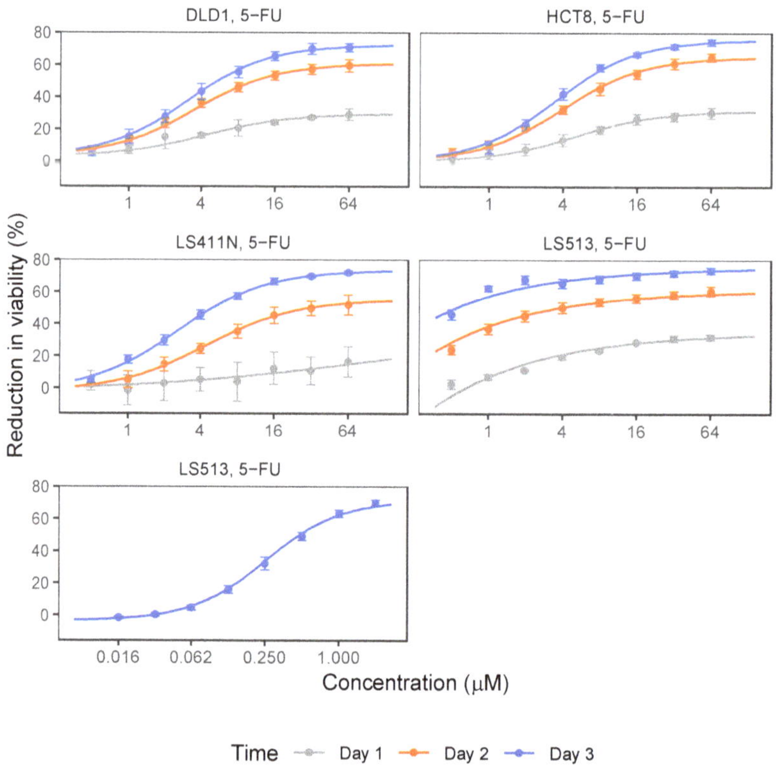

Figure 1. Effect of 5-Fluoruracil (5-FU) treatment on the DLD-1, LS411N, HCT-8, and LS513 cell lines. Points show average percent reduction of cell viability after treatment with indicated concentrations of 5-FU for 1–3 days. Error bars show standard deviation (SD). Lines show fitted dose–response curves (see Materials and Methods section). Number of biological replicates (n) for all 4 cell lines (0.5–64 µM 5-FU) = 4. For LS513 (0.015625–2 µM) $n = 3$.

Screening of the anti-cancer effect of OmeGo was performed in the range of 62.5–1500 µg/mL based on estimated DHA and EPA content in OmeGo and previous reported doses of DHA, EPA, and fish oil tested on cancer cells [36,47–49]. OmeGo treatment reduced cell viability in a time- and dose-dependent manner with up to 90% and 70% for the DLD-1 and LS513 cell lines, respectively (Figure 2, Table S2; $p < 4.9 \times 10^{-128}$, Wald tests). For DLD-1 cells, the linear area of the sensitivity curve was between 125–750 µg/mL but flattened out above 1000 µg/mL OmeGo. For LS513 cells, the sensitivity was still increasing up to 1500 µg/mL. The HCT-8 and LS411N cell lines responded much less to OmeGo treatment, with a maximum reduced viability of ~24% and ~26% after 2 days, respectively (Figure 2, Table S2; $p < 8.4 \times 10^{-51}$, Wald tests).

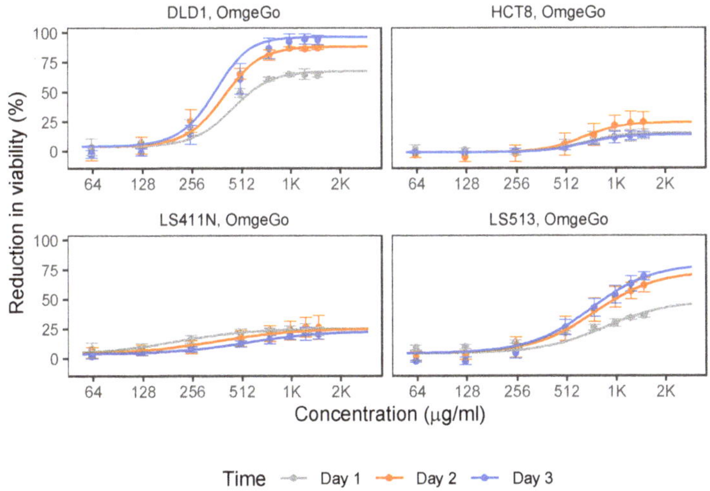

Figure 2. Effect of OmeGo treatment of the DLD-1, LS411N, HCT-8, and LS513 cell lines. Points show average percent reduction of cell viability after treatment with indicated concentrations of OmeGo for 1–3 days (DLD-1 and LS513 n = 4, LS411N and HCT-8 n = 5). Error bars show standard deviation (SD). Lines show fitted dose–response curves (see Materials and Methods section).

The concentrations of 5-FU and OmeGo that gave 20%, 30% and 50% of the maximal measured effect on cell viability (IC20, IC30, and IC50) after 3 days were estimated for all cell lines (Table 1). The IC50 values for 5-FU treatment of DLD-1, HCT-8, and LS411N cells ranged from 4.6 µM to 5.9 µM (Table 1). The initially estimated 5-FU IC20–IC50 values for LS513 cells were below the concentrations tested due to high sensitivity, and the data did not fit the model well. However, the estimated IC values (IC20 = 0.005 ± 0.00, IC30 = 0.013 ± 0.00) guided the choice of concentrations for an additional screening of LS513 cells using lower concentrations of 5-FU (0.0156–2.0 µM, 3 days, Table 1, Figure 2), resulting in an IC50-value of 0.4 µM for this cell line.

Table 1. Estimated values for IC20, IC30, and IC50 ± standard error (SE) for CRC cell lines treated with 5-FU and OmeGo for 3 days.

Cell Line	Days	5-FU (µM)						OmeGo (µg/mL)					
		IC20	±SE	IC30	±SE	IC50	±SE	IC20	±SE	IC30	±SE	IC50	±SE
DLD-1	3	1.68	0.01	2.56	0.01	4.99	0.01	353.10	1.40	410.22	1.34	519.28	1.03
HCT-8	3	2.02	0.001	3.06	0.01	5.90	0.01	464.66	1.66	537.80	1.59	676.73	3.11
LS411N *	3	1.38	0.01	2.20	0.01	4.56	0.02	278.06	2.39	370.96	2.76	583.60	5.19
LS513	3	0.15	0.00	0.216	0.00	0.40	0.00	534.85	3.75	680.84	5.97	994.97	12.34

* For estimation of inhibitory concentration (IC20–IC50) values, the "robust" model was used for the LS411N cell line, while the "robust simple" model was used for the DLD-1, HCT-8, and LS513 cell lines, based on which model best fitted the data.

2.2. OmeGo Treatment Potentiates the Anti-Cancer Effect of 5-FU in CRC Cell Lines

For combination experiments, 5-FU and OmeGo were used in concentrations covering the IC20–IC30 ranges for all cell lines (Figure 3 and Table 1). Statistical analyses indicated a significant dose-dependent effect of 5-FU treatment for all cell lines (Figure 3, Table 2). Each unit 5-FU (µM) was estimated to reduce cell viability, with 7.7–9.8% for DLD-1, HCT-8 and LS411N cells, while viability in the highly 5-FU sensitive LS513 cells was reduced by 88.5% per µM (Figure 3, Tables 2 and S3). OmeGo treatment had a significant dose-dependent additive effect in DLD-1 and LS513 cells (Figure 3, Table 2), where each unit of OmeGo (100 µg/mL) was estimated to reduce viability by about 6%. Cotreatment with 5-FU and OmeGo had a small significant antagonistic interaction in DLD-1 and LS513 cells; however, it further reduced the cell viability for DLD-1 (p-value = 0.039) and LS513 cells ($p = 1.0 \times 10^{-3}$), respectively (Table 2, Figure S1). Based on data presented in Figure 3, combinatory treatment with the lowest [5-FU] combined with different [OmeGo] gave an increased effect of 15–46%, while the highest [5-FU] combined with different [OmeGo] increased the effect by 13–31%, compared to the respective [5-FU] alone for DLD-1 cells (Table S3). For LS513 cells, the lowest [5-FU] combined with different [OmeGo] gave an increased effect of 14–41%, while the highest [5-FU] combined with different [OmeGo] increased the effect by 10–24% (Table S3). Hence, the largest chemo-sensitizing effect of OmeGo was seen at low [5-FU].

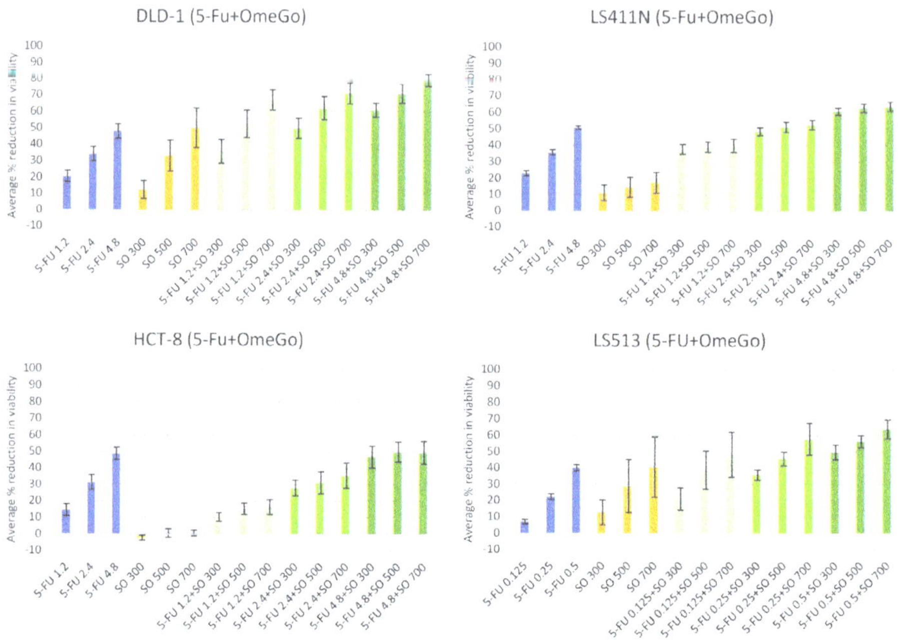

Figure 3. Effect of 5-FU (blue), OmeGo (SO = salmon oil, orange), and combinatory treatment with 5-FU + OmeGo (SO) (green) on viability of the DLD-1, LS411N, HCT-8, and LS513 cell lines. Results represent average percent reduction of cell viability (±SD) after treatment with indicated concentrations of 5-FU (µM) and OmeGo (SO, µg/mL) for 3 days (DLD-1, LS411N and HCT-8 $n = 5$, LS513 $n = 4$).

Table 2. Estimated percent (%) reduced viability (±SD) per unit treatment with 5-FU (μM), OmeGo (100 μg/mL) and combination of 5-FU + OmeGo of CRC cell lines (3 days). *p*-value < 0.05 was considered statistically significant.

Cell Line	Days	ε Intercept	5-FU			OmeGo			5-FU × OmeGo		
			Effect %	±SD	*p*-Value	Effect %	±SD	*p*-Value	Effect %	±SD	*p*-Value
DLD-1	3	8.55	8.94	0.77	1.17×10^{-26}	6.17	0.52	9.94×10^{-28}	−0.36	0.17	3.85×10^{-2}
HCT-8	3	2.82	9.82	0.79	3.80×10^{-29}	−0.02	0.53	9.67×10^{-1}	0.07	0.18	6.88×10^{-1}
LS411N	3	15.30	7.70	0.77	6.14×10^{-21}	1.23	0.52	1.90×10^{-2}	0.30	0.17	8.09×10^{-2}
LS513	3	−2.17	88.46	8.14	9.55×10^{-24}	6.29	0.57	3.64×10^{-24}	−6.10	1.84	1.00×10^{-3}

2.3. The n-3 PUFAs DHA + EPA Potentiate the Anti-Cancer Effect of 5-FU in CRC Cells

The content of DHA and EPA in 1 mg OmeGo was estimated to be 124 μM and 95.2 μM, respectively (based on information in the OmeGo certificate of analysis). Based on this, concentrations of DHA and EPA corresponding with doses of 300, 500, and 700 μg/mL OmeGo were used for combinatory treatment with 5-FU (Figure 4, Table S5). The lowest [DHA + EPA] somewhat enhanced cell viability (Figure 4, Table S6), except for LS411N cells, and hence had a less negative effect on viability compared to the corresponding concentration of OmeGo (Figures 2 and 3; $p = 9.0 \times 10^{-7}$, Student's *t*-test). The combination of the lowest [5-FU] and [DHA + EPA] reduced cell viability to a lesser extent compared to 5-FU alone for the DLD-1, HCT-8 and LS513 cells ($p < 2.1 \times 10^{-6}$, Student's *t*-test) and did not reach the level of the combinatory effect of 5-FU+OmeGo at corresponding concentrations (Figures 3 and 4; $p = 5.0 \times 10^{-10}$, Student's *t*-test). The highest [DHA + EPA] (~153 μM n-3 PUFAs, Table S5) seemed to be toxic to some cell lines (Figure 4, Table S6).

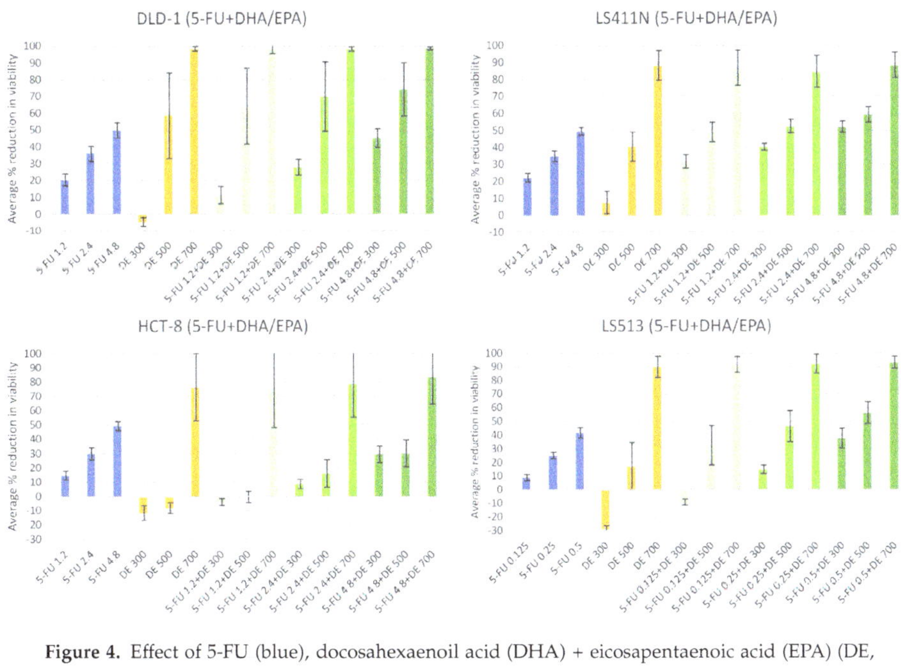

Figure 4. Effect of 5-FU (blue), docosahexaenoil acid (DHA) + eicosapentaenoic acid (EPA) (DE, orange), and combinatory treatment with 5-FU+DE (green) on viability of the DLD-1, LS411N, HCT-8, and LS513 cell lines. Results represent average percent reduction of cell viability (±SD) after treatment with indicated concentrations of 5-FU (μM) and DE (dose correlating with μM/mL OmeGo) for 3 days (DLD-1 and LS411N $n = 6$, HCT-8 and LS513 $n = 5$).

Statistical analyses indicated that DHA + EPA treatment reduced viability for all cell lines within concentrations present in the OmeGo IC20–IC30 range. Viability was reduced by 9–14% per 100 µg/mL OmeGo-correlated concentration of DHA + EPA. The 5-FU also reduced viability by 11–14% for DLD-1, HCT-8, and LS411N cells, and 150% for the highly sensitive LS513 cells, per µM 5-FU treatment (Table 3). The combinatory treatment with DHA + EPA and 5-FU had a small significant antagonistic interaction in all cell lines (Table 3, Figure S2). The effect of DHA + EPA and the combinatory treatment estimated by the linear model diverged more from the observed effects (Figure 4, Tables S6 and S7) compared to the OmeGo results, probably reflecting the less optimized dosage of n-3 PUFAs compared to OmeGo.

Table 3. Estimated % reduced viability (±SD) per unit treatment with 5-FU (µM), DHA + EPA (100 µg/mL OmeGo) and combination of 5-FU+ and DHA + EPA on CRC cell lines (3 days). p-value < 0.05 was considered statistically significant.

Cell Line	Days	ε Intercept	5-FU			DHA + EPA			5-FU × DHA + EPA		
			Effect %	±SD	p-Value	Effect %	±SD	p-Value	Effect %	±SD	p-Value
DLD-1	3	−10.86	12.45	2.07	4.32×10^{-9}	13.79	1.36	2.15×10^{-21}	−1.68	0.46	3.00×10^{-4}
HCT-8	3	−20.26	13.76	2.19	1.00×10^{-9}	9.03	1.46	1.65×10^{-9}	−1.53	0.49	1.80×10^{-3}
LS411N	3	−0.99	10.74	2.07	3.49×10^{-7}	10.60	1.36	7.47×10^{-14}	−1.40	0.46	2.20×10^{-3}
LS513	3	−33.60	150.76	21.93	2.62×10^{-11}	14.05	1.50	7.72×10^{-19}	−17.31	4.81	4.00×10^{-4}

3. Discussion

There is an increased interest in testing natural dietary compounds for potential anti-cancer effects both alone and in combination with already established cancer therapies. In this study, we found the viability of four tested CRC cell lines to be reduced by treatment with the chemotherapeutic agent 5-FU in a time- and concentration-dependent manner, which is in accordance with previous findings [50,51]. The LS513 cells were highly sensitive to 5-FU treatment compared to the other cell lines tested. This is consistent with the results by Bracht et al., who showed that LS513 cells were more sensitive to 5-FU compared to the DLD-1 and LS411N cells [52]. Testing a potential anti-cancer effect of the salmon oil OmeGo (HBC) showed that OmeGo reduced viability of two of the four tested CRC cell lines in a time- and dose-dependent manner. A combinatory treatment with 5-FU and OmeGo resulted in a further reduction in cell viability compared to 5-FU alone and hence chemosensitization of these CRC cell lines to 5-FU treatment. This indicates that OmeGo may be effective as an adjuvant or chemosensitizer together with chemotherapeutic agents to enhance the effectiveness of conventional CRC therapies.

The potential of fish oils to enhance the effect of chemotherapeutic agents like 5-FU has also been found by others. Granci et al. showed that a fish oil emulsion enhanced the cytotoxic and apoptosis-inducing effect of 5-FU in one of two CRC cell lines [33], while Jordan et al. found a fish oil-based lipid emulsion to enhance 5-FU-induced growth inhibition of CRC cells [34]. Rani and colleagues found that fish oil chemosensitized CRC cells to 5-FU treatment in animal models [24,35,53]. Studies also show the potential of the marine n-3 PUFAs DHA and EPA to enhance the anti-tumor effect and reduce cytotoxic effects of chemotherapeutics like 5-FU both in vitro in CRC cell lines and in animal models as reviewed by Hull et al. [14].

To compare the effect of OmeGo to the effect of the free omega-3 PUFAs DHA and EPA, the cells were treated with DHA and EPA concentrations corresponding with the estimated DHA and EPA levels in OmeGo. In contrast to OmeGo, the lowest DHA + EPA concentration tended to slightly stimulate cell viability in some cell lines. This was also seen for the effect of the combinatory treatment with the lowest concentration of 5-FU and DHA + EPA for DLD-1, HCT-8, and LS513 cells. The combinatory treatment reduced cell viability compared to treatment with DHA + EPA alone, but to a lesser extent than 5-FU treatment alone. When a linear model was fitted to the data, the free n-3 PUFAs were estimated to have a higher effect per unit compared to OmeGo (100 µg/mL). However, this probably reflects the extensive reduction in viability of the highest concentration of the free n-3 PUFAs, which seemed toxic to the cells. The estimated effects of DHA + EPA alone and in combination with 5-FU diverted from the observed effect, especially for the lower concentrations, indicating an additive but not linear effect for the n-3 PUFAs. Somehow, it seemed to be a threshold value for treatment with the n-3 PUFAs, with an enhanced reduction of cell viability when crossing the threshold. This is also reflected by the high standard deviations for some of the cell lines after DHA + EPA treatment. The highest dose of DHA + EPA (~150 µM) is high compared to the basal plasma total concentrations of DHA (~80 µM) and EPA (~20 µM), although such plasma concentration may be achieved by DHA/EPA and/or fish oil supplements [54]. However, as stated by Serini et al. based on in vivo results and the fact that cancer cells have different sensitivity to the cytotoxic effects of n-3 PUFAs, they never use n-3 PUFA concentrations over 30–50 µM in their experiments [55]. In contrast to OmeGo, the lower doses of n-3 PUFAs, which would correspond to typical physiological doses, did not enhance the effect of 5-FU in terms of reduced cell viability. The highest concentration of OmeGo showed a more balanced effect on cell viability and hence may be used as an adjuvant to cancer cell therapies in concentrations that are not physiologically relevant for DHA/EPA alone.

Why some cancer cells are sensitive towards n-3 PUFAs, while others are not, is still unknown. We are currently addressing this in an ongoing study where we investigate genetic differences that may affect n-3 PUFA sensitivity in cancer cells. In a previous publication from our group, we found that DHA sensitivity correlated with a specific gene expression profile, the basal levels of autophagy, and MAP1LC3B-II protein in 10 different CRC cell lines [36].The tested CRC cell lines responded very differently towards DHA treatment; the DLD-1 and HCT-8 cells were about 50% and 30% growth-inhibited by DHA (70 µM) treatment for 48 h, respectively, compared to no (or a slightly positive) effect on growth of LS411N and LS513 cells under the same conditions (assessed by cell counting) [36]. The results presented here indicate less effect of the combination of corresponding [DHA + EPA] on DLD-1 and HCT-8 cells compared to previous results with DHA treatment alone. However, the combination of DHA + EPA might have a different effect on the cells compared to DHA alone, and we previously showed that EPA has a somewhat lower effect on CRC cell lines compared to DHA [56]. The type of growth media used was the same as previously. However, we changed the type of fetal bovine serum (FBS) used, which might influence the results on n-3 PUFA sensitivity due to unknown factors such as level and type of growth factors and selenium. Selenium levels are known to vary between serum types and batches and may result in different responses of cancer cells to stress-causing agents [57]. Also, the Resazurin assay may not be directly compared with cell-counting results, as the capacity to reduce resazurin to resorufin is affected by the cells' mitochondrial enzymes and metabolic capacity [58].

Treatment with different chemotherapeutic agents like 5-FU [59] and n-3 PUFAs is known to induce oxidative stress in human CRC cells [36,60]. The highest concentration of DHA + EPA prompted a very high reduction in cell viability for all the tested CRC cell lines, which might indicate induction of a high level of oxidative stress or cytotoxicity. The corresponding dose of OmeGo (700 µg/mL) had a lesser effect on cell viability. However, OmeGo contains the natural antioxidant and liposoluble carotenoid astaxanthin, which might reduce the oxidation of the n-3 PUFAs in OmeGo and/or the possibility of inducing oxidative stress in the treated cells. Astaxanthin has both antioxidant and anti-inflammatory activity (reviewed in [61]) and may also suppress CRC metastasis [62].

We are planning a follow-up study on molecular pathways affected by OmeGo treatment in CRC cells. Pre-clinical testing of potential new treatment regimens for CRC is highly needed, and we plan to continue the exploration of the anti-cancer potential of OmeGo in pre-clinical xenograft studies in mice. Only a few clinical trials have explored the anti-cancer effect of n-3 PUFAs and marine oils on CRC. However, some studies have reported an association between increased intake of marine n-3 PUFAs after CRC diagnosis and lower CRC-specific mortality [15] and longer disease-free survival for CRC patients with a high intake of dark-meat fish after diagnosis [16]. This will be interesting to study in a randomized intervention trial for patients with CRC given OmeGo in addition to conventional CRC treatment.

4. Materials and Methods

4.1. Cell Lines, Culture Conditions, and Chemicals

The CRC cell lines DLD-1, LS411N, HCT-8 and LS513 from American Type Tissue Collection (ATTC, Rockville, MD, USA) were grown in RPMI media (Gibco A1049101, Life Technologies, Carlsbad, CA, USA) in a humidified atmosphere at 5% CO_2 and 37 °C. To the RPMI media was added fetal bovine serum (10%, Sigma #F7524, batch 0001660391, Sigma-Aldrich, Saint-Louis, MO, USA) and gentamicin (Gibco #1570049, Life Technologies). Cell lines were used up to passage ~20. Stock solution of OmeGo (Hofseth BioCare, Ålesund, Norway) was prepared in ethanol (1:8, 0.116 g/mL) and 5-FU (#548357, 50 mg/mL, Accord Healthcare AB, Harrow, UK) in phosphate-buffered saline (PBS, 0,0192 M); hence, both EtOH and PBS were used as vehicles. The OmeGo stock was stored at −20 °C, while the 5-FU stock was freshly prepared for each experiment. Stocks of DHA (Sigma-Aldrich, #D2534) and EPA (Sigma-Aldrich, #E2011) diluted in ethanol were stored at −20 °C. The dilution ratio of OmeGo in ethanol was optimized to assure a low effect of the vehicle, and the ethanol concentration did not exceed 0.75% volume/volume during treatments. For OmeGo, the same batch was used in all experiments.

4.2. Cell Treatment and Resazurin Viability Assay

Cells were seeded in 96-well trays (1500 cells/well) and incubated for 24 h before treatment with OmeGo, 5-FU, DHA, and EPA diluted in growth media in the concentrations given in the Results section. Cell viability was assessed using the Resazurin (7-Hydroxy-3H-phenoxazin-3-one 10-oxide) assay after 0, 24, 48 and 72 h (0–3 days) treatment. Media was removed and wells were washed once with PBS before adding resazurin (0.03 g/L) diluted in growth media. The resazurin stock was prepared in sterile 1 × PBS (0.15 g/L) and stored at −20 °C. Resazurin is a blue dye that is highly fluorescent when reduced to pink resorufin, which is proportional to aerobic respiration and the number of viable cells. The plates were incubated at 37 °C for 4 h before measuring fluorescence with a 544 nm excitation wavelength and a 590 nm emission wavelength using the FLUOstar Omega plate reader (BMG Labtech, Ortenberg, Germany).

4.3. Data Analysis

The average blank fluorescence signal was subtracted from the average fluorescence signal for each treatment before calculation of percent reduction of cell viability as percentage of signal compared to control. Dose–response curves were fitted to the cell viability data, and IC20, IC30, and IC50 values were estimated based on the resulting curves by using the functions drm and ED, respectively, from the R-package drc (version 4.1.3) [63]. We used the following log-logistic model to fit dose–response curves for each cell line and each treatment:

$$c + \frac{d - c}{1 + e^{b(\ln x - \ln e)}}, \quad (1)$$

where parameters *b*, *c*, *d*, and *e* are the slope, lower limit, upper limit, and IC50, respectively. Two models were fitted to the data: a full model with a common upper limit and slope, lower limit, and IC50 dependent on treatment time; and a simple model with common slope, upper limit, and IC50 and lower limit dependent on treatment time. The final choice between the full and simple models was based on which model best fitted the data. All models used Tukey's biweight function for robust fitting. The simple model was used to test for time- and dose-dependent effects. Specifically, the function linear Hypothesis from the R-package *car* was used to do a *F* statistics-based Wald test of the null hypotheses that the upper limit is equal to the lower limit for the 24 h treatment, that the lower limit for the

24 h treatment is equal to the lower limit for the 48 h treatment, and that the lower limit for the 48 h treatment is equal to the lower limit for the 72 h treatment.

For estimation of the treatment effect of 5-FU, OmeGo, DHA + EPA and combination treatments, the lmList function from the R-package nlme was used to fit the data from each cell line and treatment to the linear model:

$$\% \text{ reduced cell viability} = \beta_{5\text{-FU}} \times 5\text{-FU } (\mu\text{M}) + \beta_{SO} \times SO \; (100 \; \mu\text{g/mL}) + \beta_{5\text{-FU} \times SO} \times 5\text{-FUxSO} + \varepsilon \quad (2)$$

where 5-FU and SO are the concentrations of 5-FU and OmeGo or DHA + EPA used in the experiment, respectively. The fitted models were used to create isobolograms and estimate combination effects for selected effective doses. Combination effects were computed by using the Chou–Talalay combination index [64]. For comparing treatment effects of specific levels of OmeGo, DHA + EPA, and 5-FU, the lme function from the R-package nlme was used to fit a hierarchical linear model with treatment as fixed effect and cell-line as random effect. All statistical analyses were conducted in R (version 4.1.3).

5. Conclusions

OmeGo significantly reduced viability and potentiated the anti-cancer effect of 5-FU for the DLD-1 and LS513 CRC cell lines. Low doses of OmeGo had a higher negative effect on viability of CRC cells both alone and in combination with 5-FU compared to the corresponding lowest doses tested for DHA and EPA. Results suggest that treatment with a combination of OmeGo and 5-FU could be an alternative treatment strategy for patients with CRC. This will be further tested in pre-clinical and clinical studies.

Supplementary Materials: The following supporting information can be downloaded at: https://www.mdpi.com/article/10.3390/md21120636/s1, Table S1: Effect of 5-FU on CRC cell lines (average % reduction in cell viability (±SD)); Table S2: Effect of OmeGo on CRC cell lines (average % reduction in cell viability (±SD)); Table S3: Effect of combinatory treatment with OmeGo and 5-FU (3 days) on CRC cell lines (average % reduction in cell viability (±SD)); Table S4: Estimated effect of combinatory treatments of 5-FU and OmeGo in indicated concentrations; Table S5: Concentration of DHA and EPA (μM) corresponding to OmeGo doses (μg/mL) used for combinatory treatment with 5-FU; Table S6: Effect of combinatory treatment with DHA + EPA and 5-FU (3 days) on CRC cell lines (average % reduction in cell viability (±SD)); Table S7: Estimated effect of combinatory treatments of 5-FU and DHA + EPA in indicated concentrations (for DHA + EPA, the OmeGo correlated concentrations were used); Figure S1: Combination results from 5-FU and OmeGo treatment of DLD-1 and LS513 cells. For each cell line, the corresponding drug combination linear model was used to create OmeGo and 5-FU combination values for selected effective doses. Values are computed Chou–Talalay combination indices for selected drug combination values; Figure S2: Combination results from 5-FU and DHA + EPA treatment of DLD-1, LS411N, HCT-8, and LS513 cells. See Figure S1 for details.

Author Contributions: Conceptualization, C.H.H.P., S.A.S., A.W., E.H. and P.S.; formal analysis, P.S.; investigation, C.H.H.P. and H.S.; methodology, C.H.H.P., H.S. and P.S., resources, C.H.H.P., S.A.S., P.S. and E.H.; writing—original draft preparation, C.H.H.P.; writing—review and editing, C.H.H.P., S.A.S., P.S., H.S., E.H. and A.W.; visualization, C.H.H.P.; project administration, C.H.H.P. All authors have read and agreed to the published version of the manuscript.

Funding: This research was funded by Hofseth BioCare, Ålesund, Norway and Department of Clinical and Molecular Medicine (IKOM), NTNU.

Institutional Review Board Statement: Not applicable.

Data Availability Statement: All relevant data is given in the manuscript and Supplementary Materials.

Acknowledgments: Statistical analyses were performed at BioCore, NTNU. BioCore is funded by the Faculty of Medicine at NTNU and Central Norway Regional Health Authority. Technical advice from Per Arne Aas, IKOM, NTNU is highly appreciated.

Conflicts of Interest: The authors declare no conflict of interest. E.H. is employed by Hofseth BioCare. C.H.H.P. has a temporary auxiliary position at Hofseth BioCare, however, not related to the submitted work.

References

1. Larsen, I.K.; Møller, B.; Johannesen, T.B.; Robsahm, T.E.; Grimsrud, T.K.; Larønningen, S.; Seglem, A.H.; Gulbrandsen, J.; Jakobsen, E.; Ursin, G. *Cancer in Norway 2019—Cancer Incidence, Mortality, Survival and Prevalence in Norway*; Cancer Registry of Norway: Oslo, Norway, 2020.
2. Danckert, B.; Ferlay, J.; Engholm, G.; Hansen, H.L.; Johannesen, T.B.; Khan, S.; Køtlum, J.E.; Olafsdottir, E.; Schmidt, L.K.H.; Virtanen, A.; et al. NORDCAN: Cancer Incidence, Mortality, Prevalence and Survival in the Nordic Countries, Version 8.2. 2019. Available online: http://www.ancr.nu (accessed on 2 October 2023).
3. Osloeconomics. Kreft i Norge—Kostnader for Pasientene, Helsetjenesten og Samfunnet; Oslo Economics. 2016. Available online: https://oslocancercluster.no/wp-content/uploads/2016/10/20161004-Kreftkostnader_i_Norge-WEB.pdf (accessed on 2 October 2023).
4. Dekker, E.; Tanis, P.J.; Vleugels, J.L.A.; Kasi, P.M.; Wallace, M.B. Colorectal cancer. *Lancet* **2019**, *394*, 1467–1480. [CrossRef] [PubMed]
5. American Society of Clinical Oncology (ASCO). Colorectal Cancer: Types of Treatment. Available online: https://www.cancer.net/cancer-types/colorectal-cancer/types-treatment (accessed on 22 September 2021).
6. Vodenkova, S.; Buchler, T.; Cervena, K.; Veskrnova, V.; Vodicka, P.; Vymetalkova, V. 5-fluorouracil and other fluoropyrimidines in colorectal cancer: Past, present and future. *Pharmacol. Ther.* **2020**, *206*, 107447. [CrossRef] [PubMed]
7. D'Eliseo, D.; Velotti, F. Omega-3 Fatty Acids and Cancer Cell Cytotoxicity: Implications for Multi-Targeted Cancer Therapy. *J. Clin. Med.* **2016**, *5*, 15. [CrossRef] [PubMed]
8. Eltweri, A.M.; Thomas, A.L.; Metcalfe, M.; Calder, P.C.; Dennison, A.R.; Bowrey, D.J. Potential applications of fish oils rich in omega-3 polyunsaturated fatty acids in the management of gastrointestinal cancer. *Clin. Nutr.* **2017**, *36*, 65–78. [CrossRef] [PubMed]
9. Helsedirektoratet. Fisk Til Middag to Til Tre Ganger i Uken [Nettdokument]. Available online: https://www.helsedirektoratet.no/faglige-rad/kostradene-og-naeringsstoffer/kostrad-for-befolkningen/fisk-til-middag-to-til-tre-ganger-i-uken (accessed on 18 September 2021).
10. EFSA Panel on Dietetic Products; Nutrition and Allergies (NDA). Scientific Opinion on the Tolerable Upper Intake Level of eicosapentaenoic acid (EPA), docosahexaenoic acid (DHA) and docosapentaenoic acid (DPA). *EFSA J.* **2012**, *10*, 2815. [CrossRef]
11. Frøyland, L.; Bentsen, H.; Graff, I.E.; Myhrstad, M.; Paulsen, J.E.; Retterstøl, K.; Ulven, S.M. *Evaluation of Negative and Positive Health Effects of n-3 Fatty Acids as Constituents of Food Supplements and Fortified Foods*; Norwegian Scientific Committee for Food Safety: Oslo, Norway, 2011; 88p.
12. Murphy, R.A.; Devarshi, P.P.; Ekimura, S.; Marshall, K.; Hazels Mitmesser, S. Long-chain omega-3 fatty acid serum concentrations across life stages in the USA: An analysis of NHANES 2011–2012. *BMJ Open* **2021**, *11*, e043301. [CrossRef] [PubMed]
13. MacLean, C.H.; Newberry, S.J.; Mojica, W.A.; Khanna, P.; Issa, A.M.; Suttorp, M.J.; Lim, Y.W.; Traina, S.B.; Hilton, L.; Garland, R.; et al. Effects of omega-3 fatty acids on cancer risk: A systematic review. *JAMA* **2006**, *295*, 403–415. [CrossRef]
14. Volpato, M.; Hull, M.A. Omega-3 polyunsaturated fatty acids as adjuvant therapy of colorectal cancer. *Cancer Metastasis Rev.* **2018**, *37*, 545–555. [CrossRef]
15. Song, M.; Zhang, X.; Meyerhardt, J.A.; Giovannucci, E.L.; Ogino, S.; Fuchs, C.S.; Chan, A.T. Marine omega-3 polyunsaturated fatty acid intake and survival after colorectal cancer diagnosis. *Gut* **2017**, *66*, 1790–1796. [CrossRef]
16. Van Blarigan, E.L.; Fuchs, C.S.; Niedzwiecki, D.; Ye, X.; Zhang, S.; Song, M.; Saltz, L.B.; Mayer, R.J.; Mowat, R.B.; Whittom, R.; et al. Marine omega-3 Polyunsaturated Fatty Acid and Fish Intake after Colon Cancer Diagnosis and Survival: CALGB 89803 (Alliance). *Cancer Epidemiol. Biomark. Prev.* **2018**, *27*, 438–445. [CrossRef]
17. Anti, M.; Armelao, F.; Marra, G.; Percesepe, A.; Bartoli, G.M.; Palozza, P.; Parrella, P.; Canetta, C.; Gentiloni, N.; De Vitis, I.; et al. Effects of different doses of fish oil on rectal cell proliferation in patients with sporadic colonic adenomas. *Gastroenterology* **1994**, *107*, 1709–1718. [CrossRef] [PubMed]
18. West, N.J.; Clark, S.K.; Phillips, R.K.; Hutchinson, J.M.; Leicester, R.J.; Belluzzi, A.; Hull, M.A. Eicosapentaenoic acid reduces rectal polyp number and size in familial adenomatous polyposis. *Gut* **2010**, *59*, 918–925. [CrossRef] [PubMed]
19. Courtney, E.D.; Matthews, S.; Finlayson, C.; Di Pierro, D.; Belluzzi, A.; Roda, E.; Kang, J.Y.; Leicester, R.J. Eicosapentaenoic acid (EPA) reduces crypt cell proliferation and increases apoptosis in normal colonic mucosa in subjects with a history of colorectal adenomas. *Int. J. Color. Dis.* **2007**, *22*, 765–776. [CrossRef] [PubMed]
20. Cockbain, A.J.; Volpato, M.; Race, A.D.; Munarini, A.; Fazio, C.; Belluzzi, A.; Loadman, P.M.; Toogood, G.J.; Hull, M.A. Anticolorectal cancer activity of the omega-3 polyunsaturated fatty acid eicosapentaenoic acid. *Gut* **2014**, *63*, 1760–1768. [CrossRef] [PubMed]
21. Xie, H.; Chang, Y.N. Omega-3 polyunsaturated fatty acids in the prevention of postoperative complications in colorectal cancer: A meta-analysis. *Onco Targets Ther.* **2016**, *9*, 7435–7443. [CrossRef] [PubMed]

22. Nabavi, S.F.; Bilotto, S.; Russo, G.L.; Orhan, I.E.; Habtemariam, S.; Daglia, M.; Devi, K.P.; Loizzo, M.R.; Tundis, R.; Nabavi, S.M. Omega-3 polyunsaturated fatty acids and cancer: Lessons learned from clinical trials. *Cancer Metastasis Rev.* **2015**, *34*, 359 380. [CrossRef] [PubMed]
23. Tu, M.; Wang, W.; Zhang, G.; Hammock, B.D. Omega-3 Polyunsaturated Fatty Acids on Colonic Inflammation and Colon Cancer: Roles of Lipid-Metabolizing Enzymes Involved. *Nutrients* **2020**, *12*, 3301. [CrossRef]
24. Rani, I.; Kumar, S.; Sharma, B.; Prasad, R.; Kaur, S.; Sharma, P.; Agnihotri, N. Elucidation of underlying molecular mechanism of 5-Fluorouracil chemoresistance and its restoration using fish oil in experimental colon carcinoma. *Mol. Cell Biochem.* **2021**, *476*, 1517–1527. [CrossRef]
25. Calviello, G.; Di Nicuolo, F.; Serini, S.; Piccioni, E.; Boninsegna, A.; Maggiano, N.; Ranelletti, F.O.; Palozza, P. Docosahexaenoic acid enhances the susceptibility of human colorectal cancer cells to 5-fluorouracil. *Cancer Chemother. Pharmacol.* **2005**, *55*, 12–20. [CrossRef]
26. Yang, T.; Fang, S.; Zhang, H.X.; Xu, L.X.; Zhang, Z.Q.; Yuan, K.T.; Xue, C.L.; Yu, H.L.; Zhang, S.; Li, Y.F.; et al. N-3 PUFAs have antiproliferative and apoptotic effects on human colorectal cancer stem-like cells. *J. Nutr. Biochem.* **2013**, *24*, 744–753. [CrossRef]
27. Vasudevan, A.; Yu, Y.; Banerjee, S.; Woods, J.; Farhana, L.; Rajendra, S.G.; Patel, A.; Dyson, G.; Levi, E.; Maddipati, K.R.; et al. Omega-3 fatty acid is a potential preventive agent for recurrent colon cancer. *Cancer Prev. Res.* **2014**, *7*, 1138–1148. [CrossRef] [PubMed]
28. Zhuo, Z.H.; Zhang, L.M.; Mu, Q.T.; Lou, Y.R.; Gong, Z.H.; Shi, Y.J.; Ouyang, G.F.; Zhang, Y. The effect of combination treatment with docosahexaenoic acid and 5-fluorouracil on the mRNA expression of apoptosis-related genes, including the novel gene, in gastric cancer cells. *In Vitro Cell. Dev. Biol. Anim.* **2009**, *45*, 69–74. [CrossRef] [PubMed]
29. De Carlo, F.; Witte, T.R.; Hardman, W.E.; Claudio, P.P. Omega-3 Eicosapentaenoic Acid Decreases CD133 Colon Cancer Stem-Like Cell Marker Expression While Increasing Sensitivity to Chemotherapy. *PLoS ONE* **2013**, *8*, e69760. [CrossRef] [PubMed]
30. Ocal, O.; Naziroglu, M. Eicosapentaenoic acid enhanced apoptotic and oxidant effects of cisplatin via activation of TRPM2 channel in brain tumor cells. *Chem. Biol. Interact.* **2022**, *359*, 109914. [CrossRef] [PubMed]
31. Dupertuis, Y.M.; Boulens, N.; Angibaud, E.; Briod, A.S.; Viglione, A.; Allémann, E.; Delie, F.; Pichard, C. Antitumor Effect of 5-Fluorouracil-Loaded Liposomes Containing n-3 Polyunsaturated Fatty Acids in Two Different Colorectal Cancer Cell Lines. *AAPS PharmSciTech* **2021**, *22*, 36. [CrossRef] [PubMed]
32. Hardman, W.E.; Moyer, M.P.; Cameron, I.L. Dietary fish oil sensitizes A549 lung xenografts to doxorubicin chemotherapy. *Cancer Lett.* **2000**, *151*, 145–151. [CrossRef] [PubMed]
33. Granci, V.; Cai, F.; Lecumberri, E.; Clerc, A.; Dupertuis, Y.M.; Pichard, C. Colon cancer cell chemosensitisation by fish oil emulsion involves apoptotic mitochondria pathway. *Br. J. Nutr.* **2013**, *109*, 1188–1195. [CrossRef]
34. Jordan, A.; Stein, J. Effect of an omega-3 fatty acid containing lipid emulsion alone and in combination with 5-fluorouracil (5-FU) on growth of the colon cancer cell line Caco-2. *Eur. J. Nutr.* **2003**, *42*, 324–331. [CrossRef]
35. Rani, I.; Sharma, B.; Kumar, S.; Kaur, S.; Agnihotri, N. Apoptosis mediated chemosensitization of tumor cells to 5-fluorouracil on supplementation of fish oil in experimental colon carcinoma. *Tumour Biol.* **2017**, *39*. [CrossRef]
36. Samdal, H.; Sandmoe, M.A.; Olsen, L.C.; Jarallah, E.A.H.; Hoiem, T.S.; Schonberg, S.A.; Pettersen, C.H.H. Basal level of autophagy and MAP1LC3B-II as potential biomarkers for DHA-induced cytotoxicity in colorectal cancer cells. *FEBS J.* **2018**, *285*, 2446–2467. [CrossRef]
37. Hofseth BioCare. OmeGo® Delivers All the Nutritional Benefits of Consuming Fish. Available online: https://hofsethbiocare.com/products/salmon-oil (accessed on 19 August 2022).
38. Hofseth BioCare. Cardio Salmon Oil—Nutritional Content. Available online: https://www.amazon.com/Hofseth-BioCare-Salmon-Capsules-Vitamin/dp/B0BQRVD4G8#immersive-view_1702498410332 (accessed on 3 February 2023).
39. Higuera-Ciapara, I.; Felix-Valenzuela, L.; Goycoolea, F.M. Astaxanthin: A review of its chemistry and applications. *Crit. Rev. Food Sci. Nutr.* **2006**, *46*, 185–196. [CrossRef] [PubMed]
40. Framroze, B.; Heggdal, H. An in vitro study to explore the modulation of eosinophil effector function in human allergic peripheral blood eosinophils using enzymatically extracted salmonid oil. *Funct. Foods Health Dis.* **2020**, *10*, 357–367. [CrossRef]
41. Bargut, T. Fish oil has beneficial effects on allergen-induced airway inflammation and hyperreactivity in mice. *PLoS ONE* **2013**, *8*, e75059. [CrossRef] [PubMed]
42. Sen, N.; Framroze, B. The Effect of Dietary Oil Capsules on Reducing Serum Concentrations of Oxidized Low Density Lipoprotein-β2-Glycoprotein-I Complex. *J. Nutr. Food Sci.* **2013**, *3*, 225. [CrossRef]
43. Abe, Y.; Sakuyama, N.; Sato, T.; Kishine, K.; Nagayasu, K.; Nakatani, A.; Kitajima, M.; Watanabe, T.; Nishimura, K.; Ochiai, T.; et al. Evaluation of the 5 fluorouracil plasma level in patients with colorectal cancer undergoing continuous infusion chemotherapy. *Mol. Clin. Oncol.* **2019**, *11*, 289–295. [CrossRef] [PubMed]
44. Fang, L.; Jiang, Y.; Yang, Y.; Zheng, Y.; Zheng, J.; Jiang, H.; Zhang, S.; Lin, L.; Zheng, J.; Zhang, S.; et al. Determining the optimal 5-FU therapeutic dosage in the treatment of colorectal cancer patients. *Oncotarget* **2016**, *7*, 81880–81887. [CrossRef] [PubMed]
45. Violette, S.; Poulain, L.; Dussaulx, E.; Pepin, D.; Faussat, A.M.; Chambaz, J.; Lacorte, J.M.; Staedel, C.; Lesuffleur, T. Resistance of colon cancer cells to long-term 5-fluorouracil exposure is correlated to the relative level of Bcl-2 and Bcl-X(L) in addition to Bax and p53 status. *Int. J. Cancer* **2002**, *98*, 498–504. [CrossRef] [PubMed]

46. de la Cueva, A.; Ramirez de Molina, A.; Alvarez-Ayerza, N.; Ramos, M.A.; Cebrian, A.; Del Pulgar, T.G.; Lacal, J.C. Combined 5-FU and ChoKalpha inhibitors as a new alternative therapy of colorectal cancer: Evidence in human tumor-derived cell lines and mouse xenografts. *PLoS ONE* **2013**, *8*, e64961. [CrossRef]
47. Sam, M.R.; Esmaeillou, M.; Shokrgozar, M.A. Fish-Oil-Derived DHA-mediated Enhancement of Apoptosis in Acute Lymphoblastic Leukemia Cells is Associated with Accumulation of p53, Downregulation of Survivin, and Caspase-3 Activation. *Nutr. Cancer* **2017**, *69*, 64–73. [CrossRef]
48. Xue, M.; Wang, Q.; Zhao, J.; Dong, L.; Ge, Y.; Hou, L.; Liu, Y.; Zheng, Z. Docosahexaenoic acid inhibited the Wnt/beta-catenin pathway and suppressed breast cancer cells in vitro and in vivo. *J. Nutr. Biochem.* **2014**, *25*, 104–110. [CrossRef]
49. Jing, K.; Song, K.S.; Shin, S.; Kim, N.; Jeong, S.; Oh, H.R.; Park, J.H.; Seo, K.S.; Heo, J.Y.; Han, J.; et al. Docosahexaenoic acid induces autophagy through p53/AMPK/mTOR signaling and promotes apoptosis in human cancer cells harboring wild-type p53. *Autophagy* **2011**, *7*, 1348–1358. [CrossRef] [PubMed]
50. Zhao, Q.; Long, Y.; Cheng, W.; Huang, Y.; Li, J.; Li, Y.; Li, X.; Guo, X.; Li, Y.; Li, G.; et al. Visfatin inhibits colon cancer cell apoptosis and decreases chemosensitivity to 5-FU by promoting the SDF-1/CXCR4/Akt axis. *Int. J. Oncol.* **2022**, *60*, 75. [CrossRef] [PubMed]
51. He, L.; Zhu, H.; Zhou, S.; Wu, T.; Wu, H.; Yang, H.; Mao, H.; SekharKathera, C.; Janardhan, A.; Edick, A.M.; et al. Wnt pathway is involved in 5-FU drug resistance of colorectal cancer cells. *Exp. Mol. Med.* **2018**, *50*, 101. [CrossRef] [PubMed]
52. Bracht, K.; Nicholls, A.M.; Liu, Y.; Bodmer, W.F. 5-Fluorouracil response in a large panel of colorectal cancer cell lines is associated with mismatch repair deficiency. *Br. J. Cancer* **2010**, *103*, 340–346. [CrossRef] [PubMed]
53. Rani, I.; Vaiphei, K.; Agnihotri, N. Supplementation of fish oil augments efficacy and attenuates toxicity of 5-fluorouracil in 1,2-dimethylhydrazine dihydrochloride/dextran sulfate sodium-induced colon carcinogenesis. *Cancer Chemother. Pharmacol.* **2014**, *74*, 309–322. [CrossRef] [PubMed]
54. Serini, S.; Piccioni, E.; Merendino, N.; Calviello, G. Dietary polyunsaturated fatty acids as inducers of apoptosis: Implications for cancer. *Apoptosis* **2009**, *14*, 135–152. [CrossRef]
55. Serini, S.; Fasano, E.; Piccioni, E.; Cittadini, A.R.; Calviello, G. Dietary n-3 polyunsaturated fatty acids and the paradox of their health benefits and potential harmful effects. *Chem. Res. Toxicol.* **2011**, *24*, 2093–2105. [CrossRef]
56. Schonberg, S.A.; Lundemo, A.G.; Fladvad, T.; Holmgren, K.; Bremseth, H.; Nilsen, A.; Gederaas, O.; Tvedt, K.E.; Egeberg, K.W.; Krokan, H.E. Closely related colon cancer cell lines display different sensitivity to polyunsaturated fatty acids, accumulate different lipid classes and downregulate sterol regulatory element-binding protein 1. *FEBS J.* **2006**, *273*, 2749–2765. [CrossRef]
57. Karlenius, T.C.; Shah, F.; Yu, W.C.; Hawkes, H.J.; Tinggi, U.; Clarke, F.M.; Tonissen, K.F. The selenium content of cell culture serum influences redox-regulated gene expression. *Biotechniques* **2011**, *50*, 295–301. [CrossRef]
58. Vega-Avila, E.; Pugsley, M.K. An overview of colorimetric assay methods used to assess survival or proliferation of mammalian cells. *Proc. West. Pharmacol. Soc.* **2011**, *54*, 10–14.
59. Fu, Y.; Yang, G.; Zhu, F.; Peng, C.; Li, W.; Li, H.; Kim, H.G.; Bode, A.M.; Dong, Z.; Dong, Z. Antioxidants decrease the apoptotic effect of 5-Fu in colon cancer by regulating Src-dependent caspase-7 phosphorylation. *Cell Death Dis.* **2014**, *5*, e983. [CrossRef] [PubMed]
60. Pettersen, K.; Monsen, V.T.; Hakvag Pettersen, C.H.; Overland, H.B.; Pettersen, G.; Samdal, H.; Tesfahun, A.N.; Lundemo, A.G.; Bjorkoy, G.; Schonberg, S.A. DHA-induced stress response in human colon cancer cells—Focus on oxidative stress and autophagy. *Free Radic. Biol. Med.* **2016**, *90*, 158–172. [CrossRef] [PubMed]
61. Bjorklund, G.; Gasmi, A.; Lenchyk, L.; Shanaida, M.; Zafar, S.; Mujawdiya, P.K.; Lysiuk, R.; Antonyak, H.; Noor, S.; Akram, M.; et al. The Role of Astaxanthin as a Nutraceutical in Health and Age-Related Conditions. *Molecules* **2022**, *27*, 7167. [CrossRef] [PubMed]
62. Kim, H.Y.; Kim, Y.M.; Hong, S. Astaxanthin suppresses the metastasis of colon cancer by inhibiting the MYC-mediated downregulation of microRNA-29a-3p and microRNA-200a. *Sci. Rep.* **2019**, *9*, 9457. [CrossRef] [PubMed]
63. Ritz, C.; Baty, F.; Streibig, J.C.; Gerhard, D. Dose-Response Analysis Using R. *PLoS ONE* **2015**, *10*, e0146021. [CrossRef]
64. Chou, T.C.; Talalay, P. Generalized equations for the analysis of inhibitions of Michaelis-Menten and higher-order kinetic systems with two or more mutually exclusive and nonexclusive inhibitors. *Eur. J. Biochem.* **1981**, *115*, 207–216. [CrossRef]

MDPI AG
Grosspeteranlage 5
4052 Basel
Switzerland
Tel.: +41 61 683 77 34

Marine Drugs Editorial Office
E-mail: marinedrugs@mdpi.com
www.mdpi.com/journal/marinedrugs

www.ingramcontent.com/pod-product-compliance
Lightning Source LLC
Chambersburg PA
CBHW061454210926
51850CB00008B/1715
9783725866083